Chest Wall Surgery
Volume 2

Verses Kindler Publication

Verses Kindler Publication
Website: www.verseskindlerpublication.com

Chest Wall Surgery: Volume 2
By: Mr. Wenlin Wang
ISBN: 978-93-47494-21-5
1st Edition
Price: INR 5000/$70

Disclaimer

This book is intended solely for educational and scholarly purposes. It is written for qualified healthcare professionals and assumes a foundational knowledge of medical and surgical practice. The content is not intended to provide medical advice, establish a standard of care, or replace independent clinical judgment, professional training, or institutional protocols.

The editors and contributors have made every reasonable effort to ensure that the information presented is accurate and consistent with accepted practice at the time of publication. However, medical knowledge, surgical techniques, device availability, and regulatory requirements evolve continuously. The editors, contributors, and publisher make no representations or warranties regarding the completeness, accuracy, or applicability of the content and disclaim responsibility for any adverse outcomes resulting from the use or interpretation of information contained in this book.

All surgical procedures described should be performed only by appropriately trained and credentialed clinicians in properly equipped clinical settings, with appropriate patient selection, informed consent, and adherence to applicable local regulations and institutional guidelines. Readers are strongly encouraged to consult current literature, manufacturer instructions, and regulatory guidance before applying any technique or using any device described herein.

References to specific products, devices, instruments, or commercial entities are provided for informational purposes only and do not constitute endorsement or recommendation by the editors, contributors, or publisher. All trademarks and registered trademarks are the property of their respective owners.

Clinical images, case descriptions, and patient-related information included in this book have been anonymized or reproduced with appropriate permission in accordance with ethical standards. Any resemblance to identifiable individuals is unintentional.

Editor's Introduction

Chest wall Surgery has gradually evolved to include the management of complex, secondary, and acquired conditions that affect both form and function. While advances in Surgical techniques and perioperative care have expanded the range of treatable conditions, the management of these advanced pathologies remains less standardized and often more technically demanding.

This volume was developed to address that need. Building on the foundation established in Volume 1, *Chest Wall Surgery* Volume 2 brings together current understanding and Surgical approaches related to complex chest wall disorders in a structured and clinically relevant manner. The goal is not only to describe operative techniques, but also to place them within a broader clinical context that supports sound decision-making in challenging scenarios.

The chapters address a wide range of conditions, including complex and secondary thoracic deformities, congenital heart disease associated with chest wall abnormalities, post-cardiac Surgery deformities, and reoperative cases. In addition, this volume includes rare conditions such as sternal cleft and straight back syndrome, along with dedicated sections on trauma, oncologic conditions, and advanced reconstruction.

Both traditional and contemporary Surgical approaches are discussed, with attention to indications, technical considerations, perioperative management, and clinical outcomes. Where newer methods are presented, they are discussed alongside established practices to allow readers to evaluate their role in clinical practice.

As in Volume 1, this book reflects the collective experience of contributors working across different healthcare settings and Surgical environments, reflecting the complexity and variability inherent in advanced chest wall Surgery.

This volume is intended for Surgeons managing complex chest wall conditions, as well as trainees seeking a focused reference in advanced practice. Each chapter is designed to stand independently, allowing the book to function as both a comprehensive resource and a practical reference.

We hope that this volume will further consolidate current knowledge, support thoughtful Surgical decision-making, and contribute to the continued development of chest wall Surgery as a defined area of Surgical practice.

Wenlin Wang
Rajkamal Vishnu
Editors

Preface

Chest Wall Surgery- Volume 2 focuses on the management of complex and advanced conditions of the chest wall that extend beyond primary deformity correction. These include secondary and post-Surgical deformities, reoperative cases, congenital anomalies, trauma, oncologic conditions, and reconstruction.

While Volume 1 addresses the fundamental principles and commonly encountered conditions, this volume is directed toward clinical situations that are often less straightforward. Many of these cases involve altered anatomy, previous Surgical interventions, and variable patterns of disease, making standard approaches less reliable. As a result, Surgical management in these settings requires careful planning, flexibility in technique, and sound clinical judgment.

The purpose of this volume is to present these conditions in a structured and practical manner. The emphasis is not only on describing operative techniques, but also on understanding when and how to apply them. In complex chest wall Surgery, outcomes depend as much on decision-making as on technical execution, and this perspective is reflected throughout the chapters.

The scope of the volume includes complex and secondary thoracic deformities, deformities associated with congenital heart disease and prior cardiac Surgery, and reoperative cases. In addition, less common conditions such as sternal cleft, localized deformities of the sternum and ribs, and straight back syndrome are discussed. Although these conditions are not frequently encountered, they require specific considerations and tailored approaches.

The later sections address acquired conditions, including trauma and oncologic disease, as well as the principles of chest wall reconstruction. Advances in stabilization techniques, Surgical planning, and reconstruction have expanded the options available to Surgeons, but they have also introduced new challenges in selecting the most appropriate approach for each patient.

The content reflects the experience of contributors working in different clinical environments and managing a wide range of chest wall pathology. This diversity is intentional and reflects the realities of practice, where patient factors, institutional resources, and Surgical experience all influence decision-making.

This volume is intended to complement Volume 1 and to serve as a focused reference for Surgeons managing complex chest wall conditions, as well as for trainees seeking a deeper understanding of advanced Surgical practice. Each chapter is designed to be read independently, allowing the book to function both as a comprehensive resource and as a practical reference in day-to-day clinical work.

We hope that this volume will contribute to a clearer and more structured approach to complex chest wall Surgery and support thoughtful, consistent, and effective patient care.

Rajkamal Vishnu
Editor
Cleveland Clinic, Cleveland, USA
[01- 2025]

Index

Chapter 6: Chest Wall Infections

CHAPTER 2
PART 2

CHEST WALL DEFORMITIES

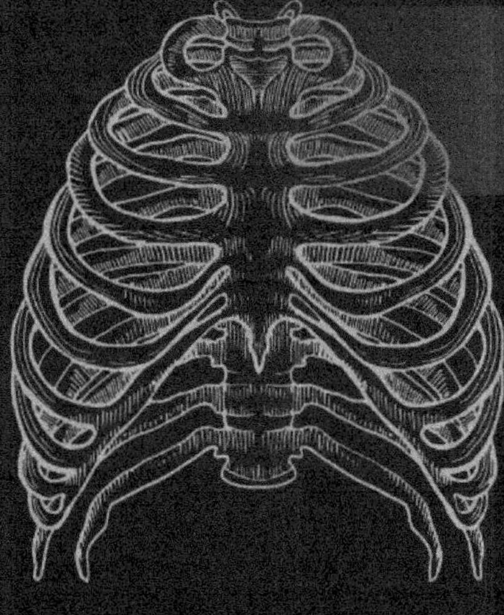

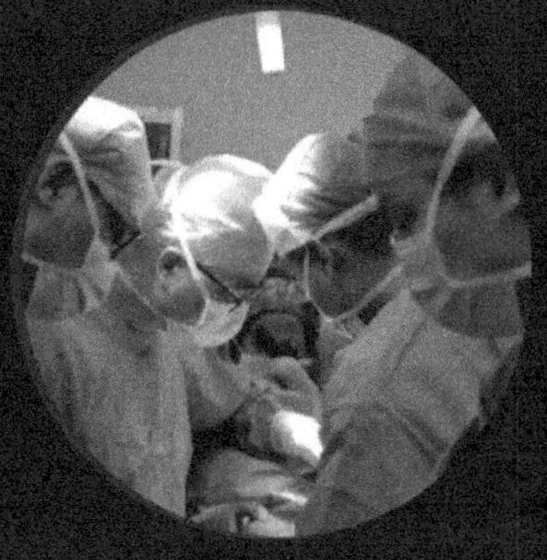

Section 17

COMPLEX CHEST WALL DEFORMITY

All chest wall deformities can generally be classified into two main categories: **protrusion deformities and depression deformities** [1]. In reality, many deformities are not purely protrusions or depressions, but may involve both at the same time [2]. Such deformities may be due to specific conditions, such as Wenlin chest, Poland syndrome, or asphyxiating thoracic dystrophy (Jeune syndrome), but more often they are simply independent combinations. These combinations are quite random, without a specific pattern, and are not a distinct disease. To better understand and treat these deformities, we group them together as a special category called complex chest wall deformities [3,4].

1.Basic Concept

Complex thoracic malformations are combinations of two basic malformations, and because of the variety of combinations, they are not strictly speaking a separate disorder, but rather a number of disorders. The pathogenesis of these diseases is complex and it is difficult to identify their true causes.
Morphologically, composite malformations can be divided into three basic types (Fig. 2-17-1) [3-5]: the first is a malformation in which the bumps and depressions are distributed up and down, the second is one in which the bumps and depressions are distributed left and right, and the third is one in which the bumps and depressions are irregularly distributed. The morphology of the three types of malformations varies significantly, but all of them have the two most basic types of malformations

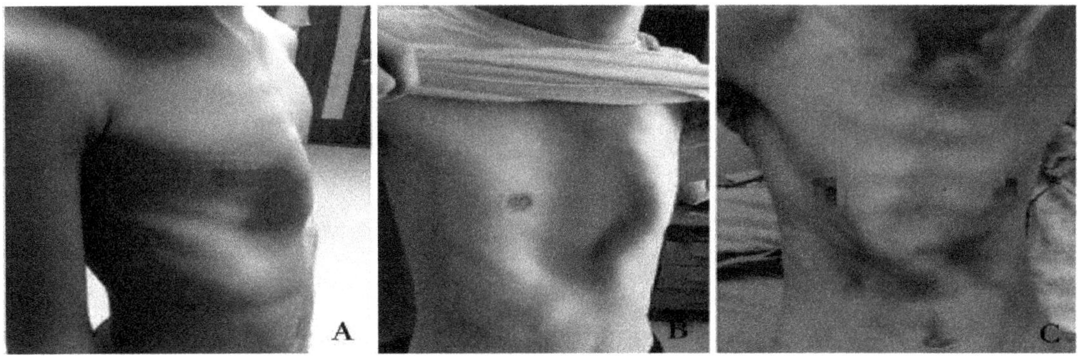

Figure 2-17-1 Three basic types of compound malformations (A. Convexities and depressions up and down; B. Convexities and depressions left and right; C. Convexities and depressions irregularly distributed)

The main problem with compound malformations is in the appearance, with the chest wall having a distinctly abnormal appearance, which is the underlying reason for most patients' visits. Symptoms may occur due to the presence of depression if the depression causes significant compression of the heart and lungs. The bulge does not produce compression and does not produce symptoms.

The diagnosis of compound malformations is mainly based on visual observation. Imaging studies can be helpful in clarifying the details of the malformation and its relationship to the heart, lungs, and other organs. The indication for surgery for this type of patient depends mainly on the patient's own feelings. If the patient feels that the deformity is unsightly or uncomfortable, surgery is needed; if the patient feels that the deformity is neither unsightly nor uncomfortable, surgery can be avoided.

2. Surgical Treatment

A complex deformity involves two basic deformities, and to achieve complete treatment, both deformities must be addressed simultaneously. Since the two deformities are entirely independent, they can theoretically be corrected separately. However, if their interrelation is not considered, the surgical outcome may be affected.

The anterior chest wall is an integrated structure whether it is a depression or a protrusion, both occur within this whole, so they are closely related. When operating on the depression, for example, by pushing it up from below the lifting force is transmitted through the chest wall to the protruding area, making the protrusion more pronounced. This requires that the protrusion must be treated at the same time. Likewise, if the protrusion is corrected first, for example, by pressing it down, the compressive force will also be transmitted through the chest wall to the depression, making the depression deeper. Correcting one deformity will aggravate the other. If they are corrected at different times, it can lead to serious consequences. If they are corrected at the same time, it creates opposing forces between the two treatments, making each correction more difficult. Therefore, surgery for a complex deformity is by no means a simple sum of two separate procedures, but rather an organic integration of both surgeries [5,6]. During this process, the surgical details must be well designed; only then can good results be achieved; otherwise, surgical success is difficult to guarantee.

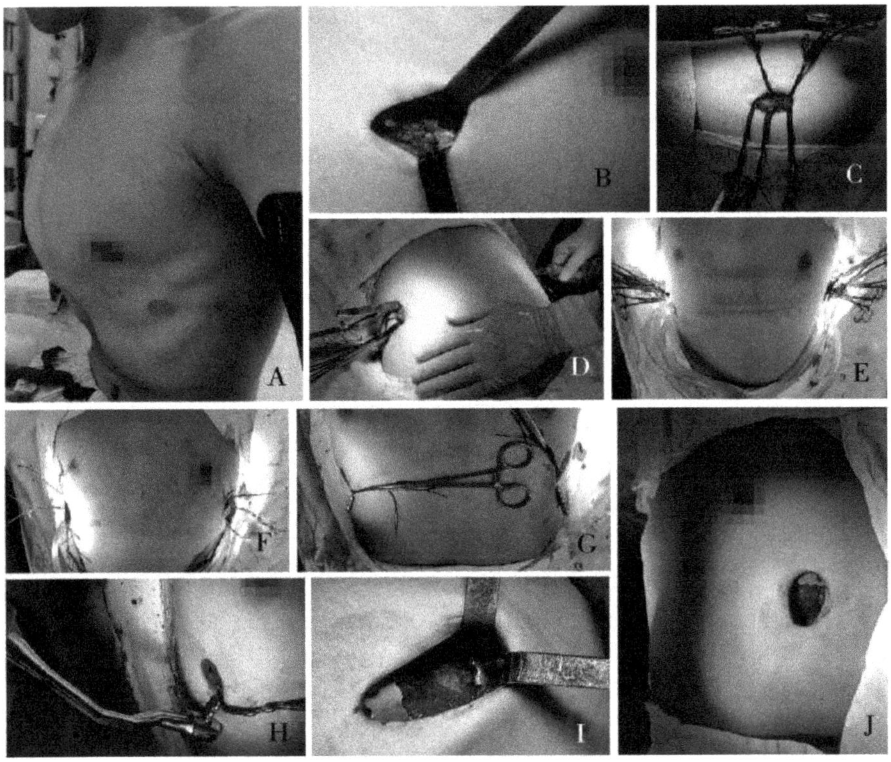

Figure 2-17-2 Sandwich procedure for a composite deformity (both the Wenlin procedure and the Wung procedure are used during the operation. A. Thoracic appearance of the deformity; B. Incision in the lateral chest wall, with the rib associated with the lateral chest wall used to secure the plate; C. Placement of wire retractor wires across the ribs, 5 in total, for securing 2 plates for the Wenlin procedure and 1 for securing the plate for the Wung procedure; D. Successive threading of plate guides into the plate tunnels and the thoracic cavity; introduction of the plate guides; E. Introduction of 3 plate guides into the plate tunnels and the thoracic cavity; F. Introduction of 2 plates into the plate tunnels with the plate guides, with the plate guides in place; and F. Introduction of 2 plates into the plate tunnels with the plate guides. E. Introduce 3 plate guides into the plate tunnel and chest cavity; F. Introduce 2 plates into the plate tunnel with plate guides and fix the plates to complete the fixation of Wenlin's surgical plates; G. Place the 3rd plate into the chest cavity with plate guides, with the plate located in the deep depression of the anterior chest wall; H. Flip the 3rd plate over to hold up the depression and then fix it to the ribs; I. Position of the plates after fixation of the plates; J. Appearance of the chest wall after fixation of all plates, with deformity largely disappearing. The deformity has almost disappeared.

(i) Sandwich Surgery

This procedure is designed for complex deformities in which the protrusion and depression are distributed vertically (Figure 2-17-2) [2,7–10]. The specific method includes two parts: the Wenlin procedure for the protrusion and the Wung procedure for the depression. The Wenlin procedure is performed through a lateral chest wall incision, using one or two steel bars. The Wung procedure is also performed through a lateral chest wall incision, and generally one steel bar is sufficient. Of course, if the depressed area is large or the deformity is complex, two steel bars can be used as well

When two procedures are performed at the same time, they are bound to affect each other during the operation. The relationship between the two procedures needs to be handled appropriately; if handled correctly, they will provide each other with favourable conditions. If not handled properly, it will bring trouble to the operation of both sides. Therefore, some details of the operation need extra attention: (1) In the process of specific implementation, generally through an incision Do not make separate cuts, as this will reduce the efficiency of the cuts. (2) Pay attention to the order of operations. Since all the operations are done through one incision, if you do not pay attention to the order, it will lead to confusion and cause great trouble for the operation. (3) Take care of each other. No matter which deformity is corrected first, it will aggravate the severity of the other deformity and make the other operation more difficult. It is for this reason that it is necessary to take both operations into account at all times during the operation, and to proceed in a gradual manner in order to obtain a good result.

The Meiji operation is an operation performed for both deformities. By the nature of the operation, the operation for the bulge can be considered as an orthopaedic treatment for chicken breasts, but the operation for the depression is more complex and very different from the operation for funnel chest. Funnel chest is the most common depressed deformity in which the depression is a pit with a central depression surrounded by a bulge. In a compound deformity, on the other hand, the depression is usually not a typical pit, but may be a variety of depressions. Especially when the bulge is flattened, the depression may take on a variety of shapes. The Nuss procedure for such depressions is a very demanding procedure. If the details of the technique are not mastered properly, it will be difficult to achieve a satisfactory result. Specific details including the number, length, curvature, placement and fixation of the plates are directly related to the orthopaedic results, and therefore should be well-designed during the operation to ensure the successful completion of the operation.

Sandwich surgery is so named because the operation is performed like a sandwich, i.e. two plates are clamped to the chest wall from both sides to normalise the deformed chest wall. On the face of it, this is a good image, but if you look into it, you will find that this is not the case: in the Wenlin procedure, the plates are positioned completely on one side of the chest wall, and in a true sandwich, the plates on the other side would also be positioned completely on the inside of the chest wall. In the Nuss procedure, the plate is not completely medial, but only partially medial to the chest wall. This is not a true sandwich. Since it is not a sandwich, the surgery is inevitably flawed in theory. In the Wenlin procedure, the force that compresses the medial bulge is loaded on the ribs of the lateral chest wall through a steel plate, causing the ribs here to be lifted. In the Nuss procedure, however, the force supporting the median depression is loaded on the ribs of the lateral chest wall through a steel plate. This force is a downward compressive force in the opposite direction of the force in the Wenlin procedure. When the ribs of the lateral chest wall are simultaneously subjected to forces in two different directions, their effects may cancel each other out. If the force is too great and the ribs are brittle, the ribs may be pulled apart, resulting in a fracture. Once a fracture occurs, the surgery is bound to fail. Therefore, the so-called sandwich procedure, when performed with the Wenlin procedure and the Nuss procedure, is potentially problematic because the Nuss procedure does not operate entirely on the inside of the chest wall. In order to effectively avoid this risk, the basic principle of the operation is to spread the stresses as much as possible. There are various ways of distributing the stresses, including increasing the number of plates or increasing the force area, which can help to eliminate these disadvantages. However, since the number of plates is limited and the area subject to stress is also subject to a number of factors, it is not easy, but definitely not impossible, to completely eliminate such disadvantages. There is a reliable way to eliminate them completely, and that is not to use this kind of surgery at all.

In sandwich surgery, there is only one operation for the bulge and that is the Wenlin procedure. However, in addition to the Nuss procedure, there is also the Wang procedure, which provides an alternative to the Nuss procedure for the treatment of composite deformities. However, since the plate of the Wang operation is located on the same side of the chest wall as the plate of the Wenlin operation, the operation can no longer be called a sandwich operation, but a completely new combination.

The Wang operation is performed from the surface of the depression, which is completely different from the Nuss operation, and has both. It has clear advantages, but also has its own defects. Therefore, the actual operation needs to be chosen according to the actual situation. Regardless of whether it is the Nuss procedure or the Wang procedure, as long as the indications for the procedure are properly understood, good surgical results can be achieved.

(ii) Willine Surgery

In compound thoracic deformities, there is sometimes a right-to-left distribution of bumps and depressions, i.e., one side of the chest wall is raised and the other is depressed. This deformity is similar to an asymmetrical chicken chest or funnel chest, but the signs of the bumps and depressions are more pronounced, making it a composite deformity rather than an asymmetrical stand-alone deformity.

Theoretically, a sandwich operation for this deformity would have the same potential for good results. However, this is tantamount to treating two asymmetrical deformities at the same time, the Wenlin procedure for the asymmetrical chicken breast and the Nuss procedure for the asymmetrical funnel chest. In both cases, the operation is more difficult, which definitely increases the overall difficulty of the operation. In addition, due to the parallel arrangement of the convexities and depressions, the plates for both procedures need to be placed on the same flat surface, which will cause the plates to interfere with each other, which is not conducive to the operation. Therefore, this deformity is not suitable for sandwich surgery.

After observing this deformity, we finally designed a special procedure, the Willine procedure [5,11]. The original design of the procedure was still to operate on both basic deformities at the same time. However, in order to perform the operation more efficiently, we combined the two operations into one and performed the orthopedics through the same plate. This procedure is performed by making incisions in the chest wall on both sides, placing steel wire guides at the ribs where the plates are fixed, and constructing the plate tunnels; the tunnels on the convex side are located on the surface of the bony structures, and the tunnels on the depressed side are located on the deeper surface of the bony structures, and the tunnels on both sides converge next to the sternum on the depressed side; after the tunnels are completed, the guide tubes of the plates are placed by means of the guides, and then the plate is inserted, firstly lifting up the chest wall on the depressed side, and then pressing on the opposite side. The plate is then inserted to lift the chest wall on the depressed side and then compress the chest wall on the opposite side of the convexity. Finally, the ends of the plate are fixed, the incision is closed, and the procedure is completed.

It is clear that the Willine procedure has the following advantages [5] |(1)Extremely efficient. This procedure combines two basic operations into one surgery, without increasing the difficulty or adding extra steps, yet fulfills the purpose of both surgeries, making it highly efficient. (2) Saves steel bars. Generally, whether using the Wenlin procedure or the Nuss procedure, separate steel bars are needed for each. However, the Willine procedure combines the two, significantly reducing the number of steel bars required. Fewer steel bars not only lower surgical costs but also keep the surgical field cleaner and make the operation easier. (3) Simple operation. The Willine procedure is a combination of two surgeries, but its actual operation is equivalent to half of the Wenlin procedure and half of the Nuss procedure, so it is much simpler. It is especially worth noting that this procedure does not require the use of a thoracoscope at all, which greatly lowers the threshold for performing the surgery. (4) Safe operation. In a standard sandwich procedure, the involvement of the Nuss procedure means its inherent risks must be faced. Although the Willine procedure includes elements of the Nuss procedure, the steel bar does not pass through the mediastinum, which actively avoids the most dangerous part of the Nuss procedure, making the operation much safer. (5) Ideal results. Complex deformities with left–right distribution are generally difficult to correct satisfactorily by other methods. The Willine procedure directly addresses both deformities, and usually Good results can be obtained

The advantages of the Willine procedure are quite clear, but it also has some shortcomings [5]: (1) The correction on the depression side is sometimes not ideal. When operating on the depression side, the structure supported by the steel bar may involve only a few ribs rather than the entire depressed chest wall, which may affect the correction of the depression. (2) When there is significant asymmetry in the force applied on both sides, it can increase the difficulty of the procedure, placing higher demands on surgical detail.

To address these shortcomings, the following points should be noted during the procedure [5]:(1) When operating on the depression side, as many ribs as possible should be lifted to ensure the most satisfactory correction of the depressed side of the chest wall;(2) If conditions allow, the number of steel bars can be increased to achieve a more complete correction of the depression; (3) Before the surgery, the length, shape, and fixation position of the steel bars must be carefully planned to achieve the best possible correction of the deformity

(iii) Other Procedures

Complex deformities are not single deformities, so surgery for them is a major test of a surgeon's skills. In practice, focusing closely on the specific characteristics of the deformity and choosing the appropriate procedure is key to achieving correction. However, if a surgeon only considers a limited number of procedures, it will not help achieve an optimal correction. To achieve better corrective results, these special deformities need to be viewed with a broader and wider perspective. Of course, this also requires deep reflection on surgical techniques to develop more possible solutions.

The Willine procedure combines the Wenlin procedure and the Nuss procedure, with the Nuss procedure targeting depression. We know that, apart from the Nuss procedure, the Wang procedure can also be used for depression correction. So, is it possible to design a procedure that combines the Wenlin procedure and the Wang procedure at the same time? This is absolutely possible. The core idea of switching from the Nuss procedure to the Wang procedure is simply moving the steel bar from inside to outside. In the Willine procedure, this change is very easy to achieve, so a completely new procedure is born: using a single operation to perform both the Wenlin and Wang procedures simultaneously [5,12–14]. The specific method is to create tunnels on the surface of both the protrusion and depression, using the same steel bar: performing the Wenlin procedure on the protrusion side and the Wang procedure on the depression side. This design is entirely feasible and can yield excellent results. However, if we look at this new combination from a higher level, it actually reverts to the Wenlin procedure only the fixation position on the depression side is rather special. This perspective is quite thought-provoking. As everyone knows, the Wenlin procedure is specifically designed to correct protrusions. Why can a left–right distributed complex deformity also be corrected by such a procedure? Could it be that the target is essentially the same type of deformity? After this reflection, if we carefully compare this complex deformity with a simple protrusion-type deformity, we can quickly see their connection. This complex deformity can completely be regarded as an asymmetric protrusion deformity. Looking at it from another angle, this surgery can also be seen as a Wang procedure with added fixation for the protrusion side. As we know, the Wang procedure is used for correcting depressions. When this combination is viewed as a Wang procedure, the nature of the deformity also changes; could it be regarded as a depression deformity? This view is reasonable because, in this case, the deformity can be seen as an asymmetric depression deformity. Earlier we specifically noted that left–right distributed complex deformities should not be seen as asymmetric pectus carinatum or pectus excavatum because they clearly differ in nature. However, if the related technical details are properly handled, the treatment methods do overlap to some extent at the very least, this conceptually offers more options. This precisely illustrates flexible understanding and application (Figure 2-17-3).

As can be seen from the above analysis, compound malformations, although they all consist of different simple malformations, give a completely different picture of the nature of the malformations if one looks at the main features or analyses the malformations from a macroscopic point of view. These realisations are of great significance and play an extremely important role in the diagnosis and treatment of malformations. If one thinks along these lines, a flexible understanding and design of the surgery can yield unexpected results.

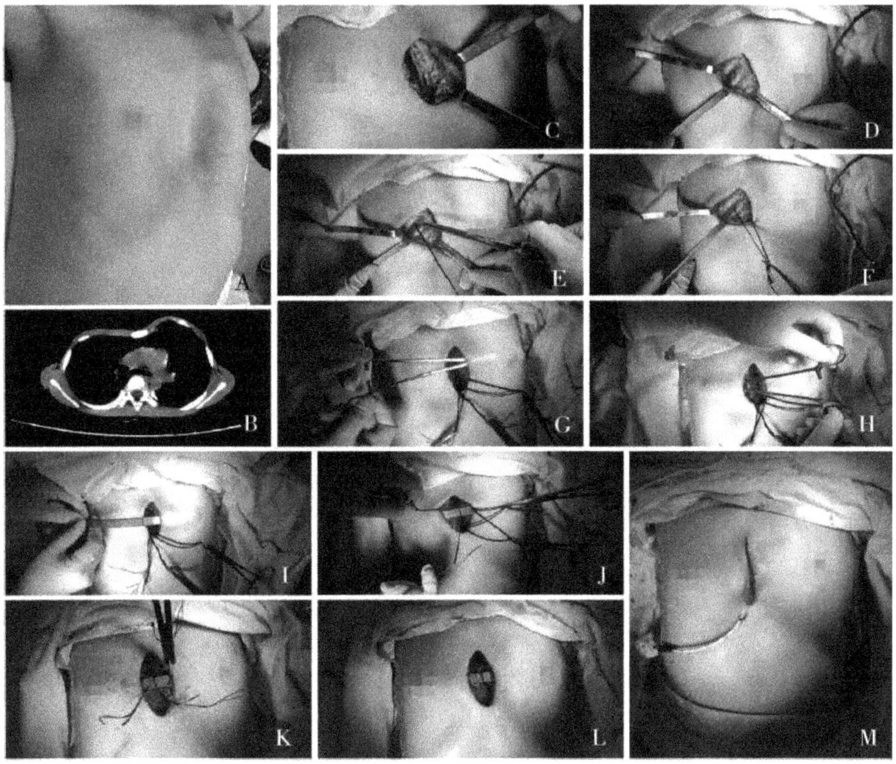

Figure 2-17-3 Compound deformity of left-right alignment after cardiac surgery, which is actually equivalent to asymmetric funnel chest, is corrected by Wang's procedure (A. Asymmetric deformity of the anterior chest wall, with the left side high, the median depression, and the right side low, and the old surgical scar can be seen in the middle of the chest wall. D. Free the bony surface of the right chest wall; E. Place the wire guide wire around the ribs with right-angle pliers; F. Place the wire guide wire around the ribs; G, H. Use long curved pliers to make a tunnel for the plate to both sides of the chest wall; I. Place the plate; J. Introduce the wire with the wire guide wire; K. Tighten the wire to fix the plate; L. Finish fixation of the plate; M. Close the incision and place a drainage in the field of the operation. (End of surgery)

To sum up, compound thoracic deformity is a special category of deformity, and since it is not a particular disease, the surgical treatment is relatively complicated, and the choice of surgical method needs to be decided according to the specific features of the deformity. In practice, only by keeping in mind the intrinsic characteristics of the two basic deformities and looking at the deformities from a broad perspective can we find the most appropriate surgery and ultimately achieve orthopaedic success. If one fails to recognise the inherent connection between the deformities and always looks at each deformity in isolation, one will choose a certain fixed type of operation uniformly, and the result is bound to be unsatisfactory.

REFERENCES

[1] Wang, W. L., C. M. Chen, X. J. Li, et al. 2018. "Overall Classification Method of Thoracic Deformities." *Chinese Journal of Clinical Thoracic and Cardiovascular Surgery* 25 (11): 981–985.
[2] Wang, W. L. 2021a. "Severe Pectus Carinatum Surgery in Young Women: Wenlin Procedure and Wung Procedure." *Thoracic Deformity Surgery Expert*, March 14.
[3] Wang, W. L. 2020a. "Understanding Issues of Complex Deformities." *Thoracic Deformity Surgery Expert*, February 24.
[4] Wang, W. L. 2018a. "Discussion on Surgical Methods for Complex Thoracic Deformities." *Thoracic Deformity Surgery Expert*, August 3.
[5] Wang, W. L. 2021b. "Wenlin Procedure for Complex Thoracic Deformities." *Toutiao*, November 7.
[6] Wang, W. L. 2020b. "Treatment Issues of Complex Deformities." *Thoracic Deformity Surgery Expert*, February 25.
[7] Wang, W. L. 2019a. "Sandwich Procedure for Severe Complex Deformities." *Thoracic Deformity Surgery Expert*, August 9.
[8] Wang, W. L. 2019b. "Sandwich Procedure for Severe Complex Deformities." *Thoracic Deformity Surgery Expert*, March 23.
[9] Wang, W. L. 2018b. "Sandwich Procedure and Modified Sandwich Procedure." *Thoracic Deformity Surgery Expert*, July 30.
[10] Park, H. J., and K. S. Kim. 2016. "The Sandwich Technique for Repair of Pectus Carinatum and Excavatum/Carinatum Complex." *Annals of Cardiothoracic Surgery* 5 (5): 434–439.
[11] Wang, W. L. 2018c. "Minimally Invasive Technique for Mixed-Type Asymmetric Thoracic Deformity." *Surgical Case Reports* 1 (2): 1–2.
[12] Wang, W. L. 2019c. "Minimally Invasive Surgery for Complex Thoracic Deformity after Cardiac Surgery." *Thoracic Deformity Surgery Expert*, April 30.
[13] Wang, W. L. 2017a. "Treatment of Asymmetric Complex Thoracic Deformities." *Thoracic Deformity Surgery Expert*, November 17.
[14] Wang, W. L. 2017b. "Successful Surgery for Severe Complex Thoracic Deformity Today." *Thoracic Deformity Surgery Expert*, August 18.

Thoracic deformities can be divided into two types of deformities, primary and secondary, in terms of their onset. Primary deformities are those that occur in the thorax without a clear cause. In general, most of the deformities encountered in clinical practice are primary. Secondary deformities are those that occur after a definite cause. These causes can be trauma, surgery, infection, or other factors that directly contribute to the development of the deformity[1-4]. To determine whether a thoracic deformity is a secondary deformity, three elements need to be clarified: (1) whether there is an etiological cause; (2) whether the etiological cause occurred before the deformity; and (3) whether there is a causal relationship between the etiological cause and the deformity. Only when these three elements are clear can a secondary thoracic deformity be identified. In terms of the nature of the deformity, there is no fundamental difference between secondary and primary deformities, both of which are manifested as abnormalities in the shape of the thorax [1]. Such anomalies have all the attributes of common thoracic deformities, and can be either proptosis, concavity, or complex deformities. However, due to the presence of a clear etiology, these deformities have their own characteristics. The treatment of these deformities is clearly different from that of primary deformities.

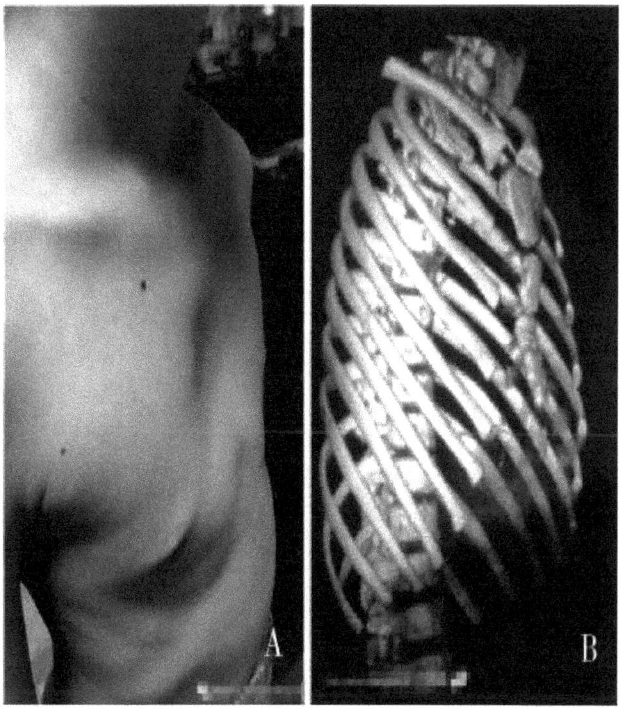

Figure 2-18-1 Funnel chest due to trauma (A. median depression deformity of the anterior chest wall; B. fracture of the sternum with depression of the surrounding structures)

1. Pathogenesis

The causes of secondary thoracic deformities are clear but varied, and each causative factor may lead to thoracic deformity through a different mechanism, so it is important to analyse the mechanism in conjunction with the cause of the disease. Trauma itself is a very complex pathogenetic factor, and the mechanism of secondary deformity varies greatly depending on the nature and severity of the trauma [5,6]. For example, severe crush injuries, falls, impact injuries, or sharp force injuries may result in secondary thoracic deformities, but the mechanisms are clearly very different (Figure 2-18-l). When the chest wall is damaged by various injuries, the chest wall may be damaged in a number of ways

Following damage to structures, particularly bony structures, if the injury is not treated in a timely manner or if it is not treated appropriately, the bony structures will heal abnormally, ultimately leading to abnormalities in the overall appearance and shape of the thorax (Fig. 2-18-2). While this is the general mechanism of secondary thoracic deformity due to trauma, the specific mechanism of bony structural damage may vary from cause to cause.

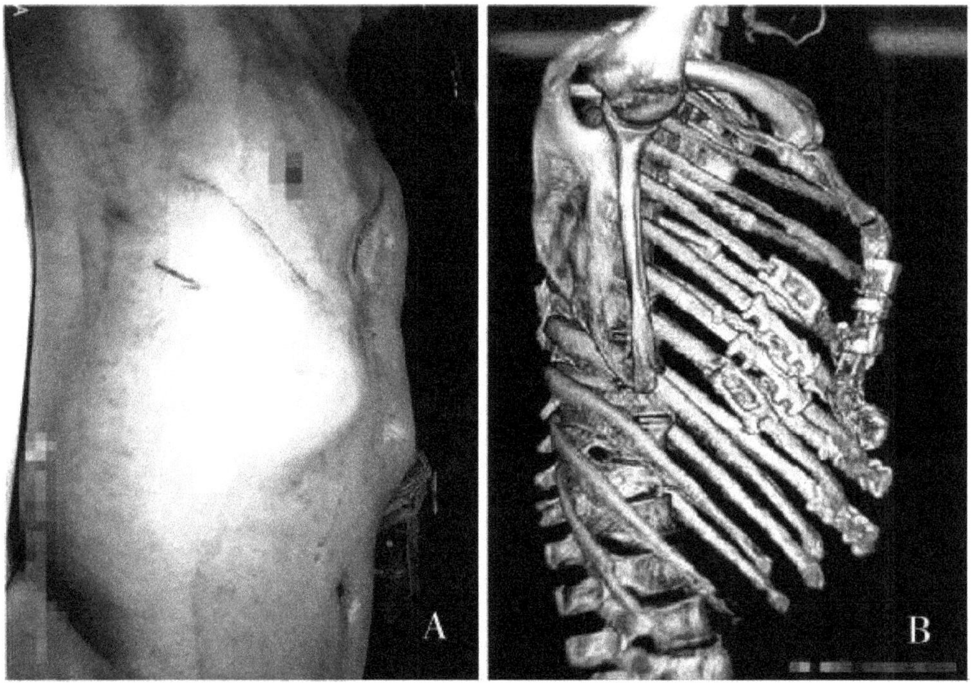

Figure 2-18-2 Deformity due to inadequate posttraumatic fixation (A. depressed anterior chest wall deformity; B. multiple fractures of the anterior chest wall, including ribs, rib cartilage, and sternum, for which fixation was unsatisfactory despite surgical fixation procedures, resulting in postoperative anterior chest wall deformity)

Surgically induced deformities are mainly those secondary to various thoracic surgeries. These surgeries can be generalised thoracic surgery, cardiac surgery or various surgeries on the chest wall. The specific nature of the surgery varies and can lead to deformities through different mechanisms.

Malformations due to general thoracic surgery are commonly seen in neonatal surgeries, such as early lung cystadenoma resection or diaphragmatic hernia repair, both of which can induce funnel chest [7-9]. The pathogenesis of thoracic deformities due to these two types of surgery has been described in detail in

other chapters, where the weakness of the chest wall and the action of external forces are the two necessary factors for the formation of the deformity.
Secondary thoracic deformities after cardiac surgery can be either protruded or depressed [10,11]. Sternal deformity is known as pectus excavatum and depressed deformity is known as funnel chest. Both deformities are actually related to the weakness of the chest wall and external forces. After cardiac surgery, the stability of the thorax is compromised. If the chest wall is very soft, it may move forward to form a proptosis when subjected to constant positive pressure from the heart. Conversely, if it is pulled by fibrous structures from the mediastinum, a depressed deformity may develop.
Secondary thoracic deformities can also occur secondary to a traditional chest wall surgery, such as thoracoplasty also known as thoracic revision surgery. This is a type of surgery that actively causes deformity. The goal of the surgery is to eliminate the dead space in the chest cavity by artificially collapsing the chest wall. Thoracic revision surgery was once a more common procedure widely used for refractory pulmonary
Tuberculosis, lung abscesses, and bronchopleural thinning are treated. Thoracic collapse deformity is the target of the procedure, and such a characterisation is different from all other procedures.
Surgery of the chest wall leading to secondary thoracic deformities can also be corrective surgery for thoracic deformities, such as open surgery for chicken breast. When all the rib cartilage on both sides is removed, the development of the thorax is compromised and secondary thoracic dysplasia occurs after surgery, a deformity that is typical of secondary thoracic deformities.
Secondary deformities following chest wall surgery can also be seen after other types of chest wall procedures, such as thoracic deformities following fracture fixation surgery (Figure 2-18-3), chest wall deformities caused by chest wall tumor resection, and deformities resulting from chest wall infection surgeries; all of these are relatively common secondary thoracic deformities. The main reason these surgeries ultimately lead to thoracic deformities is that, after lesion removal, the chest wall reconstruction does not meet normal standards.

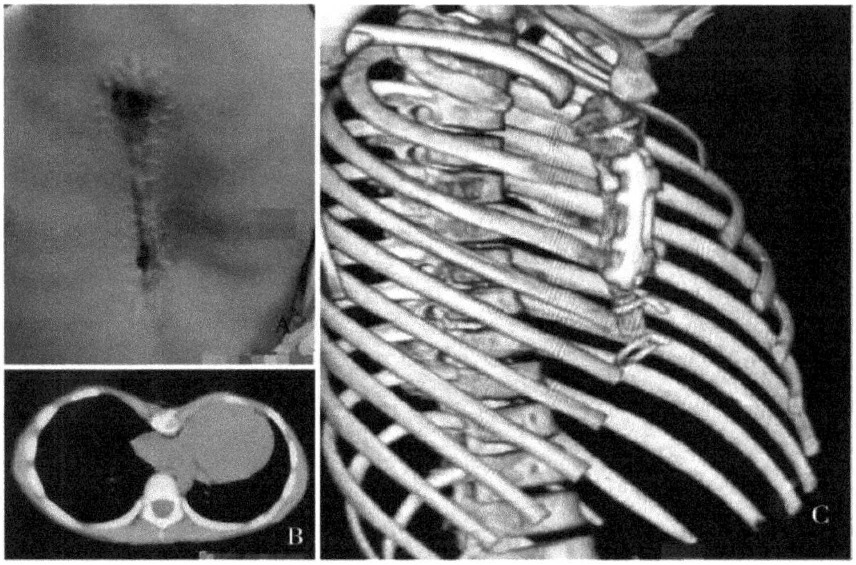

Figure 2-18-3 Deformity due to failure of sternal fracture fixation (the child's original disease was congenital heart disease, and during the implementation of cardiac surgery, the sternum was fractured due to excessive traction, and the sternum was fixed during the process of chest closure, which resulted in postoperative thoracic deformity due to improper fixation methods. a. Appearance of the chest wall, which shows a clear concave deformity; b. CT cross-sectional view showing the concave anterior chest wall and cardiac compression; c. Three-dimensional reconstruction (showing sternal fracture as well as fixation material, depression of the lower sternum)

Infections leading to thoracic deformities mainly come from chronic pyothorax, when the pleural fibrous plate is thickened, it can pull on one side of the chest wall causing the chest wall to collapse as a whole, resulting in secondary thoracic deformities (Figure 2-18-4) [12-14].

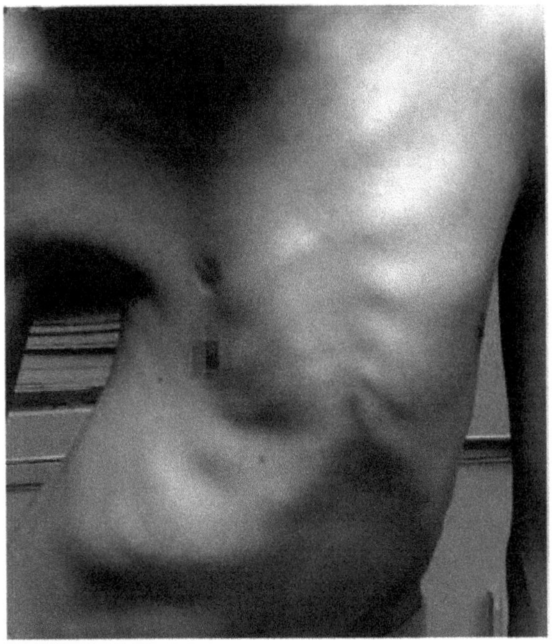

Figure 2-18-4 Secondary chest wall deformity caused by empyema. The main feature is collapse of one side of the chest wall with significant spinal scoliosis.

Secondary deformities caused by other factors can be seen in barrel chest following chronic respiratory diseases [15], and also in thoracic deformities caused by long-term hypoxia in high-altitude regions. The pathogenesis of these deformities is related to the extra work performed by the respiratory muscles due to prolonged hypoxia. When this extra work continues, the chest wall may change shape under muscular traction, eventually forming a barrel chest. In addition to all the causes mentioned above, various other causes of secondary thoracic deformities can also be seen in clinical practice. The common feature of these deformities is that a specific cause leads to an abnormal chest wall shape; the deformity may not be typical and often presents in a very complex manner (Figure 2-18-5) [16].

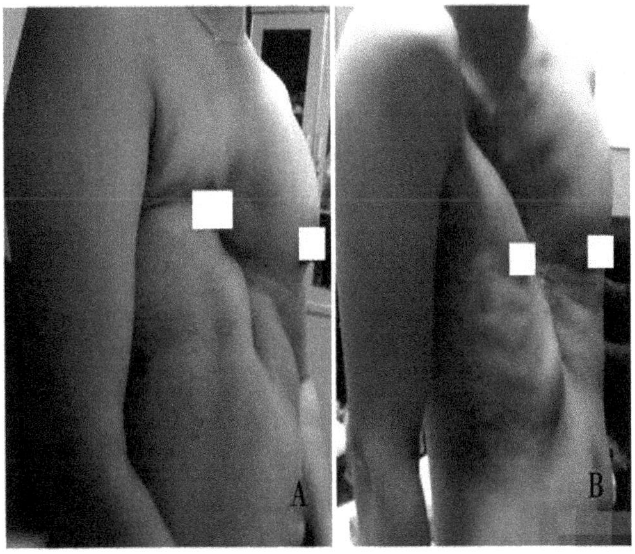

Figure 2-18-5 Secondary thoracic malformations due to abortion during fetal life (A. Young female with malformation of the right breast and pectoralis major muscle and severe destruction of bony structures; B. Young male with a large longitudinal grooved depression in the anterior chest wall)

2. Pathological features

Secondary thoracic deformities are essentially the same in nature compared to primary thoracic deformities. However, secondary thoracic deformities due to certain factors may be more complex and severe [1-4]. For example, thoracic deformities secondary to trauma are more severe in structure and shape than normal thoracic deformities [5,6], and those secondary to surgery are more severe [7-11]. These deformities can be of different types, the majority of which are of the depressed type, with the raised type being less common, although some morphologically complex deformities may exist. In terms of localised structures, most of these deformities have more severe localised lesions. The lesions are not only present in the chest wall structures themselves, but may also be present in the periphery. There is often connective tissue proliferation or severe adhesions on the inner side of the chest wall, and in some cases there are even foci of infection or other obvious primary lesions. The presence of these lesions complicates the pathology of secondary thoracic deformities and makes surgery much more difficult.

3. Clinical presentation

Secondary thoracic deformities have a clear causative agent, which allows patients to exhibit signs and symptoms of the primary disease in addition to the clinical manifestations of the deformity itself [1]. For example, in trauma-induced thoracic deformity, in addition to the symptoms that may be caused by the deformity itself, the patient may have significant localised pain, which is a symptom associated with the trauma, as well as severe systemic symptoms. These are clinical manifestations specific to trauma. In another example of thoracic collapse that occurs in chronic pyothorax, the patient will have a combination of significant symptoms of pyothorax. The clinical presentation of secondary thoracic deformities may be more complex and severe than that of primary thoracic deformities. It is for this reason that surgical treatment is more necessary

4. Inspection

The examination of secondary thoracic deformity consists of two aspects, the first is the examination related to thoracic deformity, and the second is the examination of the primary disease, the specific examination items and means need to be decided according to the characteristics of the deformity and the nature of the primary disease. The main purpose of the thoracic deformity examination is to clarify the overall shape of the deformity and the characteristics of the local lesion, while the examination of the primary disease is to clarify the current status of the disease and its possible impact on surgery. In patients with this type of deformity, an enhanced CT of the chest can be used as a necessary examination. If conditions permit, a three-dimensional reconstructive examination may be considered to provide a comprehensive view of the focal areas (Fig. 2-18-6).

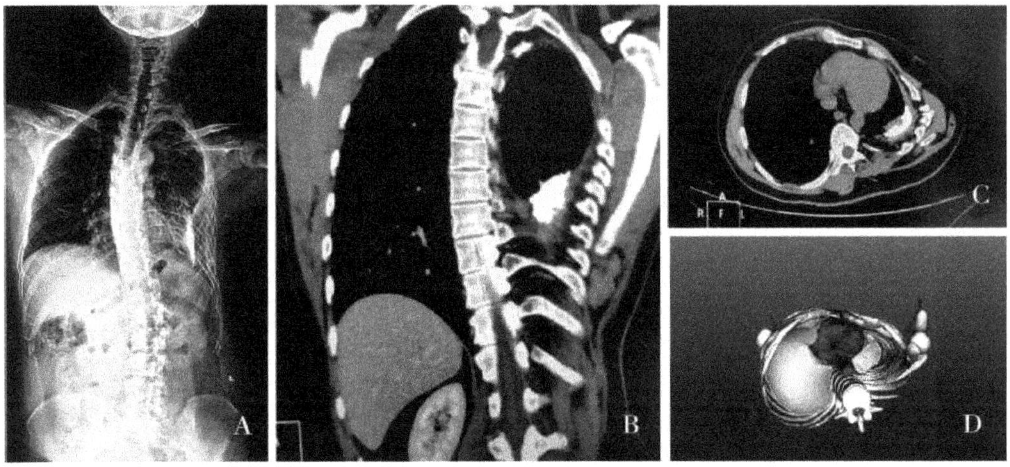

Figure 2-18-6 Imaging of secondary thoracic deformity (A. CT scan showing left intrathoracic lesion, left chest wall collapse, and scoliosis; B. CT coronal view showing intrathoracic lesion, left chest wall collapse, and scoliosis; C. CT cross-sectional view showing right-to-left asymmetry of the chest wall, left intrathoracic lesion, and left chest wall collapse; and D. Three-dimensional reconstruction showing left chest wall collapse)

5. Diagnosis and differential diagnosis

The diagnosis of secondary thoracic deformity is not difficult when the cause is clear and the shape of the deformity is obvious. However, the diagnosis must be based on two aspects [1-4]: the nature of the thoracic deformity and the nature of the primary disease. The former is easier, while the latter is sometimes more difficult. For example, in a patient with traumatic thoracic deformity, the chest wall may have been traumatised at an early age, but if the deformity occurs many years later, it is difficult to establish a causal relationship between the two, and it is not easy to make a final diagnosis.

Secondary thoracic deformities should be differentiated from primary deformities in combination with other pathologies. For example, a thoracic deformity following lung surgery should be a typical secondary deformity. However, a flat chest combined with a spontaneous pneumothorax is a primary deformity, and even after surgery for a spontaneous pneumothorax, the flat chest of such a patient remains a primary deformity, not a secondary deformity. There is also a very special case of post-cardiac surgery funnel chest. In this case, the funnel chest can be caused by the cardiac surgery, but it can also exist before the cardiac surgery. The latter is the case of primary funnel chest in combination with heart disease. This is a case where the funnel chest was not corrected at the same time as the cardiac surgery, so the patient continues to have a funnel chest after the surgery. Such a funnel chest is a primary deformity unrelated to cardiac surgery. However, the effects of cardiac surgery make the treatment of funnel chest pain difficult.

A similar situation can be seen in chicken chest after cardiac surgery. Chicken chest can exist before or after cardiac surgery. While the former is a primary chicken chest, the latter is a secondary chicken chest.

6. Indications for Surgery

In general, surgery for secondary thoracic deformities is not fundamentally different from that for primary thoracic deformities, so the basic principles are the same when talking about indications for surgery. Overall, surgery should be left to the patient and family to decide. If it is felt to be unsightly or uncomfortable, surgery is needed. If it is neither unsightly nor uncomfortable, surgery is not needed.

In the case of secondary thoracic deformities, the symptoms tend to be more pronounced due to the presence of a primary disease, so surgery is more often than not required. However, both factors must be taken into account when implementing the specific treatment. In addition to the deformity itself, the primary disease must also be considered. If the primary disease is too severe to be cured or carries a high risk, surgery cannot be performed easily. In addition, some thoracic deformities are compensatory lesions, such as secondary barrel chest, which are contraindications to surgery and cannot be treated surgically. Also, there are thoracic deformities that have a therapeutic role, such as chest wall collapse due to thoracic revision surgery. If the primary lesion in the lungs is still present, the collapse of the chest wall cannot be actively eliminated, and this should also be considered a contraindication to chest wall surgery.

7. Surgical treatment

Secondary thoracic deformities come in a wide variety of shapes, and the choice of surgical approach depends on the characteristics of the deformity. However, regardless of the complexity of the deformity, it can be classified using a holistic classification, which can provide directional guidance for the surgery to be performed successfully.

(1) Principles of Surgery

Secondary deformities are associated with the presence of a primary disease, which inevitably makes surgery more difficult if it is performed. When the primary disease and thoracic deformity are operated at the same time, it puts special requirements on the surgery. Because secondary deformities are more complex, the following principles need to be observed when performing surgery [1-4]: 1) Minimally invasive surgery is not indispensable, and open surgery can be considered when necessary. Some secondary deformities may appear to be simple deformities, but the underlying structures may be very complex. For example, in a funnel chest secondary to trauma, the bony structures may be abnormally thickened, and even have large bone scabs forming. Such structures cannot be treated by minimally invasive surgery in any case. Instead, open surgery is required, which is almost exclusively effective. In the case of thoracic deformity secondary to resection of a chest wall tumour, the primary surgery is itself an open surgery, and if the thoracic deformity is corrected, it is even more necessary to use an open surgery rather than minimally invasive surgery. (2) Thoracoscopy is not possible without it, and more often than not, the surgery needs to be done under direct vision. Due to the presence of the primary disease, there may be severe adhesions in the thoracic cavity, and the operation for the lesion in the thoracic cavity cannot be done through Thoracoscopy. If there is a need for localised orthopaedics, direct vision surgery will be the only reliable option. For example, in the case of thoracic deformities resulting from septicothorax surgery, such surgery is performed on the body surface, and when correction is performed by open surgery, not only is there good visualisation, but complete removal of the lesion is guaranteed. At this point, if Thoracoscopy is used, it becomes an absolute of tiredness. (3) Combining contouring and reconstruction, using a variety of surgical techniques. In some special deformities, the basic shape of the bony structure is destroyed, and it is difficult to obtain good results if only shaping is considered. It is necessary to use reconstructive methods in conjunction with surgery to rebuild the necessary structures in order to achieve a good result. Such a situation exists in almost every serious secondary thoracic deformity surgery, and it is almost impossible to proceed without knowing the reconstruction technique. (4) The primary disease must be treated at the same time. The primary cause of secondary thoracic deformity may also affect the patient, so in the course of treatment, not only must the deformity be treated, but also the primary cause must be treated, so that the disease can be completely cured. For example, if the thoracic deformity is caused by trauma, it may be accompanied by damage to the thoracic organs in addition to damage to the chest wall, in which case the damage to the organs in the thoracic cavity must be dealt with first, and then the correction of the thoracic deformity can be carried out. In the case of thoracic deformity caused by pyothorax, the removal of pyothorax is the first operation that must be completed, which is the basis for the success of deformity correction.

(2) Surgical approach

Surgery for secondary thoracic deformity consists of a two-part operation [1-4]: one is the management of the primary disease; the other is the correction of the thoracic deformity itself. The two parts of the operation are interrelated and indispensable, and must be given equal attention.

(i)Treatment of the primary cause

Secondary thoracic deformities all have a definite cause, and all result from a specific etiology of the deformity. However, the form in which these etiologies exist at the time of performing thoracic deformity surgery can vary greatly. In the case of trauma, it can be a long time ago or it can be a recent trauma, both of which can cause secondary thoracic deformities, but the form of the trauma is obviously different, and therefore the principles and methods of management are different. The same is true for secondary thoracic deformities caused by tumours. The tumour may be untreated or resected. The primary disease at this point obviously also differs markedly. The specific form in which the primary tumour exists varies, as does the manner in which the surgery is performed. When performing surgery, it is necessary to make specific analyses according to the specific conditions of the primary disease and design the most appropriate surgical method, which is the most basic principle of dealing with the primary disease.

(ii) Correction of thoracic deformities

Secondary thoracic deformity has a special shape and complex structure, so when performing the surgery, it is not possible to only perform plastic surgery, but to consider reconstruction at the same time, and these two methods are the most basic methods of treating secondary thoracic deformity.

(1) Plastic surgery. Secondary thoracic deformities, however complex, have general features of thoracic deformity which are similar to those of the primary thoracic deformity and can therefore be corrected by general plastic surgery. Such an operation is relatively simple and can be performed minimally invasively if there are no factors that particularly affect the operation. If minimally invasive surgery is difficult, risky, or simply not possible, open surgical contouring may be considered (Fig. 2-18-7)

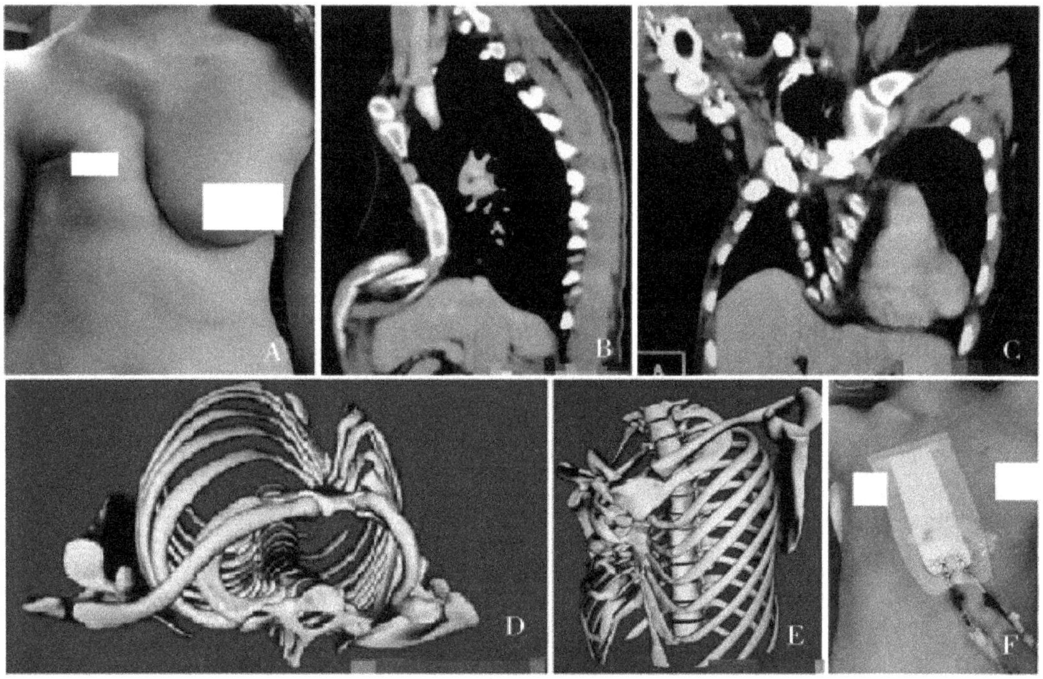

Figure 2-18-7 Plastic surgery for secondary thoracic deformity (A. The right chest wall soft tissue and bony structures have obvious deformity; B. CT sagittal view shows severe deformity of the bony structures of the anterior chest wall; C. CT coronal view shows a severe deformity of the anterior chest wall, with the heart located in the left thoracic cavity; D, E. Three-dimensional reconstruction shows a severe deformity of the thoracic contour; F. Orthopedics treatment was completed using a comprehensive surgical approach, with the deformity essentially disappearing after the operation.

(2) Reconstructive surgery.Some thoracic deformities have serious local lesions, which cannot be operated by ordinary shaping means, and then it is necessary to cut off or excise the local deformity, and then reconstruct the local structure to obtain a satisfactory shape.

Reconstructive surgery is generally a very complex procedure. It is not the same as reconstruction of a primary lesion. For example, in reconstructive surgery of the chest wall after resection of a tumour in the chest wall, if the tumour has not been operated on, the reconstructive surgery of the chest wall can be completed at the same time as the resection of the tumour, and the reconstructive surgery is relatively simple; however, if the reconstructive surgery is completed after the resection of the tumour, the difficulty of the operation will be significantly increased.

Among the reconstructive surgeries for secondary thoracic deformities of various causes, the most difficult surgery is reconstructive surgery for chest wall collapse secondary to pyothorax. This lesion itself has a long history of severe lesions in the chest cavity, chest wall collapse, narrowing of the intercostal space, shortening of the ribs, and scoliosis, making reconstructive surgery extremely challenging. In order to complete the surgery, the following key points need to be noted: 1) The intrathoracic lesions must be completely removed. The patient may have abscesses, fibrous plate thickening, and calcification in the chest cavity, and these lesions must be completely removed, or else the reconstruction of the chest wall will be affected. (2) Complete reconstruction of one side of the chest wall must be performed. The patient's chest wall collapse often involves all the ribs, and for the collapse to be eliminated, manipulation must be done on each rib to place it in the correct position and length.

Lengthening, firm fixation, and ultimately complete normalisation of the appearance of one side of the chest wall. (3) To use effective materials for reconstruction. To complete the reconstruction operation, it is necessary to have suitable materials, which are the most basic requirement for reconstruction surgery. For rib and rib cartilage reconstruction, Matrix RIB (Fig. 2-18-8) or other materials can be used (Fig. 2-18-9). If a defect in the sternum is involved, digital materials may be considered for reconstruction. (4) Adequate cleansing and drainage are required. Abscessed chest is inherently an infectious lesion, and for satisfactory postoperative recovery, it is important to complete the relevant intraoperative operations; otherwise, it will cause the infection to spread, which will not only fail to achieve the goals of the surgery but also bring about a variety of complications.

Compared with general plastic surgery, reconstructive surgery is more destructive and more difficult to operate. The reconstruction will be even more difficult if the treatment of the original disease is taken into account. It is precisely because of this difficulty that extra attention must be paid to the details of the operation in order to ensure the success of the surgery.

8. Prognosis

Secondary thoracic deformities are often quite severe. Since the primary disease is still present, both the primary condition and the thoracic deformity must be treated simultaneously, which means the surgical difficulty is significantly increased and poses a major challenge for every surgeon. Because of this increased complexity, the success rate of surgery for secondary thoracic deformities is certainly lower than that for primary thoracic deformities. However, as long as the surgical principles are strictly followed, these procedures can ultimately be successful.

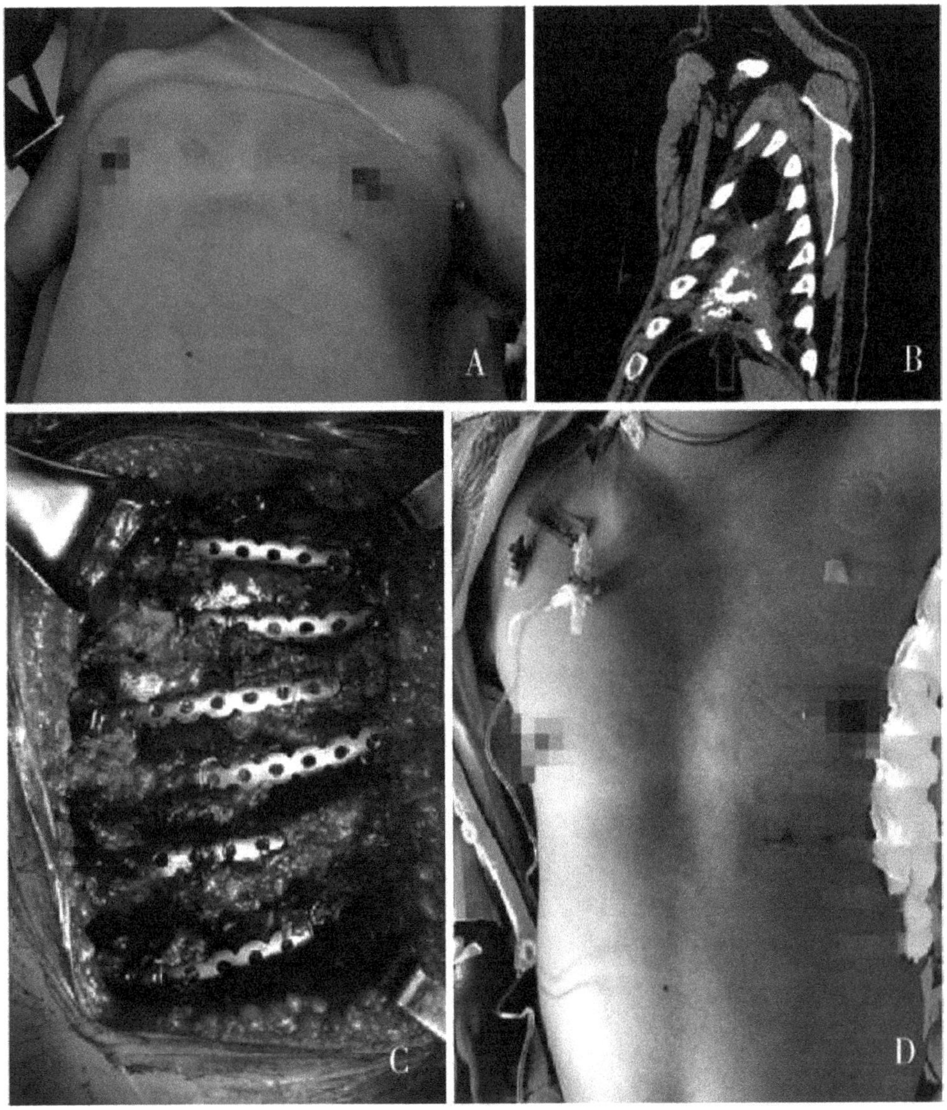

Figure 2-18-8 Reconstruction of secondary thoracic deformity due to pyothorax (A. Collapse of the left chest wall with left-right asymmetry; B. CT sagittal view showing left intrathoracic lesion; C. Removal of the intrathoracic lesion and reconstruction of the chest wall with Matrix RIB; D. Postoperative appearance of the thoracic contour, which is essentially back to normal

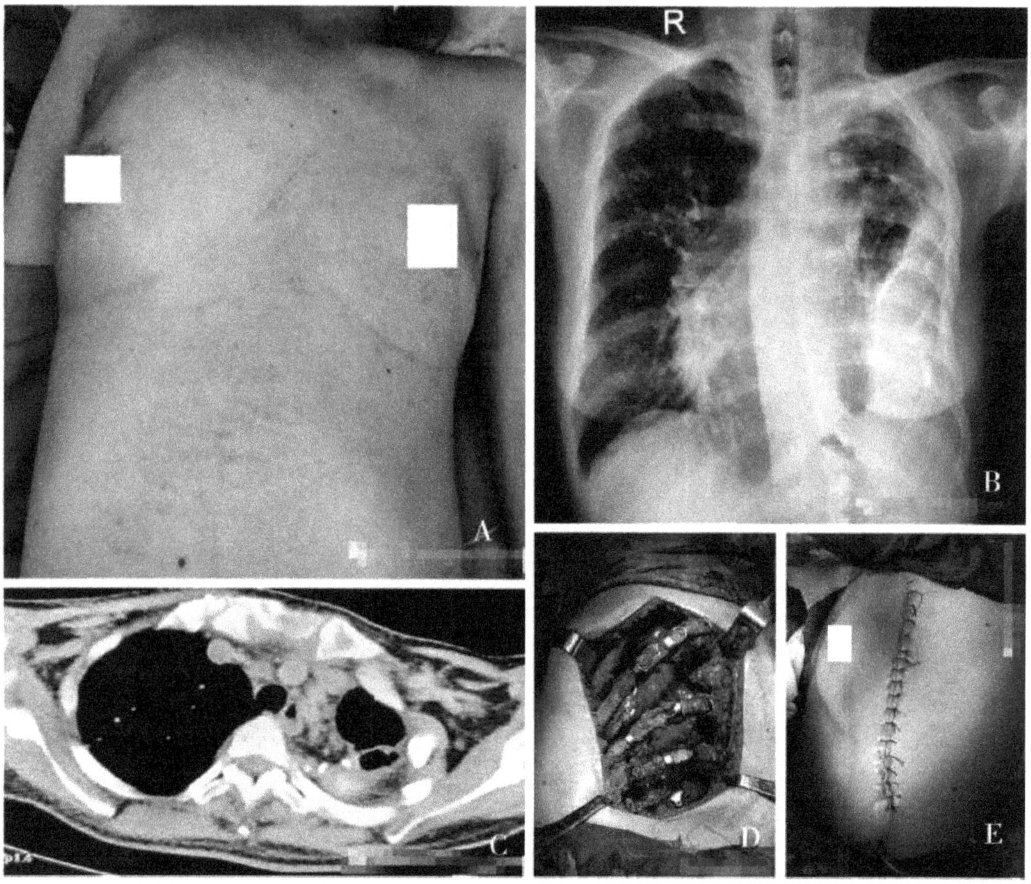

Figure 2-18-9 Reconstructive surgery for secondary thoracic deformity due to pyothorax (A. Appearance of the chest wall with a collapsed left chest wall; B. Frontal view X-Ray showing a significant left intrathoracic lesion, a collapsed left chest wall, and a scoliotic spine; C. CT cross-section showing a left intrathoracic lesion and a collapsed left chest wall; D. Removal of the left intrathoracic lesion and reconstruction of the thorax with a rib grafting plate; and E. Postoperative chest wall)

REFERENCES

[1] Wang, W. L. 2021a. "Secondary Thoracic Deformities." *Thoracic Deformity Surgery Specialist*, September 21.

[2] Wang, W. L. 2019a. "Secondary Funnel Chest (1)." *Thoracic Malformation Surgery Specialist*, December 13.

[3] Wang, W. L. 2019b. "Secondary Funnel Chest (2)." *Thoracic Deformity Surgery Specialist*, December 14.

[4] Wang, W. L. 2019c. "Secondary Funnel Chest (3)." *Thoracic Deformity Surgery Specialist*, December 16.

[5] Wang, W. L. 2020a. "Traumatic Funnel Chest." *Thoracic Deformity Surgery Specialist*, September 20.

[6] Wang, W. L. 2019d. "Wang Surgery for Secondary Deformity Completed at the Fifth Affiliated Hospital of Southern Medical University." *Thoracic Deformity Surgery Specialist*, August 8.

[7] Wang, W. L. 2020b. "Principles of Funnel Chest Formation after Neonatal Thoracic Surgery." *Thoracic Deformity Surgery Specialist*, November 23.

[8] Wang, W. L. 2021b. "Wang's Surgery for Secondary Funnel Chest after Lung Cystadenoma." *Thoracic Deformity Surgery Specialist*, March 8.

[9] Wang, W. L. 2020c. "Mechanism of Funnel Chest Formation after Surgery for Congenital Diaphragmatic Hernia." *Thoracic Deformity Surgery Specialist*, November 24.

[10] Wang, W. L. 2020d. "Wang Procedure for Postoperative Funnel Chest in Congenital Diaphragmatic Hernia." *Thoracic Deformity Surgery Specialist*, October 31.

[11] Wang, W. L. 2021c. "A Very Low-Level Error: A Specific Thoracic Deformity after Cardiac Surgery." *Thoracic Deformity Surgery Specialist*, January 22.

[12] Wang, W. L. 2021d. "MatrixRIB Chest Wall Reconstruction Surgery Secondary to Unilateral Chest Wall Collapse." *Thoracic Deformity Surgery Specialist*, July 10.

[13] Wang, W. L. 2020e. "Surgery in Gansu Today: MatrixRIB Reconstructive Surgery for Secondary Thoracic Deformity." *Thoracic Deformity Surgery Specialist*, November 6.

[14] Wang, W. L. 2019e. "Xining: Secondary Thoracic Deformity Surgery after Sepsis." *Thoracic Deformity Surgery Specialist*, August 30.

[15] Pierce, J. A., and R. V. Ebert. 1958. "The Barrel Deformity of the Chest, the Senile Lung and Obstructive Pulmonary Emphysema." *American Journal of Medicine* 25 (1): 13–22.

[16] Wang, W. L. 2020f. "Secondary Surgery for Severe Thoracic Deformity." *Thoracic Deformity Surgery Specialist*, December 27.

CONGENITAL HEART DISEASE COMBINED WITH THORACIC DEFORMITY

Most thoracic malformations are congenital, and since they are congenital, the lesions may not be limited to the thorax alone, and many patients with thoracic malformations may have congenital lesions in other parts of the body. Of these, congenital heart disease is the most common comorbidity [1]. The pathogenesis of thoracic deformity itself is unclear, as is the pathogenesis of congenital heart disease, and there may be some common mechanism at work when the two are combined. If the two diseases are studied together, it may be more conducive to the elucidation of their mechanisms.

1. General Concepts

Among all kinds of thoracic deformities, the thoracic deformity that is most likely to be combined with congenital heart disease is funnel chest, in addition to other types of deformities, such as flat chest can also be combined with this kind of disease, but the combination of heart disease in chicken chest is relatively rare, which may be related to the pathogenesis of chicken chest. This may be related to the pathogenesis of pectus excavatum. Most people believe that pectus excavatum is associated with acquired factors, whereas congenital factors are the most common cause of heart disease, so the combination of the two is rare. Combined with thoracic anomalies, the preexisting congenital heart disease can be the common atrial septal defect or ventricular septal defect, and occasionally, there are other rare malformations, and some patients will be combined with Marfan syndrome [2,3], which is an extremely serious preexisting heart disease.

2. Hazards

In most cases, there is no functional abnormality, so there are no obvious symptoms, and the main harm comes from the thoracic deformity. There are many types of thoracic deformities, and the main harm comes first from the appearance, which is the common harm of all thoracic deformities. In addition to the cosmetic risk, there is also a physiological risk, which comes mainly from the compression of the chest wall depression. In the case of raised deformities, there is no such hazard, whereas in the case of depressed deformities, if the compression is severe, it can affect the functioning of the heart and lungs, leading to a range of symptoms. In a small number of patients, the heart can be directly affected by the severity of the preexisting disease, and the risk to cardiac function is even more severe in the case of a depressed deformity.

3. Clinical manifestations

Mild forms of preexisting heart disease can have no symptoms in the early stages. If the lesions are severe, symptoms may appear at an earlier age. When a depressed type of malformation is combined with preexisting heart disease, the depression directly presses on the heart, which is itself defective, and the symptoms of heart disease are then

The symptoms are readily apparent. As a result, thoracic malformations combined with CHD present earlier and are more severe than in patients with isolated CHD.

4. Inspection

When thoracic malformations are suspected to be combined with preexisting heart disease, a number of special investigations are required. The first is an examination of the thoracic deformity. This examination is not significantly different from the independent examination of thoracic malformations. The most basic means of cardiac examination is auscultation [4]. If a murmur is detected, further investigations are necessary, and in this case, the most important examination is a cardiac ultrasound and, if necessary, an angiogram.

5. Diagnosis and differential diagnosis

Diagnosis is not difficult when the two diseases are present alone. However, the combination often results in a missed diagnosis. Thoracic deformities are abnormalities in the appearance of the thorax, which are easy to detect and unlikely to be missed. Depressed malformations can be associated with a heart murmur, which can lead to a missed diagnosis of cardiac disease if auscultation is not performed, or if the nature of the murmur is not investigated [4]. Missed diagnosis of heart disease is very harmful to patients and must be avoided as much as possible. The easiest way to avoid a missed diagnosis is to pay attention to auscultation. Once a heart murmur is detected, regardless of the nature of the murmur, cardiac ultrasonography should be performed, which is the most effective way to eliminate the missed diagnosis of heart disease.

Differential diagnosis is required in cases of thoracic malformations combined with a functional heart murmur. In this case, there is no organic pathology of the heart, and the heart murmur comes from a change in the shape of the heart due to compression of the chest wall. The nature of the murmur can change depending on the position. The diagnosis can be made by cardiac ultrasound.

6. Surgical treatment

(1) Indications for surgery

Surgery for simple thoracic deformities is primarily a decision for the patient and family. If there are no obvious symptoms or if there is no higher demand for appearance, surgery may not be considered. However, preeclampsia is a condition that must be operated on. When a thoracic deformity is combined with a pre-existing heart condition, surgery is usually required. There are exceptions, however, if the heart disease itself has developed into a contraindication to surgery.

(2) Surgical strategy

Thoracic deformity combined with congenital heart disease is a very specific combination, and due to the various factors involved in the treatment process, three different surgical strategies are possible [5]: (1) simultaneous surgery for both diseases; (2) surgery for congenital heart disease only, without thoracic deformity; and (3) surgery for thoracic deformity only, without congenital heart disease.

(1) Treatment efficiency is improved, so that the patient suffers less pain and the economic burden is reduced. Separate thoracic deformity surgery and cardiac surgery are both necessary surgeries. Completing the surgery in two separate operations not only increases the workload and the time of disease treatment, but also significantly increases the patient's pain, and in addition, the two surgeries will add a lot of extra costs. In addition, the two surgeries will cost the patient a lot of extra money. It can be seen that performing the two surgeries separately is an extremely unfavourable choice for the patient. If the two surgeries can be combined into one, the advantages are self-evident. (2) the two surgeries can facilitate each other and are more conducive to surgery. The presence of thoracic deformities can inconvenience the performance of cardiac surgery. For example, the depression of the funnel chest will increase the risk and difficulty of opening the chest when opening the chest, will increase the difficulty of revealing the chest during surgery, and will interfere with cardiac resuscitation after closing the chest because of the presence of compression. If only cardiac surgery is performed without correction of the funnel chest, all the effects of the funnel chest will be present throughout the cardiac surgery, which is undoubtedly an extremely unfavourable factor for cardiac surgery. However, if the operation for the funnel chest is performed at the same time, the risks can be reduced by using the specialised techniques of chest wall surgery to open the chest; when the incision is opened, the deformity of the chest wall can be performed first, which makes exposure extremely easy; and when the chest is closed, the correction of the deformity can be performed at the same time, which will completely eliminate the effect of the deformity on the heart after the operation. The completion of these operations will undoubtedly greatly facilitate the performance of cardiac surgery. Similarly, cardiac surgery will

also facilitate the operation of the funnel chest. A leaky chest is usually treated by minimally invasive surgery, whether it is the Nuss procedure or the Wang procedure, and the biggest problem is in fact the exposure, which is difficult because of the small incisions in both procedures. However, if the heart surgery is done at the same time, it is equivalent to making a large auxiliary incision in the centre. This allows all operations on the funnel chest to be done through the large incision, and the operation becomes absolutely straightforward. At this point the risks of the operation are completely eliminated, the difficulty is reduced and the thoracic deformity becomes an extremely simple and easy to perform minor operation. It can be seen that when both surgeries are performed at the same time, they can be convenient for each other. (3) Avoiding the various risks and difficulties of a second operation. When surgery for thoracic deformity and congenital heart disease is done separately, surgery for the other disease is equivalent to a second surgery. At this point, there are various challenges, and the risks and difficulties of the surgery are significantly increased. If the surgeries are done at the same time, the hassle of a second surgery can be completely avoided and the patient will receive the most satisfactory treatment.

In summary, there are many benefits to treating both diseases at the same time. Therefore, as long as conditions permit, simultaneous surgery should be performed actively. However, in clinical practice, concurrent surgery is not common, and most patients receive only one of the surgeries but not the other. This situation is mainly related to some special reasons [5]: 1) Many hospitals are unable to perform two surgeries at the same time. Cardiac surgery and thoracic deformity surgery are not ordinary surgeries and require a high level of technical expertise. Cardiac surgery itself requires a high level of comprehensive technology, and many hospitals do not have the ability to perform cardiac surgery. Thoracic deformity surgery is even more specialised, and even large general hospitals may not have the capacity to perform thoracic deformity surgery. If a hospital cannot perform both types of surgery at the same time, it will not be able to perform the surgery at the same time. This is an objective limitation. (2) Many hospitals do not have the doctors to perform both surgeries at the same time. In the traditional disciplinary structure, cardiac surgery and thoracic surgery belong to the same speciality, cardiothoracic surgery, and this structure has institutional advantages for the simultaneous implementation of the treatment of both diseases. However, with technological advances in the discipline, cardiothoracic surgery has been separated into thoracic surgery and cardiac surgery at higher level hospitals. This structure is clearly not suitable for performing thoracic deformity surgery and cardiac surgery at the same time. The cardiothoracic surgery departments of lower-level hospitals remain together, which should be the most appropriate structure for the simultaneous treatment of both diseases, but the standard of cardiac surgery and thoracic surgery in such departments is often not high. Since the standard is not high, it will likely become impossible to safely and smoothly complete both cardiac surgery and chest wall deformity surgery. Limited technical skills directly affect the treatment outcome of the surgery. In hospitals where cardiac surgery and thoracic surgery are separate departments, although both departments have the capability to perform their respective surgeries, the division of specialties often prevents simultaneous operations. When the doctors from the two specialties are unwilling or disinclined to collaborate, only one of the surgeries can be done first. (3) Many hospitals' doctors deliberately perform only one of the surgeries. If a doctor is capable of completing both procedures at the same time, they will generally choose to do so if conditions permit. However, performing the surgery often depends on various objective factors. For example, cardiac surgery requires coordinated support in anesthesia, cardiopulmonary bypass, monitoring, and more. If these conditions are not sufficiently in place, even if the doctor is capable of performing cardiac surgery, they may voluntarily abandon it and only carry out the chest wall deformity correction instead. Some doctors also consider the risks and responsibilities of the surgery. For instance, a doctor skilled in chest wall deformity surgery may worry about the additional risks of cardiac surgery and thus decide to forgo the cardiac procedure. Likewise, a doctor experienced in cardiac surgery may choose not to do the chest wall deformity correction if they are not proficient in it or are concerned about possible surgical failure. When doctors, for various reasons, proactively forgo one of the surgeries, it becomes impossible to completely cure the patient's conditions. (4) Some doctors believe simultaneous surgeries should not be done. This often stems from a difficult compromise. For example, considering the risk of re-entering the chest during the perioperative period, some cardiac surgeons do not recommend performing chest wall deformity correction at the same time. The specific reason is that such surgery requires the placement of a metal plate. If the patient later needs a second thoracotomy or even bedside emergency treatment, the presence of the metal plate may hinder life-saving measures. Therefore, these doctors do not advocate performing chest wall deformity surgery and cardiac surgery at the same time.

Simultaneous surgery for the two conditions requires various supporting conditions, including both objective and subjective factors. If any of these conditions are not met, it is impossible to ensure the smooth execution of simultaneous surgery. However, the advantages of performing both surgeries at the same time are clear — whenever possible, every effort should be made to carry out simultaneous surgery.

(3) Surgical Methods

Congenital heart disease surgery and thoracic deformity surgery are both procedures with relatively high technical thresholds and strict requirements for surgical technique. Whether performing surgery for a single condition or carrying out simultaneous operations for both conditions, well-established surgical skills are essential. In particular, for surgeries that treat both conditions at the same time, the technical requirements are even more stringent — only with excellent surgical expertise can the success of such operations be ensured.

(i) Simultaneous surgery for both conditions

In cases of chest wall deformities combined with congenital heart disease, the most common type is pectus excavatum. When surgery for pectus excavatum is performed simultaneously with heart surgery, there are various surgical options for the cardiac procedure. In earlier years, a median sternotomy was used, and this method remains a primary surgical approach even today. With the development of minimally invasive cardiac surgery, some cardiac procedures can now be done through minimally invasive or interventional methods. In such cases, if pectus excavatum is also present, apart from trying to utilize the incision as efficiently as possible, the pectus excavatum can basically be treated as an independent procedure without many special requirements [6–8]. However, when a median sternotomy is used for the cardiac procedure, there are special considerations for the pectus excavatum repair, with different surgical options [5]: The first option is the Nuss procedure, and the second option is the Wang procedure. When performing the Nuss procedure, the surgical steps are as follows [9]: first, a midline incision is made along the sternum. The sternum is split longitudinally at the depressed area, and the incision is retracted to expose the heart, allowing the cardiac surgery to be carried out. After the cardiac procedure is completed, incisions are made on both sides of the chest wall. At appropriate positions around the depression, the thoracic cavity is entered, and an introducer is inserted through the incision on one side of the chest wall, advancing through the anterior midline incision, then enters the opposite thoracic cavity and exits through the chest wall incision on the other side. The guiding tube for the steel bar is then attached, and the guide is pulled through this pathway so that both ends of the guide emerge from the incisions on either side of the chest wall. After fully pre-shaping the bar, the sternum is routinely closed with steel wires. The steel bar is then connected to the guide tube and pulled along the prepared pathway, positioning the bar under the base of the anterior chest wall depression. The bar is then flipped to elevate the sunken chest wall. Both ends of the bar are secured, all incisions are closed, and the surgery is completed.

The Nuss procedure is a traditional minimally invasive surgery which, before the advent of the Wang procedure, was the only minimally invasive method used clinically. Using the Nuss procedure in the above operation has the following advantages:1. The steel bar is positioned behind the sternum, which helps with the healing of the midline incision; 2. The area of force supporting the chest is larger, which helps eliminate the pectus excavatum deformity; 3. The relatively long midline incision makes placing the steel bar very convenient and completely avoids the possibility of injuring the heart; 4. Since the sternum is split down the middle, the depressed area can be fully reshaped and the stress can be completely released, which greatly reduces the technical difficulty of the procedure. However, the Nuss procedure also has its disadvantages: 1. It requires additional incisions on the lateral chest wall, which inevitably increases postoperative scarring of the chest wall skin; 2. During placement of the steel bar, it must pass through both pleural cavities, which increases additional trauma and may even lead to related complications; 3. The Nuss procedure has age limitations — children under 3 years old cannot undergo the surgery. For younger children, if the surgeon does not know other procedures besides the Nuss method, the surgery cannot be performed; 4. The steel bar used in the Nuss procedure imposes a constraining effect on the thorax. If the child is in a period of rapid growth, it may affect the development of the chest after surgery.

Since its introduction into clinical practice, the Nuss procedure has long been the standard surgical method for treating pectus excavatum. However, for patients with concurrent congenital heart disease, although the Nuss procedure has certain advantages, its drawbacks are particularly significant. Therefore, if there are other options available, a more ideal surgical method should be considered.

The Wang procedure is a new surgical technique for pectus excavatum that has emerged in recent years, and it can also be considered for pectus excavatum combined with heart disease [10–12]. In actual practice, if the Wang procedure is chosen, all steps before completing the heart surgery are basically the same as those for the Nuss procedure, with the difference occurring after the cardiac operation is finished. After completing all intracardiac procedures, pre-shaping is performed first, then wires for closing the sternum are placed but temporarily left untightened. Submuscular tunnels are created on both sides along the bony structures of the chest wall. A lifting wire is placed across the sternum at the base of the depression. The steel bar is inserted through the tunnels, and then all wires — including those for fixing the sternum and lifting the depression — are tightened simultaneously. This closes the sternum and reshapes the chest wall at the same time. Once the fixation is complete, the midline incision is closed, marking the end of the surgery.

The Wang procedure itself needs to be performed through a median incision, and since the heart surgery already requires a median incision, the overlap of incisions allows for avoiding additional lateral chest wall incisions. This not only saves surgical steps but also reduces the number of postoperative scars, resulting in a better cosmetic outcome.

Moreover, having a relatively long median incision means that all steps of the Wang procedure are done under excellent direct visualization, which undoubtedly provides great convenience for the operation — it not only lowers the technical difficulty but also makes the procedure safer and the results more satisfactory. Another advantage of the Wang procedure is that it does not enter the pleural cavity, which significantly reduces surgical trauma and greatly lowers the risk of complications.

From the above analysis, it is clear that both the Nuss procedure and the Wang procedure have their own unique characteristics and advantages. In actual practice, as long as the specific features of the condition are fully considered and the surgical method is chosen accordingly, ideal results can be achieved.

(ii). Only perform congenital heart disease surgery, without performing thoracic deformity surgery

On the surface, performing only congenital heart disease surgery without addressing the thoracic deformity appears to fall solely within the scope of cardiac surgery and should not be discussed here. However, due to the presence of the thoracic deformity, even if it is treated at a different time, it can still affect the cardiac surgery. Therefore, certain issues must be discussed; otherwise, they could impact the surgery's progress.

The first issue is the technical aspect of opening the chest [5]. Cardiac surgery is mainly performed through a median sternotomy, but in patients with pectus excavatum, there is a significant depression in the anterior chest wall that directly compresses the heart, which poses major challenges for creating the incision. If the sternum is directly sawed open with a sternal saw, it may injure the heart, creating significant risk. To make the procedure safer, the surgical technique must be carefully planned. The following steps can effectively mitigate the risk of injuring the heart when sawing the sternum: (1) Fully expose the xiphoid process first, then split it or remove it entirely; (2) Carefully dissect upward along the posterior surface of the sternum from its lower end to create some space behind the sternum; (3) Use a thyroid retractor to lift the lower end of the sternum for pre-shaping, creating as much space as possible behind the sternum; (4) Dissect the deep surfaces near the costal arches on both sides close to the xiphoid process, insert thyroid retractors, and lift the chest wall to elevate the anterior chest wall as much as possible. Then first, dissect the retrosternal space and use the sternal saw to open the sternum. Throughout this process, the key principle is to enlarge the retrosternal working space, ensuring that the sawing of the sternum is done as far from the heart as possible to reduce surgical risk.

The second issue is the problem of retracting the incision [5]. After the depressed anterior chest wall is incised, the depression still remains. If a retractor is used to open the incision directly at this stage, the existing depression will inevitably affect the effectiveness of the retraction. To prevent this, pre-shaping of both

sides of the chest wall can first be performed through the median incision. Once this step is complete, the retractor can be inserted into the median sternotomy and used to steadily open the incision with continuous force, providing stable exposure for the surgery.
The third issue is the technical challenge of closing the chest [5]. After the cardiac surgery is completed, the heart is in a relatively fragile state. To safely get through the perioperative period, it requires a favorable surrounding environment. However, due to the existing chest wall depression, once the chest is closed, the heart will soon be subjected to pressure from the chest wall again. This is extremely detrimental to a heart that has just undergone the trauma of surgery. To minimize this compression, it is necessary to reshape the depressed chest wall forward before closing the chest. This serves two purposes: first, to release the local stress as much as possible; second, to alter the shape of the anterior chest wall to some extent, providing a degree of remodeling. Although this effect is limited, it can help reduce pressure on the heart as much as possible, thereby aiding the heart's recovery after surgery.
From the above analysis, it can be seen that performing only the cardiac surgery itself carries significant risks — especially when the chest depression is very severe. If the depression is not addressed simultaneously, it may directly lead to the failure of the heart surgery. Therefore, as long as conditions permit, it is best to perform both surgeries at the same time.

(iii) Only perform the chest wall deformity surgery without doing the heart surgery

The presentation of congenital heart disease (CHD) can vary greatly. for the vast majority of CHD cases, there is generally no significant cardiac dysfunction, and patients do not exhibit obvious symptoms. For these patients, if only the chest wall deformity surgery is performed, the presence of the heart condition does not increase the surgical risk or difficulty; therefore, it is essentially the same as performing an isolated chest wall deformity surgery [5]. However, if the congenital heart disease is more severe and there is cardiac dysfunction, the risk of the chest wall deformity surgery will increase. In such cases, related surgical maneuvers must be carried out with extreme caution, otherwise serious complications may arise due to the heart condition.
In general, performing only chest wall deformity surgery is not a reasonable choice. However, there is one exception: when the heart disease can be treated through interventional methods. In this case, the treatment of the heart condition and the chest wall deformity surgery do not have any conflict, so the heart condition can be left untreated during the chest wall deformity surgery, and only the chest wall deformity surgery can be performed

7. Results

At present, the cases of simultaneous surgeries reported in the literature have all achieved satisfactory surgical outcomes [2,6–8]. In our previous work, we have performed surgeries on 7 patients with congenital heart disease combined with chest wall deformities. Among them, 2 cases involved congenital heart disease with sternal cleft, which were operated on jointly with Director Chen Xinxin's team at the Guangzhou Women and Children's Medical Center [13,14]. Another 2 cases were children with congenital heart disease combined with pectus excavatum, operated on in collaboration with experts from the First Affiliated Hospital of Guangzhou Medical University [11,12]. 1 case involved a patient with Marfan syndrome, thoracic aortic dissection, and severe pectus excavatum, operated on together with experts from the First Affiliated Hospital of Guangxi Medical University (Figure 2-19-1) [3]. The remaining 2 cases of severe chest wall deformity combined with congenital heart disease were completed in our own department (Figure 2-19-2) [15]. All of these patients received satisfactory treatment

8. Prognosis

When a chest wall deformity is combined with congenital heart disease, performing simultaneous surgery provides the best possible treatment for both conditions, allowing the patient to benefit significantly and experience less suffering. If simultaneous surgery is not performed, it will not only pose major challenges for any future operations but will also subject the patient to additional pain. Therefore, for thoracic surgeons, when faced with such a combination, they must make every effort to facilitate simultaneous surgery and should never forgo the opportunity simply because they are not skilled in performing heart surgery.

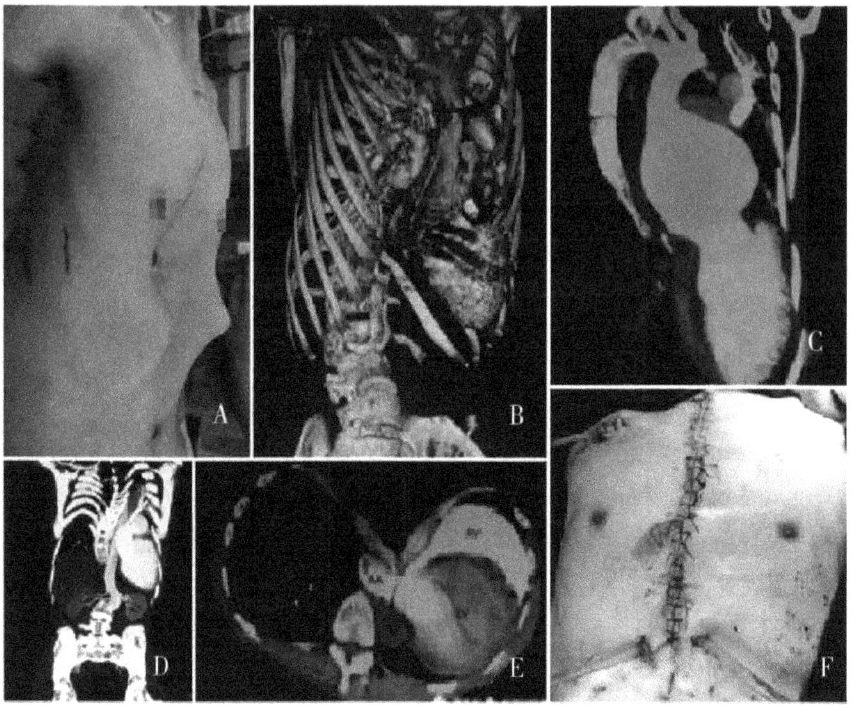

Figure 2-19-1 Simultaneous surgery for Marfan syndrome, thoracic aortic dissection aneurysm, and severe pectus excavatum (A. Appearance of the chest wall, showing severe depression of the anterior chest wall and protrusion of the costal arch; B. 3D reconstruction of the chest wall showing a severe pectus excavatum deformity of the anterior chest wall; C. Ascending aortic aneurysm and thoracic aortic dissection aneurysm; D. CT coronal view of the chest and abdomen; E. Severe anterior chest wall depression with the deepest point directly compressing the heart, forming malignant pectus excavatum; F. A median sternotomy was performed to first operate on the heart and great vessels, then the Wang procedure was used to correct the chest wall deformity, completely eliminating the deformity postoperatively.)

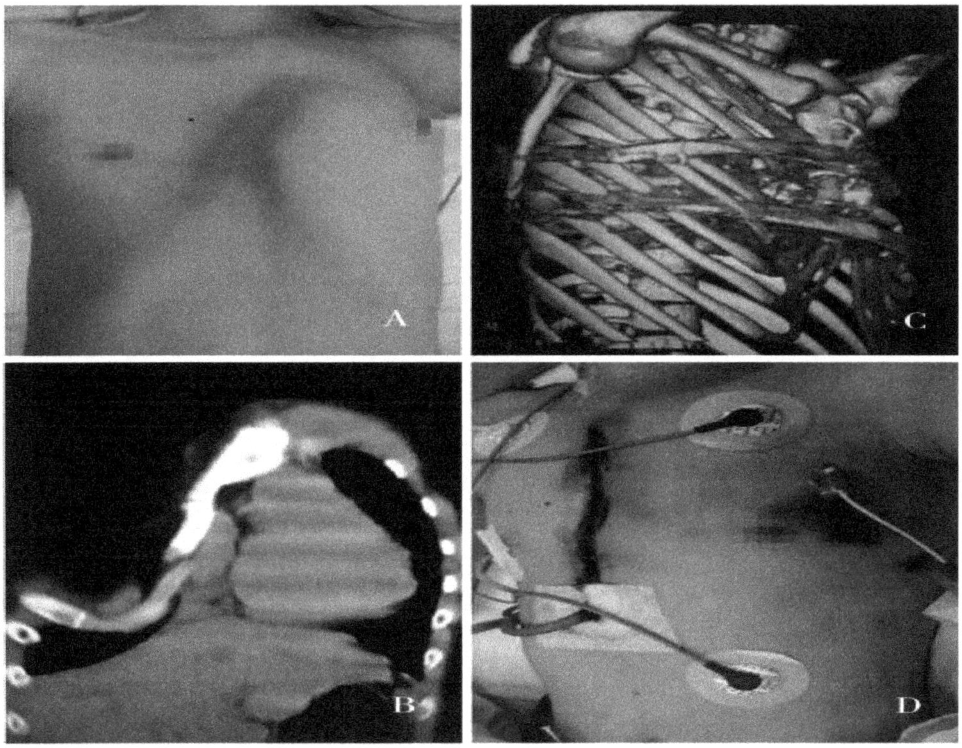

Figure 2-19-2 Severe Chest Wall Deformity Combined with Congenital Heart Disease (A. External view of the chest wall: severe anterior protrusion of the left chest wall, depression on the right side, with asymmetry between the left and right sides; B. Coronal CT image showing leftward displacement of the heart and asymmetrical chest wall deformity; C. Postoperative 3D reconstruction image: simultaneous heart surgery and chest wall deformity correction performed in one stage, with the overall chest shape basically normal after surgery; D. Postoperative external view of the chest wall appears basically normal.)

REFERENCES

[1] Wang, W. L. 2014a. "Be Alert to Babies with Chest Wall Deformities Developing Congenital Heart Disease." *Chest Wall Deformity Surgery Expert*, September 27.
[2] Nisanoglu, V., B. Battaloglu, N. Erdil, et al. 2007. "Surgical Approach for Stanford Type A Aortic Dissection in a Patient with Marfan Syndrome and Pectus Excavatum." *Texas Heart Institute Journal* 34 (2): 240–243.
[3] Wang, W. L. 2018a. "The Great Practice of the Wang Procedure: One-Stage Surgery for Severe Chest Wall Deformity Combined with Severe Heart Disease in Adults." *Chest Wall Deformity Surgery Expert*, June 16.
[4] Wang, W. L. 2014b. "Cardiac Murmurs in Chest Wall Deformities." *Chest Wall Deformity Surgery Expert*, December 30.
[5] Wang, W. L. 2021a. "Pectus Excavatum Combined with Congenital Heart Disease: Surgical Strategies and Methods." *Chest Wall Deformity Surgery Expert*, November 7.
[6] Deng, X., P. Huang, L. Yi, et al. 2017. "Hybrid Repair of Pectus Excavatum and Congenital Heart Disease: A Case Report." *Medicine (Baltimore)* 96 (51): e9503.

[7] Sun, Y., P. Zhu, and S. Y. Zheng. 2014. "Simultaneous Repair of Pectus Excavatum and Congenital Heart Disease without Cardiopulmonary Bypass or Sternal Osteotomy." *Journal of Cardiothoracic Surgery* 9: 168.
[8] Yang, G., X. Deng, Y. Yang, et al. 2019. "The Nuss Procedure for Pectus Excavatum during Atrial Septal Defect Closure through a Minimal Right Oblique Infra-Axillary Thoracotomy: A Case Report." *Medicine (Baltimore)* 98 (3): e13874.
[9] Wang, W. L. 2017. "Technical Issues in Single-Stage Surgery for Congenital Heart Disease and Chest Wall Deformities." *Chest Wall Deformity Surgery Expert*, August 1.
[10] Wang, W. L. 2018b. "The Wang Procedure: The Preferred Choice for Single-Stage Surgery Combining Heart Disease and Pectus Excavatum." *Chest Wall Deformity Surgery Expert*, June 10.
[11] Wang, W. L. 2019a. "A New Record Created at the First Affiliated Hospital of Guangzhou Medical University: Single-Stage Surgery for 'Congenital Heart Disease + Pectus Excavatum' in a 10-Month-Old Infant Weighing 6 kg." *Chest Wall Deformity Surgery Expert*, September 10.
[12] Wang, W. L. 2019b. "First Affiliated Hospital of Guangzhou Medical University: Second Surgery for Congenital Heart Disease with Pectus Excavatum Using the Wang Procedure." *Chest Wall Deformity Surgery Expert*, August 19.
[13] Wang, W. L. 2019c. "Surgical Treatment of Sternal Cleft Combined with Congenital Heart Disease." *Chest Wall Deformity Surgery Expert*, May 10.
[14] Wang, W. L. 2018c. "30-Day-Old Baby: Super Surgery (Severe Sternal Cleft with Congenital Heart Disease)." *Chest Wall Deformity Surgery Expert*, June 15.
[15] Wang, W. L. 2013. "Successful One-Stage Surgery for Congenital Heart Disease Combined with Pectus Excavatum and Pulmonary Cyst." *Chest Wall Deformity Surgery Expert*, December 20.

Section 20

THORACIC DEFORMITY AFTER CARDIAC SURGERY

After cardiac surgery, patients often develop thoracic deformities. This is considered a relatively common complication of heart surgery. Like other deformities, this condition can also affect the patient. If the impact is not severe, the patient may accept it and choose not to undergo treatment. However, if the deformity is significant, the patient may request surgery. Since the patient has already undergone heart surgery, undergoing additional surgery for a thoracic deformity will involve many specific difficulties and issues, which therefore require thorough study and consideration.

1. Pathogenesis

From a pathogenesis perspective, postoperative chest wall deformities after cardiac surgery can be categorized into three situations: 1. The patient already had a chest wall deformity before the cardiac surgery, but only the heart surgery was performed without correcting the chest deformity — in this case, the postoperative deformity is simply a continuation of the preexisting condition; 2. The patient did not have a chest wall deformity before the cardiac surgery, but developed a new deformity afterward;3. The patient had a chest wall deformity before surgery and underwent both cardiac surgery and deformity correction during the same procedure, but the correction was unsatisfactory, resulting in a significant residual deformity after surgery. Regardless of the underlying mechanism, the final outcome is the same: a chest wall deformity after cardiac surgery. A preexisting deformity can be regarded as a primary deformity, but in essence, its nature is not fundamentally different from a secondary deformity, so both can be considered secondary deformities in this context.

In terms of morphology, postoperative chest wall deformities after cardiac surgery mainly fall into two types: one is pectus excavatum (funnel chest) [1–3], and the other is pectus carinatum (pigeon chest) [4]. In addition to these two main deformities, other complex deformities may also occur, but their incidence is relatively low and they are quite rare [5,6].

Postoperative pectus excavatum after cardiac surgery is mostly due to a pre-existing chest wall depression that was not corrected and thus remained after the surgery. Ideally, the best approach would be to perform a simultaneous (combined) surgery, but due to various objective and subjective limitations, many patients undergo only the cardiac surgery without correction of the pectus excavatum, leaving the chest wall depression to persist postoperatively.

New-onset pectus excavatum after cardiac surgery is relatively rare. Its occurrence may be related to two main factors: (1) Decreased chest wall stability. Among the various structures of the anterior chest wall, the sternum is the primary load-bearing structure and plays an extremely important role in maintaining the stability of the thorax. During cardiac surgery, the sternum needs to be split along the midline. If there are problems with sternal fixation after surgery, the stability of the chest wall may be compromised, providing a structural basis for the development of a deformity. (2) Traction caused by contraction of mediastinal connective tissue. Cardiac surgery is performed entirely within the mediastinum, and significant adhesions and proliferation of connective tissue occur postoperatively. This can create a pulling force on the anterior chest wall. If chest wall stability is poor, the traction effect may lead to the development of a depression thus forming a pectus excavatum.

Postoperative pectus carinatum (pigeon chest) occurs relatively frequently and can also present in two ways: first, it may have existed before the cardiac surgery but was not treated concurrently; second, it may have newly developed after the surgery. The occurrence of pectus carinatum combined with congenital heart disease is relatively rare, but it does exist. If only the cardiac surgery is performed without addressing the pectus carinatum, the deformity will remain after the operation. Such pectus carinatum is considered a primary condition, but once it persists into the postoperative period, its nature is no longer significantly different from that of secondary pectus carinatum.

Clinically, pectus carinatum (pigeon chest) that appears after cardiac surgery is mostly a newly developed deformity. This type of deformity is more likely to occur in young children after cardiac surgery. The occurrence of pectus carinatum is also related to two factors: (1) Reduced thoracic stability. In young children, the degree of ossification of the thoracic structures is low, and the chest wall is relatively soft. After cardiac surgery, it is difficult to achieve satisfactory fixation of the sternum. If the surgical wires are tightened too much, they may cause internal fractures; if they are too loose, the fixation will be unstable. Poor sternal fixation can result in the two halves of the sternum near the incision becoming loose, compromising the overall stability of the thoracic cage. When the stability of the chest wall is compromised, any external force can lead to the formation of a deformity. (2) The effect of external force. The external force that leads to the formation of pectus carinatum is exactly opposite in direction to the force that causes pectus excavatum. This force also originates in the mediastinum but acts outward. Specifically, this force comes from the heart's own impact. The heart is an organ filled with high-pressure blood. While it is working, the internal pressure remains at a relatively high positive level. During its beating, the heart exerts a strong impact on the anterior chest wall.

Under the action of this force, if the anterior chest wall is weak, it may gradually protrude outward, forming pectus carinatum.

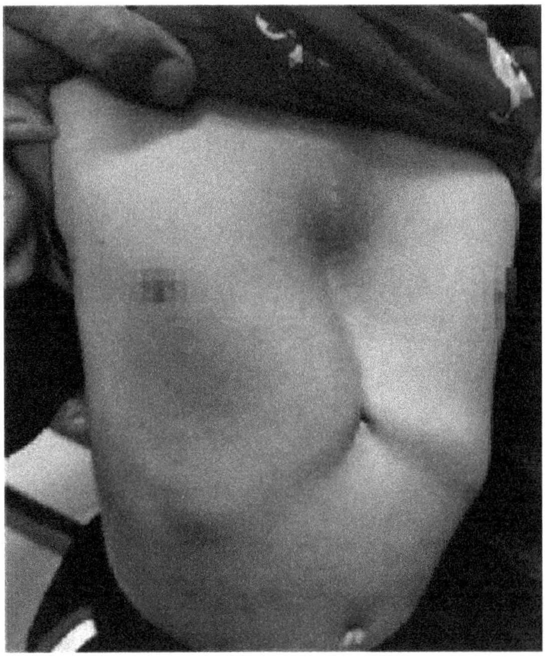

Figure 2-20-1 Funnel Chest After Cardiac Surgery

2. Pathological Characteristics

Post-cardiac surgery chest wall deformities are most commonly seen in two forms: one is funnel chest (pectus excavatum) (Figure 2-20-1), and the other is pigeon chest (pectus carinatum) (Figure 2-20-2). If a funnel chest was present before the cardiac surgery, its shape can be either symmetrical or asymmetrical. If the deformity newly develops after cardiac surgery, it is mostly a symmetrical funnel chest. The depression is located in the middle and lower part of the anterior chest wall, with an old surgical scar often visible in the midline. The longer the time after cardiac surgery, the deeper and more severe the depression may become. Pigeon chest presents similarly to funnel chest, but it is less common for pigeon chest to exist before surgery; most cases are new deformities that appear after cardiac surgery. This deformity generally centers around the surgical incision, is symmetrical on both sides, and the protrusion can be relatively localized or quite extensive. In addition to isolated funnel chest or pigeon chest, there can also be combined deformities, where both depression and protrusion exist together. This condition is relatively rare but results in a more complex deformity. The deformity can be complex, and may appear as a new deformity following a failed corrective surgery (see Figure 2-20-3)

3. Hazards

The harm caused by post-cardiac-surgery thoracic deformities is similar to that of general thoracic deformities. First, there is the cosmetic impact, and second, the functional impact. The cosmetic impact mainly comes from the appearance of the deformity itself, which is further worsened by the surgical scar from the cardiac procedure. Patients may feel self-conscious about their appearance,

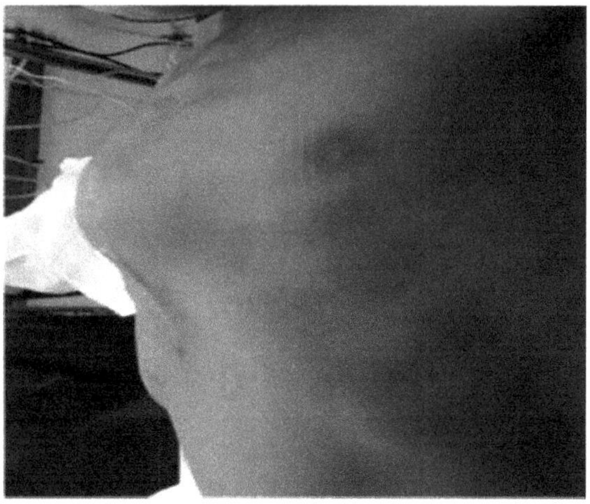

Figure 2-20-2 Pectus carinatum after cardiac surgery

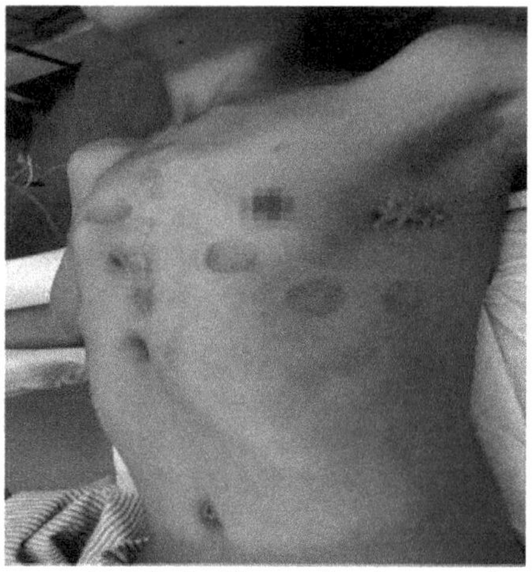

Figure 2-20-3 Funnel chest after cardiac surgery treated with the Nuss procedure — a failed surgery resulting in a complex deformity (local protrusion on the right chest wall forming an angular deformity, with a central depression)

which can lead to various psychological issues. The functional impact mainly comes from the compression caused by the depressed deformity. When the heart and lungs are compressed, related functions can become abnormal, eventually leading to various symptoms. For depressed deformities, postoperative mediastinal adhesions can pull the anterior chest wall downward continuously, which may cause the deformity to worsen over time. As the deformity worsens, the harm also becomes more severe. In addition, if the underlying heart condition was not completely resolved by the cardiac surgery, the compression from the anterior chest wall can further aggravate the existing cardiac disease.

4. Clinical Manifestations

Anteriorly protruding chest wall deformities may not necessarily present with obvious symptoms. However, in the case of depressed deformities, if the heart and lungs are compressed, the patient may develop related symptoms, such as breathing discomfort, chest tightness, and palpitations. These symptoms may worsen with physical activity. If the patient has pre-existing heart disease with cardiac dysfunction, the symptoms will be more pronounced. Additionally, patients may develop psychological issues due to concerns about their appearance, which can manifest as related symptoms.

5. Examination

The examination of thoracic deformities following cardiac surgery consists of three parts: first, the examination of the deformity itself; second, a comprehensive examination of the chest; and finally, an examination of the heart. Examination of the deformity itself forms the basis for diagnosing and treating the deformity. The overall chest examination is mainly conducted to rule out any associated intrathoracic conditions. The cardiac examination serves both to assess the postoperative recovery of the heart itself and to understand the impact of the deformity on cardiac function. Examination of the deformity itself should begin with a physical examination, supplemented by necessary imaging studies. The overall chest examination can be performed using CT scans, which can reveal both the chest wall structure and the internal thoracic structures. The cardiac examination is mainly carried out using ultrasound. To further understand the impact of the deformity on the heart, standard imaging studies are still required.

6. Surgical Treatment

(1) Surgical Indications

Deformities after cardiac surgery occur from time to time, but whether or not surgery should be performed is highly controversial. Having already undergone cardiac surgery, many patients and their families will seek the opinion of cardiac surgeons regarding whether to operate on the deformity. However, cardiac surgeons often do not recommend surgery for thoracic deformities, mainly for the following reasons: 1. Cardiac surgeons do not perform deformity correction surgeries and are often unfamiliar with the harm caused by such deformities, so they may provide unprofessional advice. 2. Even if cardiac surgeons understand the harm caused by the deformity, they may still be reluctant to recommend surgery, as the deformity occurred following their own operation — they wish to avoid unnecessary disputes. 3. Cardiac surgeons may worry that a deformity correction surgery could affect the outcome of the heart surgery, and therefore do not recommend it.

When cardiac surgeons do not recommend surgery, many patients and their families are also unwilling to undergo surgery, for the following reasons: 1. They do not want to endure the pain of another surgery. for many patients, cardiac surgery is an unforgettable and painful experience. Such an experience leaves a deep psychological shadow, making patients extremely resistant to further operations. 2. Financial constraints make another surgery impossible. for many families, cardiac surgery already places a huge financial burden on them. If they were to undergo deformity correction surgery as well, many families would be unable to afford it and therefore choose not to proceed. 3. A sense of helpless resignation. This mindset is actually quite complex, but the general idea is: since the scar from cardiac surgery has already inevitably affected their appearance, they feel that the chest wall deformity's additional impact on appearance does not really matter. Under the influence of this mindset, patients will easily refuse surgery.

While many factors lead some patients to reject surgery, there are others who may actively seek it. In such cases, the basic principles for surgery are actually the same as for general chest wall deformities. If the patient feels that the deformity is unsightly or causes discomfort, surgery should be performed. If the patient does not feel it is unsightly or uncomfortable, surgery may be avoided. Before proceeding with surgery, it is also necessary to assess whether the heart is in a condition to withstand the procedure. Some patients may continue to have cardiac function issues after heart surgery. If the heart is not able to tolerate surgery, then surgery should not be undertaken lightly.

(2) Surgical Methods

When a thoracic deformity occurs after cardiac surgery, severe adhesions will develop in the mediastinum. In this situation, the surgery is equivalent to a repeat operation for an ordinary chest wall deformity. Because the mediastinal adhesions are extensive and severe, the risks and technical difficulty are significantly increased, requiring specialized surgical techniques to complete the treatment.

(i) Pectus Carinatum Surgery

Pectus carinatum following cardiac surgery generally presents as a midline protrusion that is symmetrical on both sides and, in most cases, is not excessively severe. The deformity can be corrected using the conventional Wenlin procedure (see Figure 2-20-4) [4]. Incisions about 1–2 cm long are first made on both sides of the chest wall, the ribs are freed, and then wire traction sutures are placed at the fixation points. A tunnel is then created along the bony structures toward the midline for placement of the steel bar, with the tunnel positioned at the highest plane of the anterior chest wall. The tunnels on both sides meet near the midline. Because the cardiac surgery incision is located at the midline of the anterior chest wall, the tunnels will pass through the midline scar, and operating through the scar does not pose any difficulty. However, to make the procedure more convenient, a small incision can be made at the midline scar to facilitate placement of the steel bar. The steel bar is inserted through the tunnel, the anterior chest wall protrusion is pressed flat, and the bar is fixed on both sides, completing the surgery.

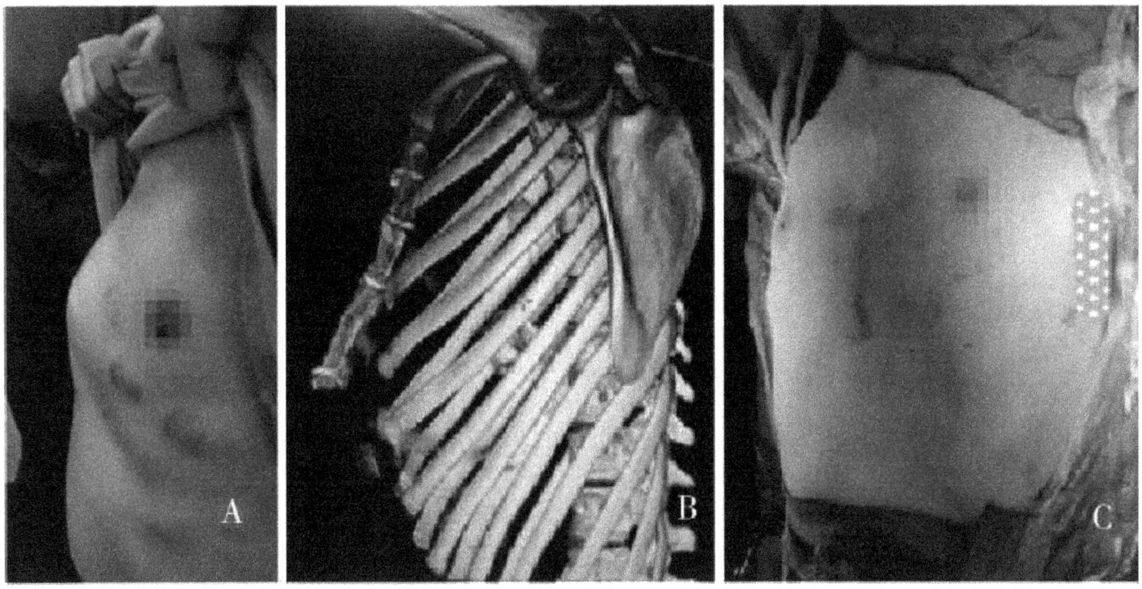

Figure 2-20-4 Wenlin Procedure for Pectus Carinatum After Cardiac Surgery (A. Anterior chest wall protrusion deformity; B. 3D reconstruction of the thorax showing significant anterior protrusion of the chest wall with an upward tilt of the lower end of the sternum; C. Deformity corrected using the Wenlin procedure, with the protrusion resolved.

The procedure described above is relatively simple and not technically demanding. However, there are two issues that require careful attention: 1. The impact on the heart during the operation. Because the anterior chest wall must be compressed, and the heart lies just beneath it, excessive or forceful compression may affect the heart. Therefore, while tightening the wires to secure the steel bar, the patient's cardiac response must be closely monitored. If the heart cannot tolerate significant compression, the procedure must be moderated — excessive compression should not be applied merely to achieve a better corrective result. 2. Possible secondary depressions. During the correction of anterior protrusion deformities, localized depressions of the anterior chest wall often occur due to the applied pressure. If left untreated, these depressions may develop into new pectus excavatum deformities. To prevent this, the localized depression must be managed. Specific methods include the Nuss procedure or the Wang procedure. However, due to the presence of mediastinal adhesions, the Nuss procedure is not ideal, as it carries higher risks and greater technical difficulty and therefore should not be the first choice. The Wang procedure, on the other hand, is performed on the anterior chest wall and does not require retrosternal dissection, making it relatively safer. Additionally, the existing cardiac surgery scar can be used for the incision, which not only facilitates the procedure but also avoids creating a new scar. Therefore, the Wang procedure offers advantages that the Nuss procedure does not and can be considered the preferred surgical option.

(ii) Pectus Excavatum Surgery

Pectus excavatum surgery after cardiac surgery differs from primary pectus excavatum repair — in effect, it is equivalent to a repeat procedure for pectus excavatum. The main risk of this surgery lies in mediastinal adhesions. Due to the extensive and widespread nature of these adhesions, the surgery places higher demands on the surgeon's skills. When selecting a surgical method, either the Nuss procedure [3] or the Wang procedure [1,2] can be considered. Before the Wang procedure was developed, the Nuss procedure was the only option, which posed significant challenges. The greatest challenge with the Nuss procedure is the placement of the steel bar. To minimize risks, special techniques must be employed; otherwise, not only is the operation difficult to complete, but it may also result in severe complications.

These techniques include the following: 1. Assistance using a midline incision. Because of the presence of retrosternal adhesions, directly placing the steel bar through the adhesions is extremely dangerous. Therefore, creating a midline incision for assistance is crucial to the success of the surgery. 2. Thorough pre-shaping. The anterior chest wall in pectus excavatum compresses the heart, creating a tight relationship between the two. When adhesions are present, operating between them becomes extremely difficult. To make the procedure as safe as possible and to facilitate the subsequent shaping, thorough pre-shaping is essential. Pre-shaping both reduces the degree of depression and releases stress, laying a solid foundation for final correction. 3. Proper coordination of steps. Separating retrosternal adhesions is the most dangerous part of the procedure. Direct dissection alone is clearly unwise; instead, it should be performed in combination with the pre-shaping steps. Likewise, when flipping the steel bar, the safest method is to coordinate it with pre-shaping. This approach effectively minimizes the impact on the heart.

The Nuss procedure has its own advantages, but for pectus excavatum after cardiac surgery, it is clearly not the best option. Due to its high degree of difficulty and risk, very few surgeons are willing to perform such an operation. Since the introduction of the Wang procedure, the surgical difficulty for this type of deformity has been greatly reduced, and the associated risks have been eliminated. As a result, the Wang procedure has gradually replaced the Nuss procedure as the preferred surgical method [1,2].

The specific steps for performing the Wang procedure are as follows: First, an incision is made at the lowest end of the scar from the initial surgery. This incision is generally located at the deepest point of the depression, near or directly in front of the xiphoid process. After exposing the xiphoid process, it is completely removed. Then, the lower end of the sternum and the adjacent costal arches are carefully freed along their surfaces, extending slightly deeper. This dissection is performed entirely under direct vision and does not require the extensive retrosternal dissection that the Nuss procedure does. Traction wires are then placed across the coastal arches, the soft tissues over the bony structures are freed, and a tunnel is created beneath the soft tissue for the placement of the steel bar. A tunnel is created, the steel bar is inserted, the traction wires are tightened to eliminate the depression, the wires are secured, the incision is closed, and the surgery is complete (see Figure 2-20-5).

Using the Wang procedure has clear advantages, specifically: 1. All steps can be completed through an incision at the site of the original midline surgical scar, without the need for any new incisions. 2. The main operative work is performed on the surface of the bony structures, away from the heart, which greatly increases safety. 3. The number of steel bars can be adjusted as needed, allowing the surgeon to easily achieve a satisfactory result. 4. The procedure does not enter the thoracic cavity, which not only reduces tissue trauma but also avoids certain related complications.

The Wang procedure was originally designed for young children with pectus excavatum. For simple pectus excavatum deformities, it is generally not recommended for patients older than 10 years of age. However, in cases of pectus excavatum following cardiac surgery, there are no age restrictions, and the procedure can be performed at any age. Because the Wang procedure has clear advantages over the Nuss procedure, it is the absolute first-choice technique for correcting pectus excavatum after cardiac surgery.

(iii) Other Surgeries

In addition to simple protrusion and depression deformities, thoracic deformities following cardiac surgery may also present with other complex deformities.

These deformities often require special surgical techniques. In addition to using a single technique as described above, it may also be necessary to combine multiple techniques to complete the procedure [5,6]. for deformities that have already undergone one unsuccessful surgery, the condition is usually more

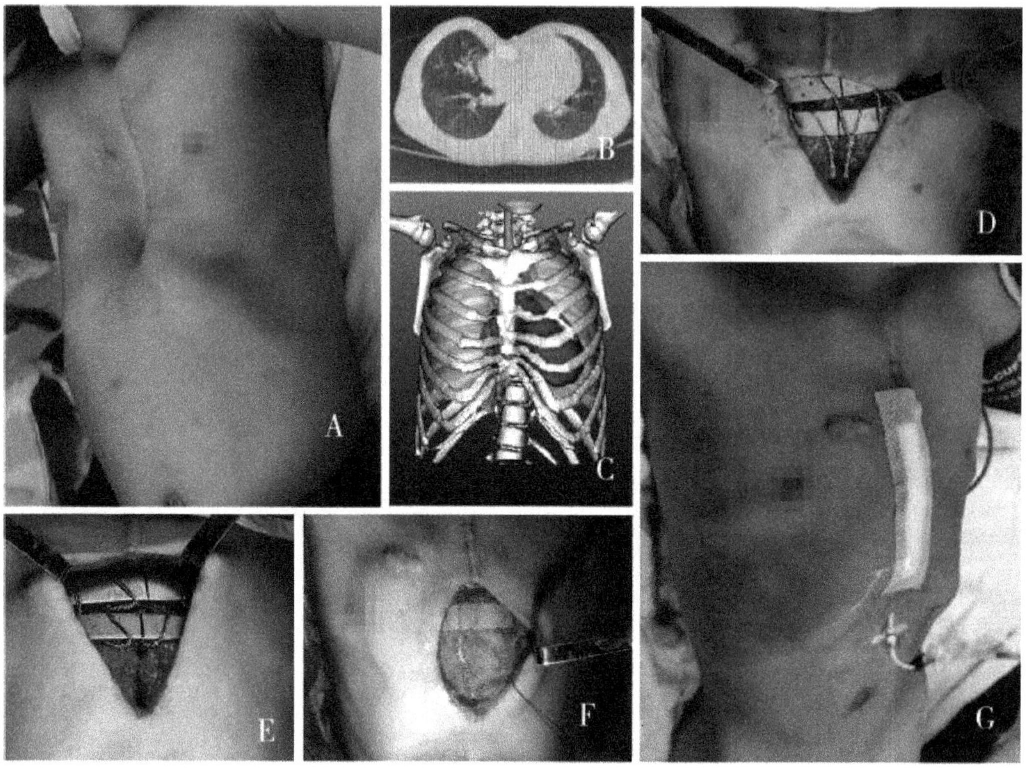

Figure 2-20-5 Wang Procedure for Pectus Excavatum After Cardiac Surgery (A. A depression deformity appears at the midline of the anterior chest wall after cardiac surgery performed through a midline incision; (B. CT cross-sectional image showing anterior chest wall depression with significant cardiac compression; (C. 3D chest reconstruction showing the anterior chest wall depression; (D. Wang procedure performed using two steel bars, with traction wires lifting and securing the bars; (E. Position of the steel bars after fixation; (F. Steel bars covered with a fibrous membrane; (G. Postoperative chest wall appearance, with the deformity completely corrected.

complex. If standard procedures cannot achieve an optimal result, open surgery may be considered. Such a procedure is the last resort, but it is not necessarily the worst option — for certain complex deformities, this type of surgery can actually produce better outcomes.

7. Prognosis

Surgery for chest wall deformities after cardiac surgery is a relatively complex type of procedure. Due to its high risks and technical difficulty, achieving a satisfactory result is not easy. However, even the most challenging surgeries have solutions. As long as the appropriate surgical method is chosen and effective surgical techniques are properly applied, success can certainly be achieved.

REFERENCES

[1] Wang Wenlin. Pectus Excavatum After Congenital Heart Disease Surgery: The Wang Procedure. Expert in Chest Wall Deformity Surgery, 28-06-2020.
[2] Wang Wenlin. The Wang Procedure for Pectus Excavatum After Cardiac Surgery. Expert in Chest Wall Deformity Surgery, 01-07-2018.
[3] Wang Wenlin. Pectus Excavatum After Cardiac Surgery: A Contraindication for the Nuss Procedure? Expert in Chest Wall Deformity Surgery, 05-11-2019.
[4] Wang Wenlin. Today's Nanning Surgery: Wenlin Procedure for Severe Pectus Carinatum After Cardiac Surgery. Expert in Chest Wall Deformity Surgery, 16-05-2020.
[5] Wang Wenlin. Minimally Invasive Surgery for Complex Chest Wall Deformities After Cardiac Surgery. Expert in Chest Wall Deformity Surgery, 30-04-2019.
[6] Wang Wenlin. The Wenlin Procedure for Severe Chest Wall Deformities After Cardiac Surgery. Expert in Chest Wall Deformity Surgery, 24-02-2021.

Patients with chest wall deformities who choose to come to the hospital for treatment do so with a strong desire for improvement. They all hope that the deformity can be completely corrected and that they can achieve a perfect chest wall appearance. However, every surgery carries uncertainties and the possibility of failure. Chest wall deformity surgery is both a therapeutic and reconstructive procedure, and its outcome is influenced by many factors. If these factors are not properly managed, they can affect the surgical result. Patients who are dissatisfied with the outcome must then face a very difficult decision — whether to undergo a second surgery. Reoperation involves treating a deformity that has already failed to be corrected once, and such a deformity is certainly different from the original one before surgery. This places even higher demands on the reoperation.

1. The Concept of Chest Wall Deformity Surgery Failure

Chest wall deformity is a special type of chest wall surgical condition, and the nature of its surgery differs from general surgery. In addition to its therapeutic aspect, reconstruction is another important aspect of this surgery. Reconstructive surgery often involves greater uncertainties, and many factors can affect the surgical outcome. Generally speaking, the results of surgery can be categorized into five types [1,2]: 1. Very satisfactory. This is the outcome that both patients and doctors hope to achieve. A very satisfactory result means the deformity is completely corrected, the chest wall appearance returns to a normal shape, and there are no unusual symptoms. If such a result can be achieved, it is the ideal outcome. 2. Some improvement. This result can leave the patient disappointed because the deformity is only partially corrected but not completely eliminated. The chest wall still appears abnormal, with only slight improvement. Such an outcome is often difficult for patients to accept. 3. No improvement. This result is also unacceptable. The shape of the chest wall after surgery remains exactly the same as before, meaning the surgery had no effect. Worse still, the patient has endured an incision and surgical trauma, suffered pain, and spent money — all without benefit. This is very hard for patients to accept. 4. Worsening of the deformity. This is a distressing outcome. The deformity not only fails to improve but becomes more severe than before surgery. 5. Death. Chest wall deformity is considered a benign condition. Although surgery for this condition carries risks, neither doctors nor patients wish to face life-threatening consequences. However, some risks are unavoidable — For example, the risk of heart injury during the Nuss procedure. This risk is almost impossible to eliminate entirely. In extremely unfortunate cases, the heart may be punctured, resulting in the patient's death. Such an outcome is undoubtedly the most terrifying one.

Among these five possible outcomes, only the first is considered satisfactory; the other four are unsatisfactory results. Given the special nature of reconstructive surgery, many people regard these four outcomes as surgical failure. Patients spend money, endure pain, and hope for a successful operation — no one wants the surgery to fail. But if it does fail, the patient must face reality. If they wish to achieve a better result, they must consider undergoing a second surgery.

2. Causes of Chest Wall Deformity Surgery Failure

A careful analysis of the reasons for chest wall deformity surgery failure reveals many contributing factors, including both objective and subjective ones, as well as factors related to the surgeon and the patient. Specifically, these can be summarized as the following factors [3–6]:

(1) Factors related to the deformity itself. Chest wall deformities come in many forms and vary in severity. Some deformities are very simple and yield good surgical outcomes. However, some deformities are quite severe or complex and lack established surgical methods. For these cases, an unsatisfactory correction is the most likely outcome. For example, in conditions such as chest wall dysplasia syndrome and asphyxiating thoracic dystrophy (Jeune syndrome), The deformity is so complex and severe that the surgery itself is extremely challenging, and achieving a completely normal chest wall is very difficult [7]. For such patients, if the postoperative result is unsatisfactory, the primary reason lies in the nature of the deformity itself, and only then should other factors be considered. Some extremely complex chest wall deformities present similar challenges. For instance, very severe pectus excavatum, pectus carinatum, or combined deformities (see Figure 2-21-1). In these cases, the surgery itself poses a significant challenge and directly affects the surgical outcome.

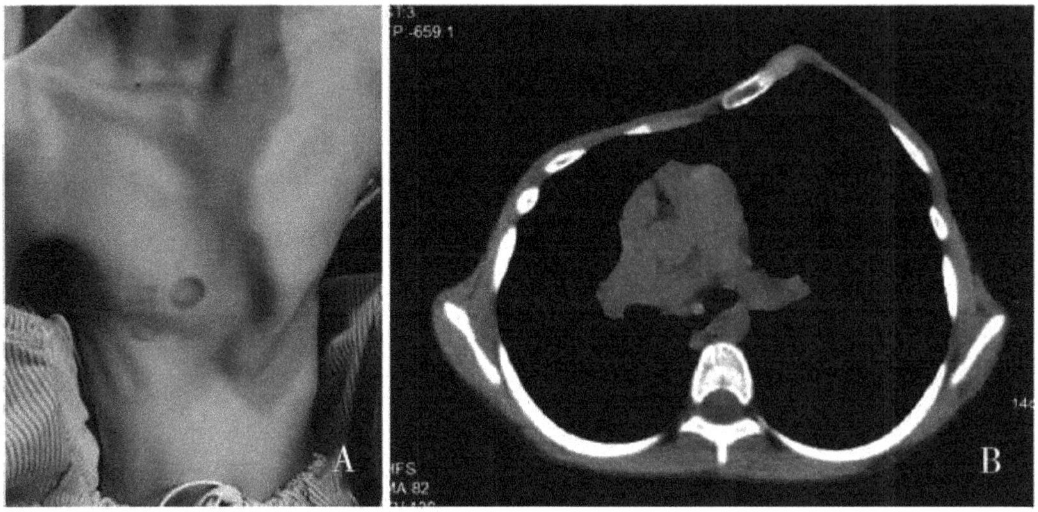

Figure 2-21-1 Severe Chest Wall Deformity (A. External appearance of the chest wall, showing an irregular and complex deformity; B. CT cross-sectional image showing both localized and overall deformity of the chest wall.)

(2) Factors related to the surgical method. Every deformity surgery goes through a process of continuous refinement, and not every surgical method is the best option. Even a procedure that is very popular at a certain time may have various shortcomings. Take the Nuss procedure as an example — it generally achieves good corrective results for typical pectus excavatum. However, in certain special cases, such as when one edge of the depression forms a sharp-angled protrusion, this procedure not only fails to correct the deformity but can actually lead to a worse outcome (see Figure 2-21-2) [8]. Other surgical methods can have similar issues. Each surgical technique has its own indications and cannot address every situation. If the surgical method is not appropriately chosen, an unsatisfactory result is inevitable. (3) Factors related to the surgeon's skill. Every deformity surgery is performed by a human being, and human factors directly affect the outcome. If the surgeon has excellent skills and can master the procedure proficiently, a good result is generally expected. However, if the surgeon's skills are or poor, this can cause serious problems (see Figure 2-21-3). A surgeon with insufficient skill is unlikely to achieve a satisfactory correction of the deformity.

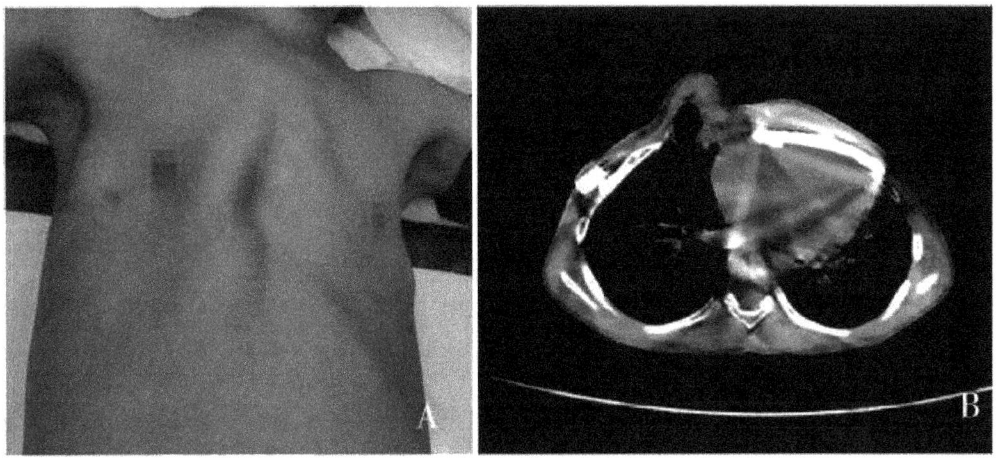

Figure 2-21-2 Severe Deformity Caused by Failed Nuss Procedure. This deformity cannot be corrected with a second Nuss procedure and must be treated with an alternative method. (A. External appearance of the chest wall; B. CT cross-sectional image of the chest showing a sharp-angled deformity on one side of the anterior chest wall, with the steel bar positioned inside the chest wall but failing to achieve correction.)

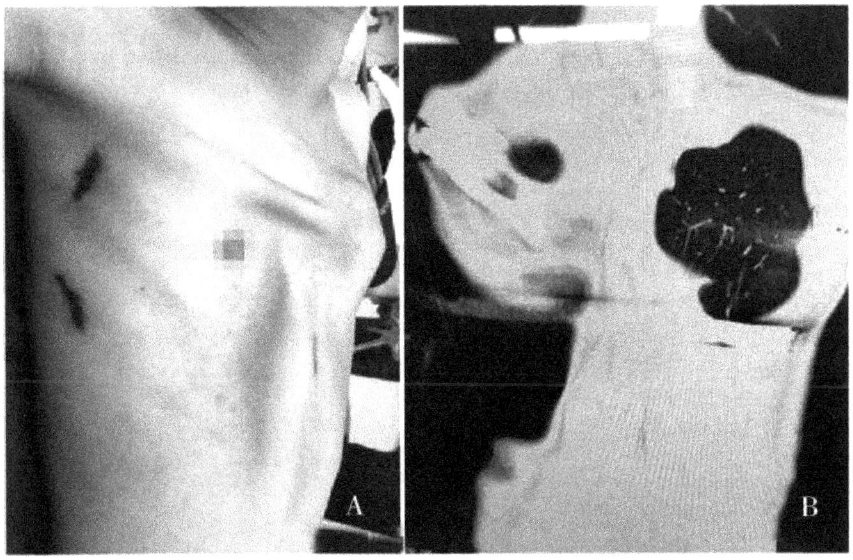

Figure 2-21-3 Severe Deformity Caused by Surgeon's Technical Error. The patient originally had typical Poland syndrome, but the surgeon misdiagnosed it as asymmetric pectus carinatum and performed a minimally invasive procedure, which failed. (A. Appearance of the failed chest wall, showing two old surgical scars and marks from the steel bar; B. Coronal CT image showing the chest wall deformity and the position of the steel bar.)

(4) Patient-related factors. In addition to the three factors mentioned above, another important factor that affects the surgical outcome is the patient's own condition and actions. During the actual procedure, the patient has little

influence over the surgical process itself, but before and after the surgery, they can significantly affect both the surgical decision-making and the final result. For example, during the preoperative phase, the patient often plays a decisive role in choosing the hospital, surgeon, surgical materials, and surgical technique — and these choices can directly impact the outcome. When it comes to selecting surgical materials or techniques to be used during the procedure, patients often express their own preferences. However, since patients typically do not fully understand the performance of the materials or the advantages and disadvantages of different surgical methods, their choices may negatively affect the result. Besides these preoperative factors, achieving a good result also depends on the patient's cooperation during postoperative recovery. If the patient does not cooperate, complications can arise that ultimately affect the outcome. For example, a patient with pectus excavatum who undergoes the Nuss procedure may disrupt wound healing or cause the implanted bar to shift if they engage in vigorous physical activity too soon after surgery, directly leading to surgical failure. These are examples of how the patient's subjective actions can affect the outcome. Apart from these, some objective patient-related factors can also influence the result, such as the patient's overall nutritional status, coexisting illnesses, the amount of soft tissue near the incision, and the local blood supply. All these can impact healing and the final result. Therefore, among the many factors that affect surgical outcomes, patient-related factors must not be overlooked.

3. Structural Characteristics of the Chest Wall After Surgical Failure

After a failed chest wall deformity surgery, the overall shape can present various deformities. To describe these shapes accurately, the best approach is to compare them with the preoperative deformity. As mentioned earlier, failed surgery can result in several possible outcomes: some improvement, no improvement, worsening, or even death. From these outcomes, it can be seen that the deformity after a failed surgery may be very severe, or it may not be too serious. It is therefore difficult to categorize failed chest walls purely by severity. However, these deformities often share certain specific structural characteristics, mainly reflected in local areas. These characteristics include [9,10]: (1) Local adhesions. After undergoing chest wall deformity surgery, adhesions usually develop. Although the chest wall is an independent structure, it has an inseparable relationship with the thoracic cavity. Surgery on the chest wall almost always affects the thoracic cavity, leading to adhesions in the surrounding area. The presence of adhesions complicates any subsequent surgery (see Figure 2-21-4A). (2) Local abnormal structures. After the initial surgery, secondary changes may occur in the local chest wall area. In addition to fibrous tissue forming in the surgical field, structures such as callus may develop, and the presence of callus can affect the performance of the next surgery (see Figure 2-21-4A). (3) Loss of important local structures. Many chest wall deformity surgeries rely on specific local structures, such as support points. A support point is typically a specific part of a rib that must meet certain requirements to function properly. Prior surgery may compromise the properties of this support point, causing it to lose its function, which can affect future surgeries (see Figure 2-21-4B). In addition, some procedures may remove parts of the chest wall, which can further complicate reoperation (see Figure 2-21-4C). (4) Development of a new deformity. The essence of corrective surgery is to reshape the deformity. The postoperative shape may be satisfactory, but if it is not, it can take on all sorts of irregular forms. In extreme cases, a completely new deformity may appear that is entirely different from the original one (see Figure 2-21-4D).

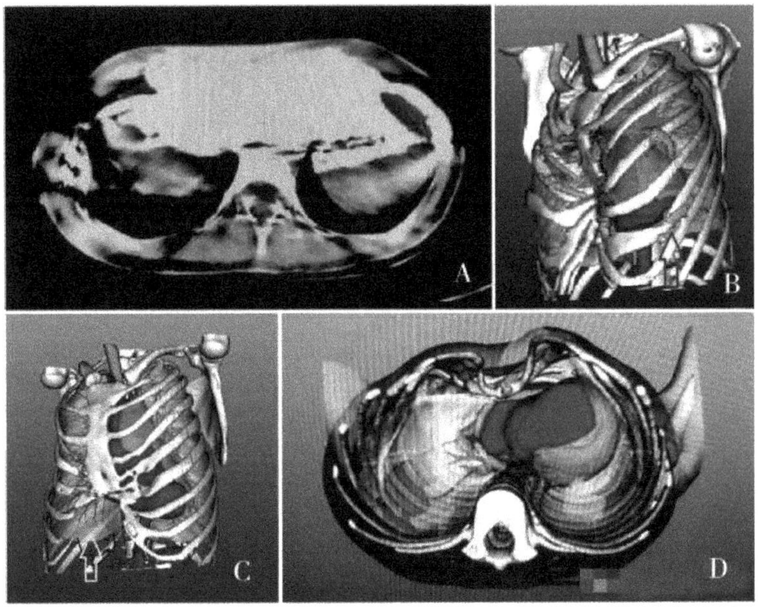

Figure 2-21-4 Structural Characteristics of the Chest Wall After Surgical Failure (A. Severe adhesions inside the thoracic cavity. Adhesions are present not only near the steel bar but also widely in other areas. B. Abnormal position of the steel bar, with the rib cut, resulting in loss of support function. C. Partial removal of the right coastal arch. D. Severe new local deformity of the chest wall.)

4. The Harms of Deformity Surgery Failure

Chest wall deformities themselves pose two types of harm to patients: psychological harm and physiological harm. After a failed chest wall deformity surgery, the chest wall remains deformed, so these two types of harm cannot be eliminated. Moreover, considering the experience of the first surgery's failure, the patient's entire physical and mental well-being will be impacted, which further aggravates both types of harm.

5. Clinical Manifestations

Chest wall deformities do not necessarily present clinical symptoms, and even after surgical failure, obvious clinical symptoms may still be absent. However, patients generally remain dissatisfied with the appearance of the deformity. This dissatisfaction with appearance can lead to psychological issues. When psychological problems become severe, they may in turn cause symptoms to develop or worsen.

6. Examinations

Before performing a repeat surgery after a failed chest wall deformity operation, some necessary preoperative examinations must be conducted. The purposes of these examinations are threefold: first, to clarify the nature of the deformity; second, to determine the severity of the deformity; and third, to exclude any possible associated diseases. As mentioned earlier, some deformities may change after the initial surgery. Once the deformity changes, the surgical approach must also be adjusted accordingly, so it is essential to assess the nature of the deformity before surgery. The severity of the deformity also plays an important role in selecting the surgical method and must be clearly understood preoperatively. Additionally, previous surgery may have affected other structures, leading to new pathological changes. The presence of such changes will influence the repeat surgery, so it is necessary to identify whether such conditions exist before the operation.

To achieve the above purposes, appropriate examinations can be performed based on the characteristics of the deformity. X-ray examination provides an overall view of the chest wall contour and reveals the shape of the bones. If there are steel bars remaining in the body from previous surgery, X-rays are a mandatory examination. To clarify the details of the lesion, CT scans can be used. Three-dimensional reconstruction can comprehensively display the condition of the deformity and lesions. If conditions permit, these examinations should be performed.

7. Diagnosis

Diagnosing the chest wall deformity itself is not difficult. If the surgery has failed, it means the deformity still exists, so diagnosis remains straightforward. When diagnosing a failed deformity after surgery, it is essential to compare it with the preoperative deformity. This comparison not only reveals the true nature of the deformity but also helps evaluate the effectiveness of the previous surgery. Additionally, when diagnosing the patient, the details of the prior surgical procedure should be studied. On one hand, this allows lessons to be learned from the surgical failure, and on the other, it provides valuable references for the subsequent surgery.

8. Surgical Treatment

(1) Surgical Indications

The goal of deformity correction is to eliminate the deformity and achieve a satisfactory chest wall appearance. If the chest wall appearance after the first surgery is unsatisfactory, the failure must be acknowledged and properly managed. Generally, there are no conservative methods to treat the deformity; achieving satisfactory results usually requires considering a repeat surgery. Undergoing repeat surgery is often a difficult decision for patients. Firstly, having experienced the previous surgery, patients may feel apprehensive and find it hard to muster the courage to undergo surgery again. Secondly, the prior surgery often entails significant financial cost, and many patients may not be able to afford another procedure. Lastly, some patients lack confidence in a second surgery, fearing it may fail again.

Patients often find it difficult to decide on undergoing a second surgery, but there are always some who are unwilling to accept the failure of the first operation and who eagerly desire a repeat surgery. As with the first deformity surgery, the decision to proceed with a second surgery ultimately must be made by the patient and their family. If they are not positive about the repeat surgery, the operation cannot proceed. Repeat surgery poses even greater challenges for doctors. After the failure of the initial surgery, the second operation must confront many new problems. Due to increased surgical risks and difficulty, combined with higher patient expectations, doctors face much greater challenges. For these reasons, very few doctors dare to perform repeat surgeries. Patients are often anxious about repeat surgery, and doctors must face new challenges, making the decision to undergo a second operation extremely difficult. In less severe failure cases, patients may choose to forgo repeat surgery. However, some failures are quite serious, not only affecting the patient's normal work and life but even threatening their life. In such cases, a second surgery is necessary.

(2) Preoperative Preparation

The preoperative preparation for repeat surgery is essentially no different from

that of a general surgery. However, considering the increased surgical risks, additional preparations are required before the operation. Furthermore, since the surgery may involve some special procedures, such as the removal of steel plates, appropriate instruments and tools should be prepared in advance.
Repeat surgery itself is a technical challenge, so preoperative preparation should especially focus on technical aspects. Key considerations include the choice of surgical method, handling of surgical details, and contingency plans for unexpected situations. Only with thorough preparation in these areas can a satisfactory surgical outcome be ensured.
The main issue to address in repeat surgery for chest wall deformities remains the deformity itself, so in essence, it is not fundamentally different from primary chest wall deformity surgery. However, because the initial surgery has caused special impacts, repeat surgery involves greater risks and significantly increased difficulty. To achieve satisfactory results, new approaches and methods must be adopted, focusing on the following key issues: (1) the surgical philosophy; (2) the technical details; and (3) the expected surgical outcomes. In recent years, chest wall deformity surgery has seen considerable progress, marked primarily by the adoption of advanced concepts such as minimally invasive surgery, which is currently the most popular approach in this field. Under the influence of this concept, open surgeries are now rarely used. However, patients requiring repeat surgery often have complex, sometimes extremely severe conditions. If surgery is still performed strictly according to popular philosophies, this will limit the application of techniques. For example, although the Nuss procedure is widely recognized as an effective surgery, it is not all-powerful (all-powerful) and is nearly ineffective for certain special deformities. If one cannot break free from conceptual constraints and is unwilling to use techniques beyond minimally invasive surgery, the operation cannot be completed successfully. Moreover, the deformities in repeat surgeries are often quite complex, and various difficulties will be encountered during surgery. Specialized surgical techniques must be employed to successfully resolve these challenges. Without these techniques, many surgeries simply cannot be completed, so extra attention must be paid to the technical details of the surgery. Besides philosophical and technical considerations, special attention must also be given preoperatively to the issue of expected outcomes. Patients who have experienced a failed surgery previously often have higher expectations for repeat surgery. If doctors cannot objectively and rationally predict surgical outcomes, it may lead to unforeseen problems after surgery.

(3) Surgical Methods

(i) Repeat Surgery for Depressed (Concave) Deformities

Depressed (concave) deformities are commonly encountered in repeat surgeries. The primary deformity in such cases may be pectus excavatum, or it may.

Depressed (concave) deformities are commonly encountered in repeat surgeries. The primary deformity in such cases may be pectus excavatum, or it may be another type. For example, some protruding (convex) deformities may become depressed deformities after excessive correction. There are three minimally invasive surgical methods for depressed deformities: the first is the Nuss procedure, the second is the Wong procedure, and the third is the Wang procedure. If there are severe adhesions deep in the depressed area, the Wang procedure can be the first choice (Figure 2-21-5) [1]. However, for depressed deformities in certain special locations, the Nuss procedure or the Wung procedure can be considered (Figure 2-21-6) [12]. In general, depressed deformities can be treated with minimally invasive surgery. If there are special local conditions that prevent a satisfactory result with minimally invasive methods, various degrees of open surgery may be considered.

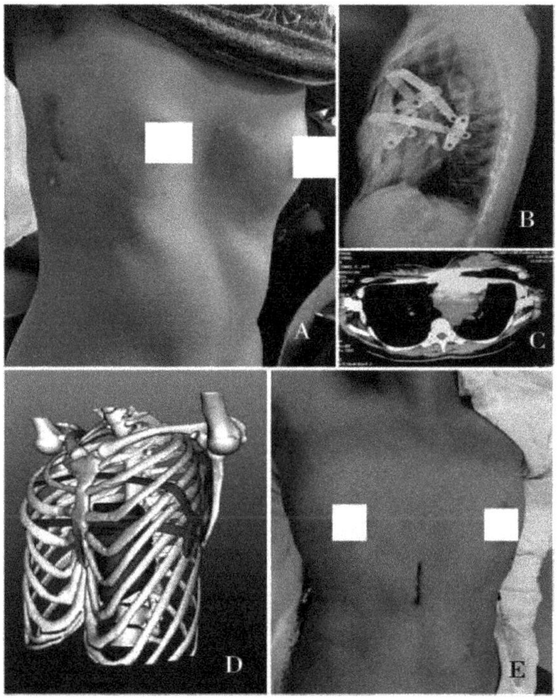

Figure 2-21-5 Wang Procedure After Failed Nuss Procedure (A. Depression of the anterior chest wall, with an old surgical scar visible on the right chest wall; B. Two steel bars inside the body, with displacement; C. CT cross-sectional image showing severe adhesions around the steel bars and cardiac compression; D. 3D reconstruction image showing the relationship between the steel bars and the depression; E. Repeat correction performed with the Wang procedure, with the postoperative chest wall appearance basically normal)

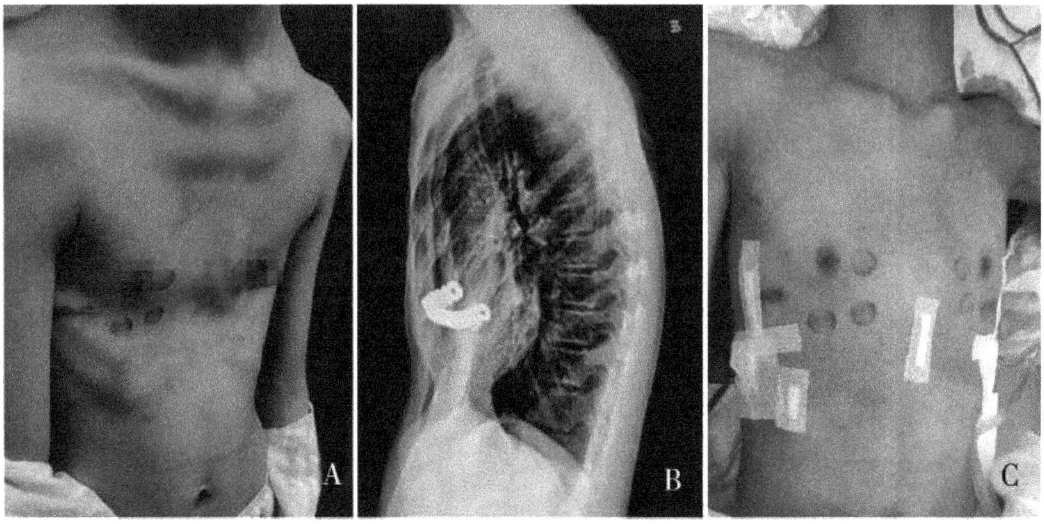

Figure 2-21-6 Wing Procedure After Failed Nuss Procedure (A. The anterior chest wall shows a groove-like depression with two old scars visible; B. X-ray shows the steel bar located above the depression, providing no support; C.

Repeat surgery performed with the Wong procedure, resulting in a basically normal chest wall appearance. 2. Revision Surgery for Protrusive Deformities
Protrusive deformities that require revision surgery generally fall into two categories: first, unsatisfactory correction of the original protrusive deformity; second, overcorrection of a depression-type deformity leading to protrusion. Regardless of the cause, a second surgery for such cases often becomes significantly more complex. In these situations, the classic Wenlin procedure [13] can still be used for correction. However, due to the impact of the previous surgery, the deformity may present more complicated issues. For example, a local sharp-angled deformity may require special pre-shaping techniques to complete the procedure successfully. Additionally, the previous surgery may have disrupted the structures used for fixation, creating challenges for re-fixation. In such cases, it is necessary to make new adjustments to address these specific details.

When performing a revision surgery, it remains crucial to pay attention to an important issue: the risk of developing a depression-type deformity. After performing the Wenlin procedure for a purely protrusive deformity, it is quite common for a secondary depression to occur. If this happens during a revision surgery, it will inevitably affect the surgical outcome. Therefore, extra caution must be taken during the operation. If depression cannot be avoided, prompt and decisive measures must be taken to correct it.

(ii) Revision Surgery for Complex Deformities

In some extreme cases, the deformity requiring revision surgery can be extremely complex, making it impossible to complete the procedure using conventional concepts and techniques alone. In such situations, a completely new surgical approach must be adopted to achieve a good outcome [14]. When performing this type of surgery, in addition to technical factors, special materials are often needed. These materials are almost crucial to the success of the procedure, so thorough preparation must be done beforehand to lay a solid foundation for a successful operation (see Figures 2-21-7 to 2-21-9)

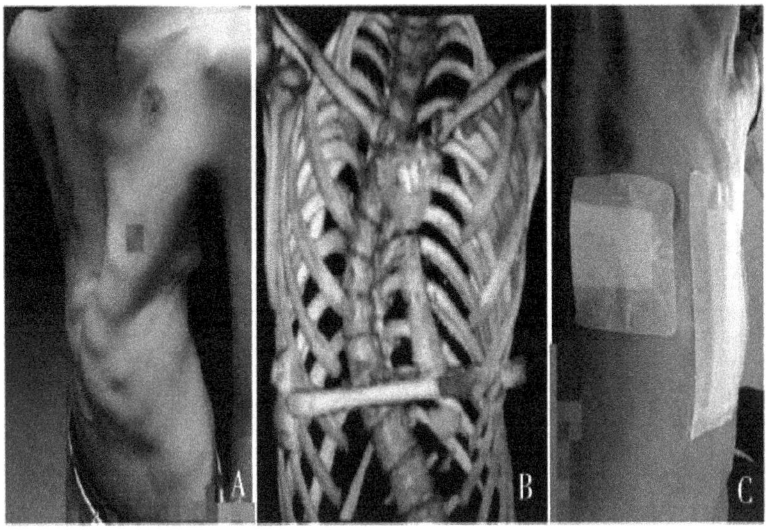

Figure 2-21-7 Extremely severe deformity caused by a failed Nuss procedure for pectus excavatum (A) Severe deformity of the anterior and lateral chest walls; (B) CT cross-sectional image showing significant anterior chest wall deformity with visible steel bar shadows; (C) CT coronal image showing severe thoracic deformity, with a central anterior chest wall depression and bilateral chest wall depressions; (D) A combined surgical approach was used for revision surgery, resulting in an almost normal postoperative chest wall appearance.

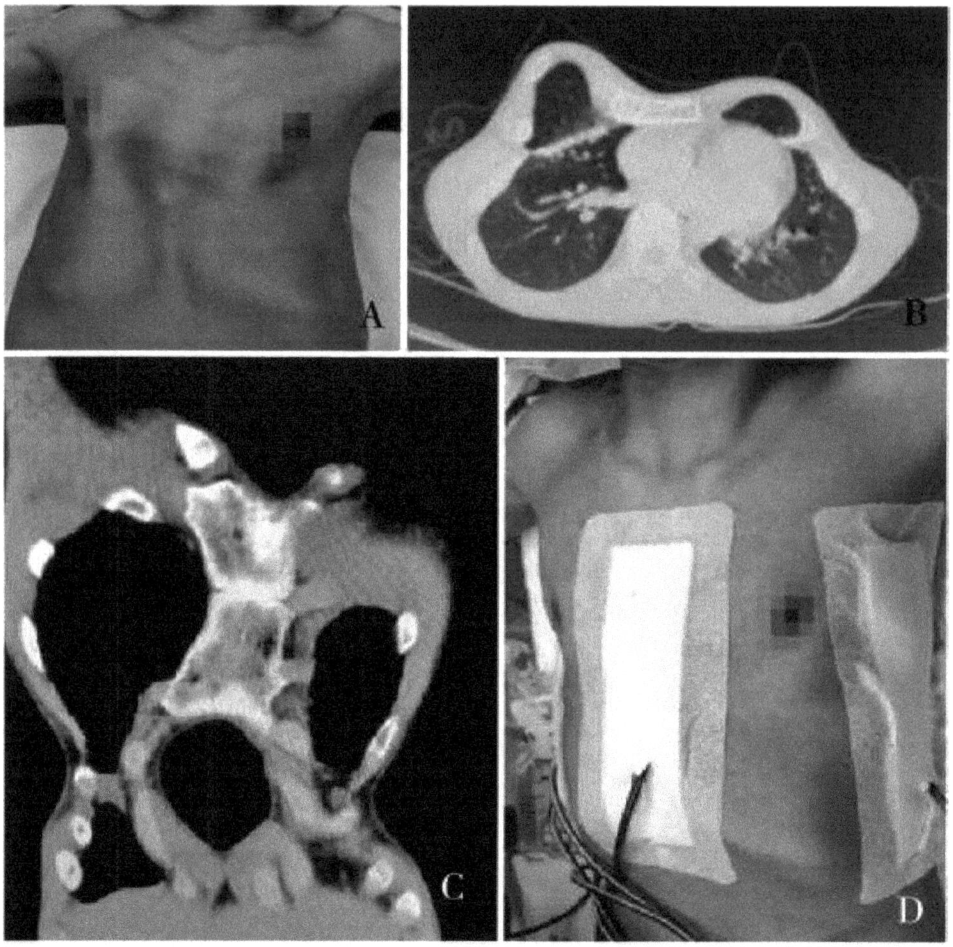

Figure 2-21-8 Severe deformity caused by a failed Nuss procedure for pectus excavatum (A) Significant deformity of the anterior and lateral chest walls, with visible old scars and traces of steel bars; (B) 3D reconstruction showing the shape of the chest wall and the position of the steel bars — marked chest wall deformity, abnormal bar placement, and visible scoliosis; (C) Steel bars removed, a combined surgical approach was performed for the revision surgery, and the deformity was almost completely corrected postoperatively.

9. Prognosis

A revision surgery targets a previously failed procedure, and because the difficulty is significantly greater than the initial surgery, it is always a major challenge. When faced with such a challenge, it is possible to achieve a satisfactory outcome if various surgical techniques are fully and skillfully applied. However, since the initial surgery failed, the repeat surgery also carries a risk of failure, and this possibility must be acknowledged mentally. To

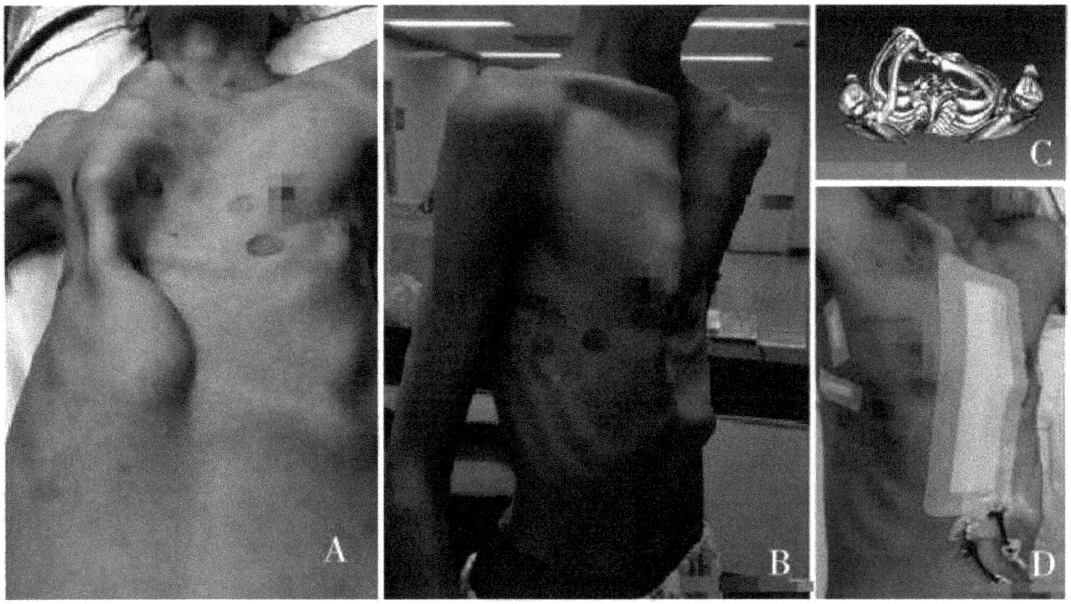

Figure 2-21-9 Extremely Severe Deformity Caused by a Nuss Procedure for Pectus Excavatum (A. Severe deformity of the anterior chest wall with a pronounced sharp-angled deformity on the right anterior chest wall; B. Obvious chest wall deformity with visible old surgical scars; C. Three reconstruction of the thorax showing severe thoracic deformity; D. A combined surgical approach was used for reoperation, and the chest wall appearance was basically restored to normal.)

increase the chances of success, every detail must be carefully managed: thorough preparation before surgery, meticulous technique during the operation, and diligent rehabilitation afterwards. Only by doing so can a good outcome be achieved.

REFERENCES

[1] Wang, W. L. 2021a. "The Five Possible Outcomes of Thoracic Deformity Surgery." *Expert in Thoracic Deformity Surgery*, September 22.

[2] Wang, W. L. 2020a. "The Dire Consequences of Failed Pectus Excavatum Surgery." *Expert in Thoracic Deformity Surgery*, November 30.

[3] Wang, W. L. 2021b. "Adverse Factors Affecting the Outcome of Thoracic Deformity Surgery." *Expert in Thoracic Deformity Surgery*, September 24.

[4] Wang, W. L. 2018. "Analysis of the Causes of Failed Groove Chest Surgery." *Expert in Thoracic Deformity Surgery*, December 18.

[5] Wang, W. L. 2020b. "Analysis of the Causes of Failed Pectus Excavatum Surgery." *Expert in Thoracic Deformity Surgery*, April 17.

[6] Wang, W. L. 2018b. "The Wang Procedure after a Failed Nuss Procedure: Why Does the Nuss Procedure Fail?" *Expert in Thoracic Deformity Surgery*, August 27.

[7] Wang, W. 2022. "Surgical Treatment of a 36-Year-Old Patient with Asphyxiating Thoracic Dysplasia." *Interactive Cardiovascular and Thoracic Surgery* 34 (1): 153–155.

[8] Wang, W. L. 2021c. “Sharp-Angled Deformity.” *Chest Wall Deformity Surgery Expert*, August 18.
[9] Wang, W. L. 2021d. “Risks and Outcomes of Secondary Surgery after Failed Pectus Excavatum Procedures.” *Chest Wall Deformity Surgery Expert*, May 5.
[10] Wang, W. L. 2016. “Clinical Analysis of 39 Cases of Secondary Pectus Excavatum Surgery.” *Chinese Journal of Clinical Thoracic and Cardiovascular Surgery* 23 (10): 1026–1028.
[11] Wang, W. L. 2020c. “The Wung Procedure after Failed Nuss Procedure.” *Chest Wall Deformity Surgery Expert*, September 6.
[12] Wang, W. L. 2020d. “A 5-Year-Old Child: Wang Procedure after Failed Pectus Excavatum Nuss Surgery.” *Chest Wall Deformity Surgery Expert*, May 25.
[13] Wang, W. L. 2020e. “The Fourth Surgery for a Pectus Excavatum Patient: Wang Procedure and Wenlin Procedure.” *Chest Wall Deformity Surgery Expert*, December 1.
[14] Wang, W. L. 2020f. “Misfortune and Fortune: A Third Operation after Two Failed Pectus Excavatum Surgeries.” *Chest Wall Deformity Surgery Expert*, October 28.

STERNAL CLEFT

Sternal cleft is an ancient condition, first described by Torres in 1739 [1]. It is an extremely rare thoracic deformity. According to available data, its incidence in newborns is only 2/100,000 [1], accounting for just 0.15 of all thoracic deformities [2]. Due to its extremely low incidence, reports of this condition both domestically and internationally are almost exclusively individual case reports. The limited number of cases makes research on this condition difficult. However, because the disease has distinct characteristics and clear clinical manifestations, many mature treatment methods have been reported. Isolated sternal clefts are rare; in most cases, it is accompanied by other conditions, which makes treatment quite complex. In addition to addressing the sternal cleft itself, treatment must also consider associated conditions, which often increase the difficulty of management.

1. Pathogenesis

Sternal cleft is a congenital condition that develops during the embryonic period. Although its exact cause remains unclear, the developmental process is relatively well understood and mainly related to abnormal sternal development. The prevailing view is that starting from the sixth week of embryonic development, the sternum begins to form from a pair of longitudinal mesenchymal structures called sternebrae, which are located on either side of the 10 anterior chest wall. The (sternal bars) move toward the midline and fuse, gradually forming the (sternal plate) around the tenth week. During this process, the mesenchymal tissue develops into cartilage tissue by the 7th week and then differentiates into 6 sternebrae[3]. Among these, 1 sternebrae develops into the manubrium, 4 into the body of the sternum, and 1 into the xiphoid process. If any part of this fusion process is disrupted, a sternal cleft may occur. Once formed, a sternal cleft becomes a permanent deformity that cannot fuse or heal on its own after birth. This defect can affect the function of the thoracic cage, leading to a series of clinical symptoms.

2.Pathological Features

The fundamental pathological change in the sternal cleft is that the sternum is completely or partially split open. Since the deep side of the sternum lies directly over the heart and great vessels—structures filled with blood and under significant positive pressure—once the sternum is split, its restraining effect on the heart and great vessels is lost. As a result, these structures may protrude through the sternal cleft to the body surface, forming ectopic organs. The most common clinical presentation is ectopia cordis. The abnormal position of the heart can lead to a series of adverse effects. In addition to malposition, congenital malformations of the heart itself are frequently present; these can range from relatively simple defects to very complex anomalies, making the overall condition more complicated and severe. For the convenience of diagnosis and treatment, some authors have proposed classifications for sternal cleft. Due to different research perspectives, there are multiple classification methods. From the standpoint of sternal structure alone, sternal clefts can be divided into complete sternal clefts and incomplete sternal clefts; the latter are further subdivided into superior sternal clefts and inferior sternal clefts (Figure 2-22-1) [3]. This classification is not only easy to understand but also aids in treatment, making it a straightforward and practical approach. Superior sternal clefts are more common and typically appear in a "U" or "V" shape (Figure 2-22-2) [4,5]. Inferior sternal clefts are relatively rare and may coexist with other thoracic deformities (Figure 2-22-3). Because most sternal clefts are accompanied by cardiac anomalies, some authors have proposed classifications that better reflect this relationship—especially to emphasize cardiac involvement. For example, Shamberger and Welch [6] classified sternal clefts into four types: cervical ectopia cordis, thoracic ectopia cordis, thoracic abdominal ectopia cordis, and sternal cleft or bifid sternum. This classification focuses on highlighting the position of the ectopic heart. Daum et al. [7] considered the relationship between sternal cleft and associated visceral anomalies and divided sternal clefts into another 4 types: (1) complete sternal cleft without other anomalies or with ectopia cordis and vascular anomalies; (2) superior sternal cleft; (3) inferior sternal cleft with Cantrell's pentalogy; and (4) sternal cleft with abdominal wall defects. This is a comprehensive classification that better reveals the connection between the sternal cleft and visceral anomalies. Hersh proposed yet another classification, also dividing sternal clefts into 4 types [5]: (1) sternal cleft without other anomalies; (2) sternal cleft with vascular anomalies; (3) true ectopia cordis; and (4) Cantrell's pentalogy. This approach views the sternal cleft as a whole, focusing on the characteristics of associated conditions. Although the sternal cleft itself is a relatively simple malformation, its associated conditions are often complex, so it is necessary to understand it from multiple perspectives. The authors mentioned above classified sternal clefts from different angles, resulting in different emphases and classification outcomes, but they share a common feature: all classification systems must address the specific structure of the sternal cleft.

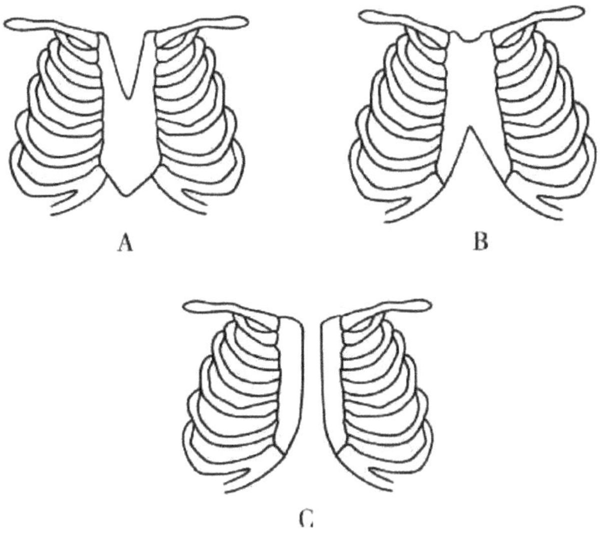

Figure 2-22-1 Classification of Sternal Clefts (A. Superior Sternal Cleft; B. Inferior Sternal Cleft; C. Complete Sternal Cleft

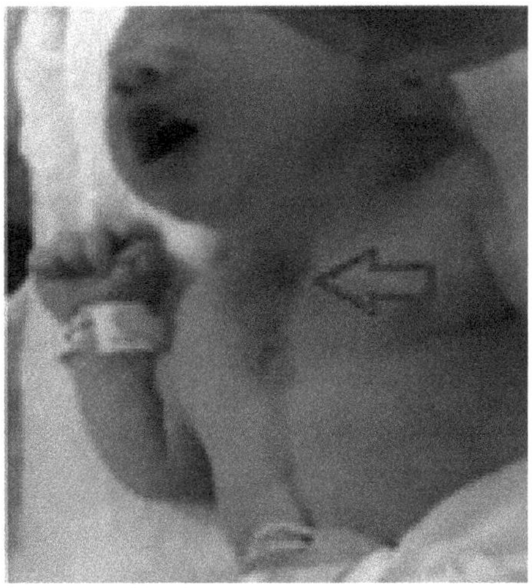

Figure 2-22-2: Child with Superior Sternal Cleft

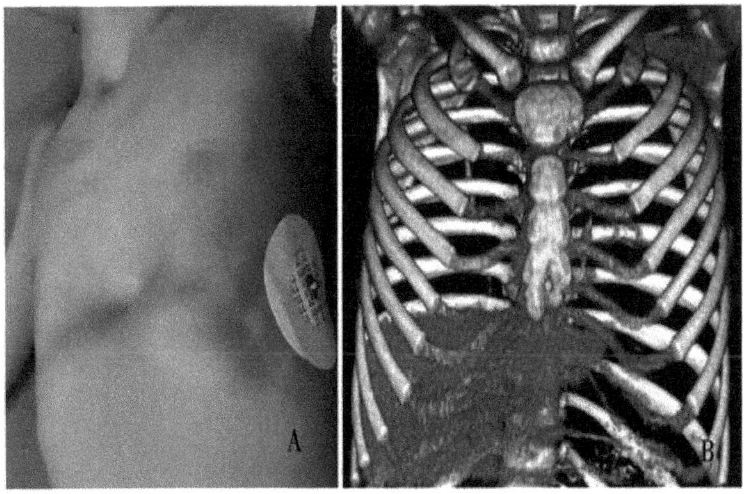

Figure 2-22-3 Inferior Sternal Cleft Combined with Pectus Excavatum in a Child (A. Noticeable depression of the anterior chest wall; B. 3-D reconstruction showing a midline cleft in the lower part of the sternum)

A complete sternal cleft is an extremely rare type in which the entire sternum is split apart — from the manubrium to the xiphoid process — leaving the sternal structures on the left and right sides separated without any bony connection. When the sternum is completely split, the integrity of the chest wall is thoroughly compromised, and various related functions are affected. This type of sternal cleft is more likely to be associated with other anomalies, such as defects of the chest muscles, absence of the pericardium, and various other visceral malformations. The presence of associated conditions makes this type of cleft even more severe. An incomplete sternal cleft refers to a partial splitting of the sternum, where the lower or upper segment remains partially fused, resulting in a superior sternal cleft or an inferior sternal cleft. The upper portion of the sternum overlies the base of the heart, mainly the roots of the great vessels. Due to its relatively fixed anatomical structure, when the upper segment splits, ectopia cordis is less likely to occur. Superior sternal clefts are more common and can occur in isolation or in combination with other anomalies. The lower portion of the sternum is anatomically distinct; it lies over the pericardium and heart, with the diaphragm attaching below and the thoracoabdominal junction nearby. When this part of the sternum splits, it often involves surrounding structures, resulting in defects of the pericardium, diaphragm, and abdominal wall. The most common manifestation of an inferior sternal cleft is Cantrell's pentalogy. This condition was first reported by Cantrell in 1958 [8] and includes five primary defects: (1) sternal defect; (2) partial absence of the pericardium; (3) anterior diaphragmatic defect; (4) midline supraumbilical abdominal wall defect with cardiac protrusion; (5) congenital heart anomalies. These basic defects illustrate that when there is a midline defect in the lower sternum, the surrounding structures are unlikely to remain intact, resulting in involvement of all adjacent structures. The incidence of Cantrell's pentalogy is extremely low, approximately 5.5/100 per million births, but the condition is critical and has a very high mortality rate, making it the most severe type of sternal cleft. The greatest danger of Cantrell's pentalogy comes from cardiac anomalies. Various congenital heart defects can occur, the most common being a ventricular septal defect, which is present in nearly every case. Next most common is an atrial septal defect, with an incidence of 34%–53%. A left ventricular diverticulum is also common, with an incidence of 20%–50%. In addition, pulmonary artery stenosis or atresia occurs in about 31.5% of cases, while Tetralogy of Fallot is less common, with an incidence of 10%–20%. The presence of heart defects not only makes the condition more severe but also greatly complicates surgical treatment. Besides Cantrell's pentalogy, a sternal cleft may also be seen in another rare condition known as PHACES syndrome, which includes posterior fossa malformations, hemangiomas, arterial anomalies, coarctation of the aorta, cardiac defects, eye abnormalities, and sternal cleft [4,9]. It is a multi-system disorder. It is a rare and complex disorder, and the sternal cleft is one of its fundamental malformations. Although a sternal cleft can be associated with various other conditions, its main lesions are macroscopic structural abnormalities, and the remaining sternal structures generally do not show significant microscopic abnormalities. In the early stages, the residual sternal structure consists of cartilage, which can gradually calcify with age and become bony tissue.

3. Hazards

The harm caused by a sternal cleft comes from two aspects: first, the impact of the cleft itself, and second, the effects of any associated organ malformations on the body. The direct harm of the cleft itself also has two main aspects: one is the impact on the integrity of the thoracic cage, and the other is the impact on organ function caused by organ displacement due to the cleft. The thoracic cage plays an important role: it not only protects the internal organs in the thoracic cavity but also participates in normal respiratory movement. When a sternal cleft occurs, the protective function of the thoracic cage is lost, and the heart and major blood vessels may bulge out toward the body surface — this is the fundamental cause of ectopia cordis. Its impact on respiratory function is multifaceted, one aspect being the possible occurrence of paradoxical respiration. Once paradoxical breathing occurs, respiratory function can be severely compromised. In addition to the direct harm of the cleft, it is often accompanied by other organ malformations, which may lead to further damage due to impaired function of those organs. Therefore, although a sternal cleft is essentially an abnormality of the sternum's structure, it often involves surrounding structures and other organs, and its harm frequently extends far beyond the sternum itself — it is not only complex but can also be very serious.

4. Clinical Manifestations

Sternal cleft is a congenital condition, so various symptoms can already be seen during the newborn period. The condition shows a clear gender difference, being more common in females [4,5]. Due to the frequent presence of associated anomalies, its clinical manifestations vary greatly. Isolated sternal clefts are extremely rare and, if not accompanied by other conditions, may present only with respiratory and circulatory system dysfunction. However, because it is often associated with other severe anomalies, the clinical presentation can be highly complex. An incomplete sternal cleft with a limited range and no obvious paradoxical respiration may have mild or no clinical symptoms. If the cleft is extensive and combined with other anomalies, significant symptoms may occur. Sternal cleft involving the lower sternum is often very severe because it usually presents as part of Cantrell's pentalogy; affected infants are critically ill, and many die shortly after birth. A complete sternal cleft may be accompanied by ectopia cordis, which severely affects cardiac function. If congenital heart defects are also present, the condition becomes even more severe.

5. Examinations

The examinations for sternal clefts mainly include three parts: first, examination of the thoracic structure; second, examination of the heart; and third, examination of other parts of the body. The purpose of examining the thoracic structure is to determine the location, shape, and size of the sternal cleft. The purpose of the heart examination is to clarify the position of the heart and any cardiac abnormalities. Examinations of other parts of the body are mainly to identify any associated conditions.

6.Variable

The most direct method for examining the thoracic cage is a physical examination, which can reveal the main features of a sternal cleft through general inspection and palpation. Imaging examinations can provide detailed information about the structure of the thoracic cage, clearly showing the location, size, and shape of the sternal cleft, as well as its relationship to other organs. The most basic imaging modality is CT (Figure 2-22-4); if conditions permit, a 3D reconstruction can also be performed (Figure 2-22-5). For cardiac assessment, echocardiography is the first choice; if necessary, cardiac angiography may be performed. Examinations of other body parts should be selected based on the specific clinical situation.

Since sternal clefts are generally congenital and such deformities are often severe, prenatal screening is important. Prenatal ultrasonography can help detect this anomaly in a timely manner [10]. However, whether to terminate the pregnancy should be determined according to the specific condition of the malformation

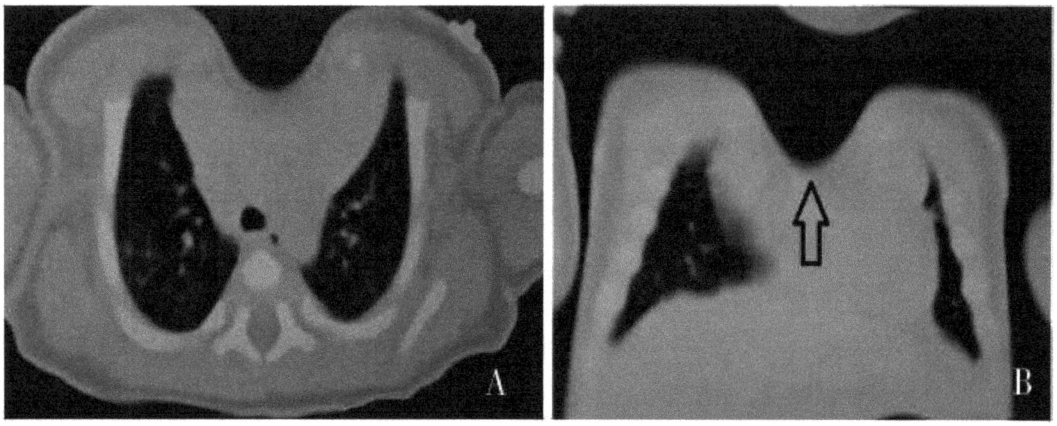

Figure 2-22-4. CT Images of a Child with Superior Sternal Cleft (A. Axial View; B. Coronal View)

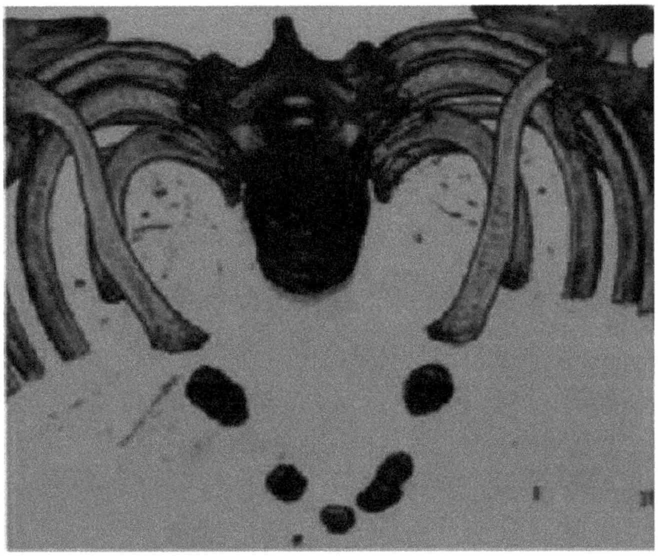

Figure 2-22-5. 3D Reconstruction of the Thoracic Cage in a Child with Superior Sternal Cleft

7. Diagnosis and Differential Diagnosis

The diagnosis of cranial cleft is straightforward: as long as there is a complete or partial split in the skull, it can be clearly identified. The challenge lies mainly in early diagnosis during the prenatal period. Once a cranial cleft is found, to ensure an accurate diagnosis, careful examination of the location, extent, and associated brain malformations is required. This helps determine the appropriate surgical plan.

The key point in the differential diagnosis of cranial cleft is to distinguish it from cranioschisis. When performing prenatal ultrasound, attention should be paid to whether there is a defect in the skull and whether brain tissue is protruding outside the skull. Cranioschisis can cause brain tissue to herniate outside the skull, which must be differentiated from cranial cleft. In a cranial cleft, the main feature is that the edges of the cleft are covered with normal skin, while cranioschisis generally lacks skin coverage on one side, with the other side connected to other structures.

8. Indications for Surgery

A cranial cleft is a severe skull deformity that seriously affects a child's health, so surgery should generally be performed as early as possible. However, the appropriate timing of surgery must be considered according to the type and extent of the defect and the general health of the child. Simple cranial clefts can usually be repaired surgically without difficulty, but complex clefts involving large defects require careful planning and technical skill. For simple cranial clefts, surgery is not technically demanding and can generally achieve good outcomes. For large or complex defects, surgery is technically challenging and may not achieve satisfactory cosmetic or functional results, or may require multiple staged procedures. These complex cases require thorough evaluation. If such staged surgical approaches are not feasible, surgery should be reconsidered.

9. Timing of Surgery

Cranial clefts are generally diagnosed during the neonatal period. When considering surgical repair, the child's general condition must be taken into account. If conditions permit, surgery should be performed as early as possible. Generally, for simple cranial clefts, surgery can be done shortly after birth, as early repair can promote normal skull development and reduce the risk of brain injury. For more complex cranial clefts, surgery should be timed carefully according to the severity of the defect and the child's growth and development. Regarding the timing of surgery during infancy, opinions vary. Some believe that early surgery promotes skull healing and reduces complications; others suggest that delayed surgery may be safer for the child's overall health. In cases where the cleft affects brain development or is accompanied by brain herniation, early repair should be considered. However, for mild cases with good skull growth, surgery can be delayed. Therefore, the timing of surgery for cranial clefts is not fixed but should be flexible. If early surgery is possible, it should be done, as early repair is generally more beneficial than delayed surgery.

10. Surgical Methods

Surgical treatment of the sternal cleft began in 1947, when Burton performed an operation on a patient with a superior sternal cleft [5]. Since then, more patients have undergone surgical repair, and numerous surgical techniques have been developed and applied in clinical practice. Overall, surgical methods can be divided into two main categories: the first is direct suture closure, and the second is reconstruction using artificial materials [11,12]. Surgery for an isolated sternal cleft is relatively straightforward, but if the defect involves the heart or other associated anomalies, the procedure becomes much more complex. Two main considerations must be addressed when performing surgery: the sequence of repairing the sternal cleft and any required cardiac surgery; the execution of the sternal cleft repair itself. When a sternal cleft is accompanied by cardiac malformations, the cardiac surgery should be completed first. If closing the sternum might adversely affect cardiac function, some recommend staging the sternal cleft repair for a second procedure. However, this staged approach has several disadvantages. Ideally, both procedures should be completed in a single operation. The key to successful sternal cleft repair is to achieve complete closure of the defect while avoiding any adverse effects.

(1) Direct Suture

If the residual sternal bones on both sides are close enough together and bringing them together will not cause significant compression of the mediastinal structures, direct suture closure can be considered. During the procedure, the residual sternal segments on both sides must first be fully mobilized. Then, they are approximated, aligned, and securely fixed in place. Once fixation is complete, the operative area must be completely covered with soft tissue to promote healing (Figure 2-22-6) [13,14].

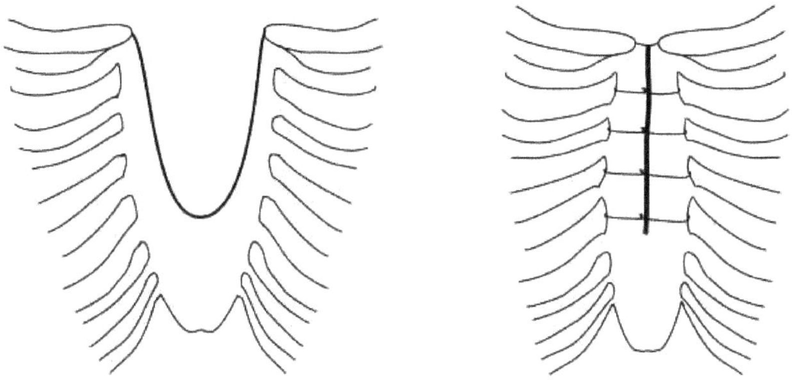

Figure 2-22-6: Schematic Diagram of Direct Closure Surgery for Superior Sternal Cleft

Direct suture is the simplest surgical method and if it can be performed, the surgery will be easily accomplished. However, there are cases where direct suturing is not possible, and these include: (1) a wide distance between the residual sternums on both sides and a large median defect that cannot be eliminated by retraction. In such cases, several special designs have been used, the main principle of which is to loosen the peripheral structures and then suture or fixate the sternum. Release of the peripheral structures can be performed either on the rib cartilage or on the rib cage. The general principle is to sever the structures without creating a significant defect and to ensure that the structures can regenerate as much as possible after the operation. (2) The residual sternum is too stiff to bring it directly together for suturing. This occurs in years

In older patients, the initial segment of the sternal cleft has typically fully ossified and become abnormally rigid, hindering the approximation of the sternal edges. To overcome this obstacle, wedge-shaped osteotomy can be performed at the initial segment, followed by closure; alternatively, the intact portion of the sternum can be completely split, with the edges trimmed and then fully sutured. Some surgeons have also cut the costal cartilages or ribs on both sides of the sternal cleft and rotated them 180 degrees toward the midline defect to suture them to the contralateral structures. These measures effectively overcome the difficulties encountered in direct closure, ultimately achieving good results [13,14]. The greatest advantage of direct closure is that the procedure is relatively simple, does not require additional materials for reconstruction, and is easier to perform. However, direct closure has its own limitations. First, suturing can sometimes be technically difficult, which may affect the quality of closure. Second, direct closure may reduce thoracic cavity volume and impair cardiopulmonary function [11,12]. Therefore, direct closure is not a perfect method, and alternative surgical approaches are necessary for certain patients.

(2) Chest Wall Reconstruction

For patients with larger defects or very rigid sternal bones, reconstruction is often the preferred surgical approach. Reconstruction of a sternal cleft is essentially the same as reconstruction for other chest wall defects: the basic principle is to repair the defect using various materials. The repair material can be autologous tissue or artificial materials. The most commonly used autologous materials are rib or costal cartilage, but bone from other parts of the body can also be used. There are various artificial materials available and the choice depends on the specific case. The basic goals of reconstruction are twofold: to eliminate the defect as completely as possible, and to restore the stability of the chest wall. To achieve these goals, there must be both appropriate surgical technique and careful selection of suitable materials. Generally, sternal cleft defects are relatively localized, so the reconstruction procedure is comparatively straightforward.

In our practice, we use a combined approach: first, the sternal cleft is reconstructed with the patient's own rib(s), and then the donor site defect in the rib area is repaired with special artificial materials [14]. The specific method is as follows: a segment of one rib, or parts of two ribs, are harvested from one side of the chest wall. The harvested rib is then divided into several sections according to the size of the sternal defect. These rib segments are placed side by side in the middle of the defect and fixed securely to the residual sternum on both sides to close the cleft. Finally, the donor site where the rib was harvested is reconstructed using MatrixRIB. We have used this method to perform reconstruction surgery on 2 pediatric patients with sternal clefts, both of whom also had congenital heart disease. First, the congenital heart defect was corrected through a median sternotomy, and then the sternal cleft was repaired, resulting in satisfactory outcomes (see Figures 2-22-7 and 2-22-8). The advantage of this method is that by using the patient's own rib for the reconstruction, it avoids the potential risks of artificial materials causing problems to the underlying heart and great vessels. It also prevents the issue of new defects forming if artificial materials need to be removed later. The rib donor site defect, repaired with artificial material, can remain in the body permanently. Even if removal is needed in the future, the local area usually has enough fibrous tissue growth to prevent adverse effects.

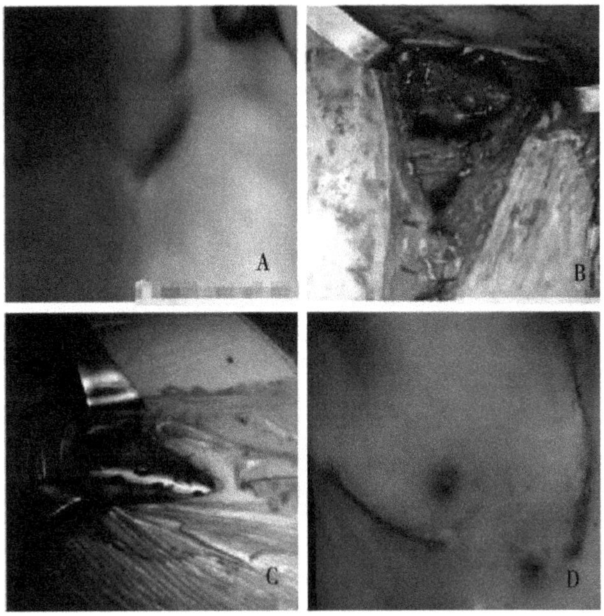

Figure 2-22-7 Simultaneous Surgery for a Child with Sternal Cleft and Congenital Heart Disease (A) Perform a median sternotomy, expose the sternal cleft, divide the residual sternum, spread the sternum apart, and prepare for cardiac surgery; (B) Establish cardiopulmonary bypass and perform the cardiac procedure; (C) Make an incision in the right chest wall and harvest segments of the right 4th and 5th ribs; (D) Use MatrixRIB to reconstruct the defect left by the removal of the right 4th and 5th ribs; (E) Divide the harvested 4th and 5th ribs into three segments and place them horizontally in the midline of the sternum, securing them firmly; (F) Close the incision to complete the surgery.

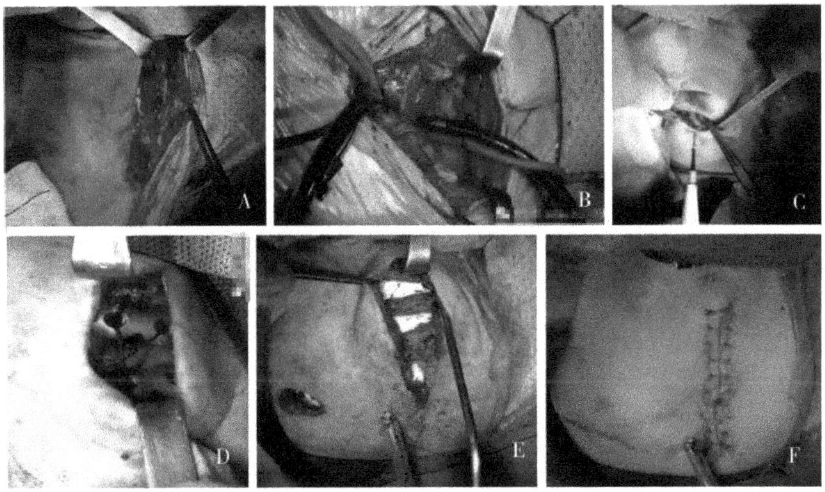

Figure 2-22-8 Simultaneous Surgery for Sternal Cleft Combined with Congenital Heart Disease in a Child (A) Appearance of the chest wall, showing partial defect in the upper part of the sternum with paradoxical breathing; (B) A median incision is made to perform the cardiac surgery. After completion of the cardiac procedure, a segment of the right 4th rib is resected, divided into three equal parts, and placed transversely between the sternal cleft for fixation; (C) The defect of the right 4th rib after resection is repaired using MatrixRIB; (D) Postoperative chest wall appearance, showing the median incision and the lateral chest wall incision.

11. Prognosis

Surgery for isolated sternal clefts is relatively straightforward, provided the procedure is performed properly. Satisfactory outcomes can be achieved in almost all cases. However, since children with sternal clefts often have other associated organ anomalies, especially complex congenital heart diseases, the treatment of these conditions directly affects the surgical results. Because cardiac surgeries require specialized cardiac surgeons and chest wall surgeons typically do not participate in these procedures, to ensure better outcomes for sternal cleft repair, close collaboration between chest wall surgeons and cardiac surgeons is essential. Only through such multidisciplinary cooperation can patients receive the optimal treatment.

REFERENCES

[1] Klein, T., M. Kellmer, T. M. Boemers, et al. 2015. "Surgical Repair of a Superior Sternal Cleft in an Infant." *European Journal of Pediatric Surgery Reports* 3 (2): 64–76.

[2] Emur, B., S. Mete, S. Beken, et al. 2020. "Complete Sternal Cleft Treatment in a Low-Birth-Weight Patient." *Turkish Journal of Thoracic and Cardiovascular Surgery* 28 (4): 684–687.

[3] Ashok Raja, J., G. Mathevan, K. Mathiatrasan, et al. 2014. "Closing the Cleft over a Throbbing Heart: Neonatal Sternal Cleft." *BMJ Case Reports* 2014: bcr2014204529.

[4] Sadeghian, N., A. Mirshemirani, and I. Sadeghian. 2014. "Sternal Cleft Associated with Patent Ductus Arteriosus, Atrial Septal Defect, and Subglottic Hemangioma: A Rarity." *APSP Journal of Case Reports* 5 (1): 6.

[5] Ravikumar, M. S., V. Palanisamy, K. Raman, et al. 2019. "Primary Closure of a Partial Superior Sternal Cleft in a 27-Day-Old Neonate: Case Report with Short Review of Literature." *Cureus* 11 (5): e4653.

[6] Alshomer, F., F. Aldaghri, N. Alohaideb, et al. 2017. "Reconstruction of Congenital Sternal Clefts: Surgical Experience and Literature Review." *Plastic and Reconstructive Surgery Global Open* 5 (11): e1567.

[7] Daum, R., and Z. Zachariou. 1999. "Total and Superior Sternal Clefts in Newborns: A Simple Technique for Surgical Correction." *Journal of Pediatric Surgery* 34 (3): 408–411.

[8] van Hoorn, J. H. L., R. M. J. Moonen, C. J. R. Huysentruyt, et al. 2008. "Pentalogy of Cantrell: Two Patients and a Review to Determine Prognostic Factors for Optimal Approach." *European Journal of Pediatrics* 167 (1): 29–35.

[9] Chaudhry, I. U. H., A. Cheema, A. Aqeel, et al. 2021. "Modified Surgical Reconstruction Technique for a Rare Isolated Congenital Sternal Cleft in a Six-Year-Old Child." *Annals of Medicine and Surgery* 65: 102280.

[10] Yuksel, M., P. Kuru, N. Ermerak, et al. 2016. "Intrauterine Diagnosed Sternal Cleft Patient and Her Management." *Journal of Visualized Surgery* 2: 48.

[11] Torre, M., G. Rapuzzi, M. Carlucci, et al. 2012. "Phenotypic Spectrum and Management of Sternal Clefts: Literature Review and Presentation of a New Series." *European Journal of Cardio-Thoracic Surgery* 41 (1): 4–9.

[12] Dogan, R., S. Uysal, U. Kumbasar, et al. 2019. "Surgical Repair of a Sternal Cleft Malformation." *Turkish Journal of Thoracic and Cardiovascular Surgery* 27 (4): 597–600.

[13] Wang, W. L. 2017. "Surgical Issues of Sternal Cleft." *I Ask Doctor*, January 7.

[14] Wang, W. L. 2018. "A Major Surgery for a 30-Day-Old Baby: Severe Sternal Cleft with Congenital Heart Disease." *Medical Science and Technology Channel*, June 14.

Localized chest wall protuberance deformity is a relatively rare, focal thoracic deformity characterized mainly by a localized protrusion of the costal cartilage or rib. Typically, it involves only a single rib or costal cartilage, while the surrounding bony structures maintain a normal shape (Figure 2-23-1) [1]. Due to this local protrusion, the thoracic appearance is abnormal, classifying it as a type of thoracic deformity. However

er, it differs significantly from common pectus carinatum and other types of anterior protrusion deformities [2,3].

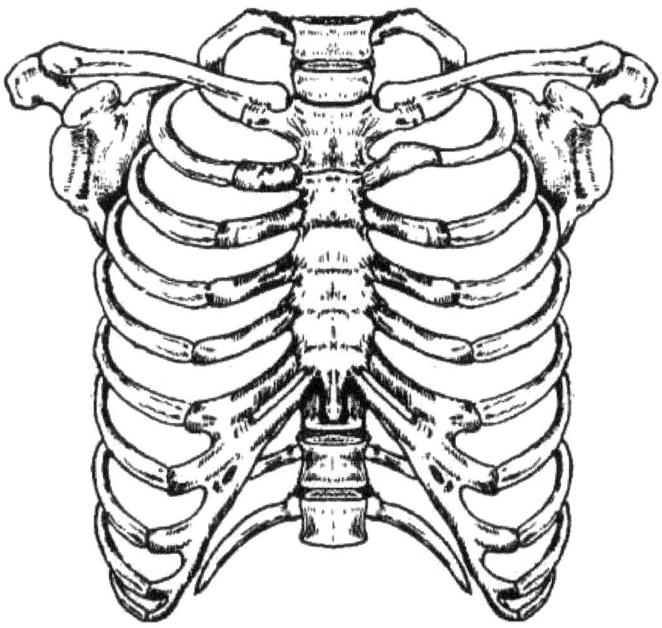

Figure 2-23-1: Localized Chest Wall Protuberance Deformity

Localized chest wall protuberance deformity is a condition we have named, and to our knowledge, it has not been reported in the literature before. Consequently, relatively few patients seek medical attention specifically for this deformity. This may be related to the level of awareness and concern about the condition. Many patients are unaware of their deformity and thus are less likely to seek medical care. Without patients presenting with this issue, doctors have fewer opportunities to encounter such cases. Since this deformity generally does not cause obvious symptoms, even patients who do visit a doctor may not have their condition recognized or treated as a true deformity. These combined factors result in limited attention to this deformity, and naturally, its reported incidence appears very low. However, incidence data do not necessarily reflect the true prevalence of the condition. In our clinical practice, we have found that such patients are not uncommon. Some of these patients experience distress and discomfort related to their condition and therefore deserve appropriate attention and care.

1. Pathogenesis

The pathogenesis of localized chest wall protrusion deformity is still unclear. It may be related to excessive growth of the costal cartilage or ribs. However, overgrowth is only a prerequisite for the formation of a protrusion; another necessary condition is a structural abnormality in the local costal cartilage or rib. If the entire rib and costal cartilage are uniform in structure and there are no internal abnormalities, then even with excessive growth, a localized protrusion will not occur. Since a protrusion exists, it indicates that there must be an inherent structural abnormality in the local rib or costal cartilage. This mechanism is actually similar to that of other anterior protrusion deformities, such as pectus carinatum [4]. Once there is a problem within the bony structure itself, external factors can take advantage of it, ultimately altering the shape of the bone and forming a deformity. The occurrence of localized chest wall protrusion deformity should be seen as the combined effect of these two factors. However, this analysis is only a hypothesis; the specific mechanism still needs further research.

2. Pathological Features

The lesions of localized chest wall protrusion deformity are limited to the costal cartilage and ribs. Lesions of the costal cartilage are confined to the anterior chest wall; rib lesions can occur along the entire length of the rib, but clinically significant protrusions are generally located on the anterior chest wall. Only protrusions in this area are easily detected and may affect the appearance of the thorax, causing distress to the patient. The localized protrusion is limited to a single rib and its costal cartilage; the surrounding bony structures are normal in shape, and the lesion does not involve the sternum or other ribs and costal cartilages[1]. From a microscopic perspective, the protrusion deformity is merely a change in shape and appearance; the internal structure is essentially normal, with no abnormal pathological structure present.

3. Harm

As a type of protrusion disorder, localized protrusion deformities generally do not compress the thoracic structures, so they do not cause any functional damage to the body. The scope of damage from localized protrusion is limited and does not significantly affect the entire structure and function of the thoracic cavity. However, its potential impact should not be ignored. In terms of appearance, if the protrusion is mild or covered by subcutaneous fat or muscle bulk, it generally does not cause visible deformity. If the protrusion is obvious, it may affect appearance, and its harmful effects are similar to other protrusion deformities, with the main issue being psychological harm. If not treated in time, it can lead to serious psychological problems.

4. Clinical Manifestations

A localized chest wall protrusion deformity does not cause compression, so it usually presents with no clinical symptoms. If the patient cares about the chest wall appearance. Are dissatisfied with the appearance and do not receive timely treatment, it may lead to psychological problems. These psychological issues can, in turn, affect the patient's physical functions and manifest as clinical symptoms. At this point, the clinical symptoms are not directly related to the deformity, and various examinations will almost never find objective pathological evidence

5. Examination

The physical signs of localized chest wall protuberance deformity are very clear. Physical examination can reveal a localized protrusion on the anterior chest wall. The protrusion may be located beside the sternum or in other areas of the anterior chest wall. The breast tissue and pectoralis major muscle may cover the protrusion, but palpation can still determine its approximate position and outline. X-rays cannot show costal cartilage lesions but can reveal abnormalities in the bony ribs. CT scans provide incomplete cross-sectional information; the ideal imaging method is three-dimensional reconstruction, which allows comprehensive and objective evaluation of the protrusion itself as well as the surrounding bony structures.

1. Diagnosis and Differential Diagnosis

The diagnosis of local chest wall bulge deformity is relatively easy. The key points of diagnosis are: (1) the rib cartilage or rib bulge is local; (2) the bulge is limited to one rib or rib cartilage; (3) the bulge does not involve the sternum. Through physical examination and related imaging examinations, the diagnosis of this deformity can be easily completed.

This diagnosis can be easily confirmed through physical examination and relevant imaging studies. Differential diagnosis is important to distinguish this deformity from certain special conditions. The first is chest wall tumors. Some chest wall tumors, especially those originating from costal cartilage or ribs, may be asymptomatic and present as localized protrusions on the chest surface, mimicking this deformity. Key differentiating points are: localized chest wall protuberance deformity is congenital and present from early childhood, becoming more apparent with age. The affected rib or costal cartilage shows only shape abnormalities without obvious thickening, and cytological examination reveals normal rib or cartilage tissue. In contrast, chest wall tumors have a short onset, rapid growth, marked local thickening, and cytology confirms tumor tissue. In most cases, differentiation is straightforward. However, if the tumor does not enlarge significantly, distinguishing the two may be difficult, with cytological examination being the only definitive method. The second differential diagnosis is mild asymmetric pectus carinatum. Pectus carinatum involves protrusion of multiple bony structures, possibly including the sternum, with a wide and large affected area. Localized chest wall protuberance deformity involves only a single rib or costal cartilage, which is the fundamental difference.

7. Surgical Treatment

(1) Indications for Surgery

As with other deformities, surgical treatment of localized chest wall protuberance deformity is primarily decided by the patient and their family. Because the deformity generally lacks significant symptoms, the decision to operate is mostly based on appearance. If the patient and family are dissatisfied with the cosmetic outcome, surgery is indicated. When deciding on surgery, one situation requires particular attention: the inability to distinguish the deformity from chest tumor, the inability to distinguish from a localized tumor. If a tumor is suspected, active surgical excision should be performed.

(2) Surgical Methods

Localized chest wall protuberance deformity is essentially an anterior protrusion deformity, so its surgical approach can refer to methods used for other protuberant deformities. Such surgeries ideally should be minimally invasive. However, because the lesion is localized, performing an open surgery directly on the site will not cause excessive damage, which provides strong justification for this approach. Therefore, surgery for localized chest wall protuberance deformity can be performed using two basic methods: open surgery and minimally invasive surgery. Both have different operative procedures but can yield good outcomes when properly executed.

(i)Open Surgery

Open surgery involves making an incision directly over the protruding area to correct the deformity. This can be implemented by two main methods: reshaping or resection.

(1) Reshaping Surgery: This method is similar to the typical reshaping procedures for other deformities, where local operations are done to eliminate the deformity and restore normal shape. Specifically, an incision is made over the protrusion to expose the lesion; then, at appropriate sites, the abnormal structure is either transected or wedge resected to destroy the original deformity. The area is then fixed to restore normal shape. This method is mature

and has been frequently used in early thoracic deformity surgeries, proving to be highly effective. For costal cartilage lesions, wedge resection followed by suturing of the cartilage can be performed. The method is simple and yields satisfactory results. For localized rib lesions, artificial materials may be used for local fixation, also producing good outcomes.

(2) Resection Surgery: One of the major characteristics of localized chest wall protuberance deformity is its localized lesion. Theoretically, complete excision of the lesion should not significantly affect chest wall appearance or function. Based on this, direct resection of the lesion can be considered. There are two specific approaches: 1. Simple excision of the protruding structure, which is the most effective way to eliminate the protrusion. However, it leaves a local chest wall defect postoperatively, making it a less ideal choice. 2. Excision followed by local reconstruction using graft materials. This method effectively eliminates the residual defect but introduces foreign materials, which may create new issues related to the implant.

Open surgery is a direct corrective procedure targeting localized chest wall protuberance deformity. It achieves definitive correction and complete elimination of the deformity. However, because the incision is made on the protrusion's surface, noticeable scars may remain. Additionally, due to the presence of the breast and pectoralis major muscle, poor exposure may necessitate a larger incision, increase surgical difficulty and result in longer scars. Therefore, direct open surgery is not always the optimal choice.

(ii) Minimally Invasive Surgery

(1) Wenlin Procedure: for all thoracic deformities, minimally invasive surgery generally involves the use of shaping materials to reshape the chest wall. For localized chest wall protuberance deformity, the specific method is the Wenlin procedure, which uses a steel bar to compress the protruding area, fixed at both ends, thereby achieving reshaping [5]. The Wenlin procedure's incisions are small, located on both sides of the chest wall, and are concealed, resulting in minimal postoperative scarring. If the procedure can completely eliminate the protrusion deformity, it should be the ideal choice. However, this type of surgery also has disadvantages. First, since the lesion area of the localized chest wall protrusion deformity is limited to only one rib or costal cartilage, this presents challenges for the placement of the steel plate. Effective placement must be exactly on the surface of the protrusion; only when positioned here can it have a good corrective effect. If the steel plate slips or if it is impossible for the plate to stay properly on the protrusion, the surgery may fail. It is clear that the key to the success of this surgery is to ensure that the steel plate can properly press on the protrusion, but the greatest difficulty with localized chest wall protrusion deformity is that it often does not easily provide the ideal conditions for the plate to exert pressure. Second, the Wenlin procedure must use a special steel plate to complete the correction, which

means there will be a foreign object inside the chest wall after the surgery. This undoubtedly affects the patient's surgical experience. Third, the Wenlin procedure involves relatively large trauma. One of the biggest advantages of the Wenlin procedure is its minimally invasive nature. However, the degree of invasiveness is a relative concept. Usually, the Wenlin procedure is considered minimally invasive because its trauma is significantly less than that of traditional open surgery. But for localized chest wall protrusion deformity, open surgery itself does not cause much trauma and is an extremely minor operation. Compared to this, the Wenlin procedure's trauma appears more significant. In this case, the Wenlin procedure no longer resembles a minimally invasive surgery but becomes a major operation. Fourth, the steel plates used in the Wenlin procedure are quite expensive, which increases the patient's surgical costs. Fifth, the steel plate needs to be removed after a certain period, which means the patient must undergo an additional surgery and bear more treatment costs. Therefore, although the Wenlin procedure is the ideal surgery for treating protrusion type deformities, it is not necessarily the ideal choice for localized chest wall protrusion deformity.

(2) Thoracoscopic resection surgery. The Wenlin procedure is a representative minimally invasive surgery, specifically designed for protrusion type deformities. However, due to its various drawbacks, other options need to be considered. Combining the most basic minimally invasive techniques of thoracic surgery, the possibility of performing the surgery under Thoracoscopy can be considered. Performing reshaping under Thoracoscopy is extremely difficult and may not be practical. However, resecting the affected area under Thoracoscopy is relatively easier. The principle of this operation is exactly the same as that of resection performed in an open state, and its advantages are obvious, making it an ideal choice. However, considering the inherent difficulty of thoracoscopic surgery itself, it places higher demands on the execution of the procedure.

In summary, the treatment of localized chest wall protrusion deformity essentially comes down to two basic surgical methods: either reshaping or resection. Both surgical methods can be performed in an open state or using minimally invasive techniques. Regardless of the method used, as long as the basic principles are followed, the local deformity can be eliminated, ultimately achieving a satisfactory outcome.

(3) Complications

In general, surgery for localized chest wall protrusion deformity is relatively simple and has a high success rate. However, because it involves some special procedures, unexpected complications can still occur. The first complication is pneumothorax. This mainly happens during open surgery but can also occur when using Thoracoscopy. The main cause of pneumothorax is insufficient evacuation of air when closing the chest. This complication is not serious and will resolve quickly with appropriate management. Performing the Wenlin procedure may also result in pneumothorax, but it is generally not severe and does not require special treatment. The second complication is bleeding. The main surgical operations for localized chest wall protrusion deformity are near the affected rib or costal cartilage. The blood vessel most likely to be injured is the intercostal artery. If the lesion is close to the sternum, there is also a possibility of damaging the internal thoracic artery.

Injury to the intercostal vessels does not usually cause severe bleeding, and hemostasis is relatively easy to achieve. However, if the internal thoracic artery is damaged and bleeding is not controlled in time, it can result in significant blood loss. If this occurs during open surgery, it is easier to manage, but if it happens during thoracoscopic surgery, it must be handled with extra caution.

The third complication is sliding of the steel plate. This mainly occurs in Wenlin procedures. As mentioned earlier, since localized chest wall protrusion deformity only involves one rib or piece of cartilage, the area for fixation is small. If conditions are not optimal, postoperative sliding of the steel plate may occur. If this happens, the surgery may fail, and the local chest wall protrusion may recur. To avoid this, some special techniques should be used during the operation. Because the lesion is far from the lateral chest wall, it is not easy to place the steel plate directly onto the affected area. At this point, the surgeon can use a finger to assist in guiding and pressing over the protrusion. First, when creating the tunnel, the surgeon's finger can guide the process so that the tunnel is precisely above the protrusion; second, when tightening the plate, the finger can press against it to help fix its position. The correct positioning of the steel plate depends on adequate local pressure. In this process, the use of the finger is particularly important. With this assistance, the chance of plate slippage is greatly reduced. Besides finger assistance, other technical details must be considered especially the fixation points of the plate. Securing both ends of the plate firmly helps prevent any tilt or displacement. However, in extreme cases, despite all efforts, the plate may still not remain fixed in place. In such cases, another extreme method may be used: making a tiny incision near the rib or calcified cartilage, locally placing a steel wire, and then fixing the plate directly on the surface of the protrusion. This method provides the most reliable fixation and fundamentally prevents the plate from slipping.

The fourth complication is local paradoxical respiration. This happens during resection surgery that removes part of the affected structure. After part of the chest wall is removed, there will inevitably be a defect. If the patient's chest wall soft tissues are thick and strong enough, paradoxical respiration usually does not occur. However, if the patient is thin and the defect area lacks sufficient soft tissue coverage or the tissue is not strong enough, paradoxical respiration may appear. Localized paradoxical respiration does not generally affect respiratory function, but it can affect appearance and thus diminish the overall surgical outcome. To prevent paradoxical respiration, the most

fundamental measure is to avoid simple excision alone. If excision cannot be avoided, as little bone structure as possible should be removed, or reconstruction should be performed to eliminate the defect.
The fifth complication is delayed wound healing. This mostly occurs in surgeries that use artificial materials, but it can also occur in other types of surgery if technical details are not handled properly.

8. Prognosis
Localized chest wall protrusion deformity is different from pectus carinatum (pigeon chest), but from an overall classification perspective, there is no essential difference, so this deformity can even be regarded as a mild form of pigeon chest. for this reason, its treatment methods share some similarities with those for pigeon chest. However, as discussed above, the surgeries for the two conditions also differ significantly in some respects. In general, surgery for localized chest wall protrusion deformity is relatively simple and safer, so the likelihood of success is higher. If the procedure is carried out strictly according to the standard protocols, good results can generally be achieved. However, because the surgery is so minor and simple, it is possible that during the operation. Paralysis of the operator's mind. Even the smallest surgery can go wrong if there is no mental attention, so giving mental attention to this particular deformity is a prerequisite for successful completion of the treatment.

REFERENCES

[1] Wang WL. Localized raised deformity of the chest wall. Thoracic Deformity Surgery Specialist, 10-6-2021.
[2] Wang WL, Long WG, Chen CM, et al. Ultraminimally invasive surgery for chicken breast. Journal of practical medicine, 2015, 31 (5): 863-864.
[3] Wang WL, Chen CH, Li XJ, et al. A holistic taxonomy of thoracic deformities. Chinese Clinical Journal of Thoracic and Cardiovascular Surgery, 2018, 25 (11): 981-985.
[4] Wang WL, Long WG, Chen CH, et al. Analysis of the pathogenesis of chicken breast. Journal of practical medicine, 2015, 31 (add): 313-314.
[5] Wang W L. Minimally invasive surgical technique for barrel chest. surgical case reports, 2018, 1 (2): 1-2.

Among the surgical diseases of the chest wall, chest wall deformity is one of the important ones. Considering the specificity of the deformity, thoracic deformity is generally treated as a chest wall deformity in clinical work. In the relevant chapters of this book, the thorax is studied as a whole, so that the term thoracic deformity refers to an abnormality in the overall appearance of the thorax. When studied in this way, the details of the constituent parts of the thorax are generally not given undue attention. This means that as long as there is no problem with the overall appearance of the thorax, it can be dismissed as a thoracic deformity. Such a viewpoint not only affects the diagnosis of thoracic deformities but also directly affects their treatment. In order to achieve a normal appearance, localized structural defects can be ignored, and sometimes even localized structures are sacrificed in exchange for a change in the overall shape. This is often done when the thorax is viewed as a whole. However, in clinical work, it is sometimes necessary to look at the problem from a different angle. For example, if more subtle structural aspects are observed, more problems may be found. The significance of these problems may be quite different from the significance when looking at the thorax as a whole, and sometimes they may seem unusual and require additional attention.

The thorax is an organic whole made up of the bony structures of the chest wall. There are three types of bony structures that make up the thorax, namely the sternum, the ribs, and the costal cartilages, but there are many more, and in general, the thorax is made up of dozens of bony structures of different sizes and shapes. If these structures are viewed as individuals, each one may have an abnormality. Such anomalies often go unnoticed, especially when the focus is only on the external shape of the thorax, and the anomalies of the individual structures are completely ignored. However, the reason that any individual structure has a normal shape is that such a shape facilitates normal physiologic function. If an abnormality in shape occurs, it will inevitably interfere with function. Abnormalities in the functioning of localized structures may be insignificant, but once these abnormalities appear to have a superimposed effect, the problem may be so severe that it eventually causes the patient to manifest symptoms. At this point the local structural abnormality can no longer be ignored and becomes a de facto disease.

This is where the study of localized structures comes in. Local structural abnormalities can take three forms: first, abnormalities of position, second, abnormalities of shape, and third, abnormalities of number. Abnormalities of position are those in which the bone is in an inappropriate position, abnormalities of shape are those in which the appearance of the bone itself is in question, and abnormalities of quantity are those in which the number of structures is different from the normal number. When the thorax is viewed as a whole, these three abnormalities do not necessarily make sense. However, when viewed in relation to localized structures, they become pathological abnormalities, also known as deformities.

The sternum is relatively fixed in position and unlikely to vary in number, so that the main problem is an abnormality of shape. There are several ribs, each of which may show abnormalities of position and shape, and the total number may be abnormal, so that the deformity of the ribs themselves is a very complex problem. The costal cartilage forms an inseparable whole with the ribs and can be viewed as part of the rib, and is not discussed separately here.

1.True sternal angle

The names mentioned in the literature include (2-24-1) true sternal angle variant, costal sternal prominence, suprasternal prominence, anatomical sternal angle, sternal stalk chair angular prominence, and anatomical variant of the ribs and sternum [1-3]. The fact that there are so many names for the same deformity does not mean that the researcher paid much attention to this deformity, but only shows the randomness of the study. This arbitrariness is understandable in view of the specialization of the researchers. They come from anatomy, imaging, or clinical specialties, and different specialties may have different perceptions of the same disease, so arbitrariness is inevitable. From another point of view, the fact that different specialties may have different views shows that the malformation itself is not a particularly serious malformation. The fact that the abnormality is not serious and can even be ignored inevitably affects the attitude of the researcher

True sternal angulation is uncommon, with an incidence of 0.61.0 per 1,000 [1], and some authors have suggested an even lower incidence of 1 in 10,000 [3], which suggests that this deformity is in fact extremely rare. When a deformity is difficult to recognize clinically, studies are necessarily limited, which undoubtedly affects the understanding of the deformity.

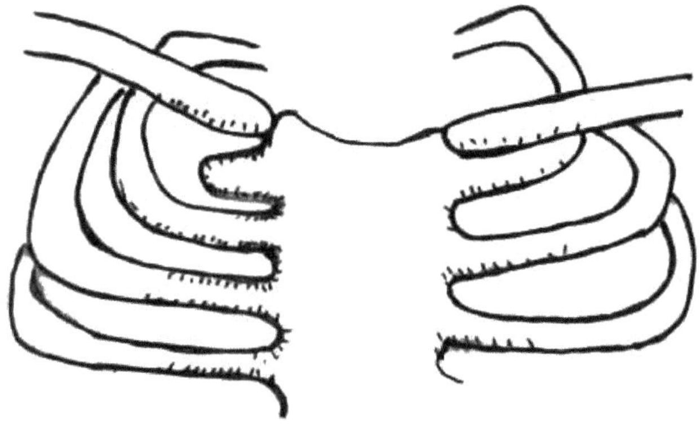

Figure 2-24-1 True sternal angle (abnormal bony prominence between the right sternoclavicular joint and the first rib cartilage below the sternoclavicular joint, with the 1 rib and all the ribs below it pushed downward, and the left rib in a normal position).

The true pathogenesis of the true sternal horn is not known and the exact mechanism is only speculative. It has been suggested that the deformity is due to overgrowth of the secondary ossification center of the sternum [1,3,5]. Physiologically, the sternal styloid is directly connected to the clavicle and the 1 rib cartilage, and there is no extra structure at the margin of the sternal styloid. In pathological conditions, the edge of the sternal styloid protrudes laterally to form a bony prominence, which is known as the true sternal horn. The protuberance is located between the clavicle and the 1st rib cartilage, and the base is attached to the sternal styloid as a single unit, with the distal end free. This suggests that the true sternal horn is derived directly from the sternal styloid and is the result of a variant of the sternal styloid.

The true sternal horn may appear on one side of the sternal styloid or on both sides at the same time, but the shape of the two sides is not necessarily the same, and it may be triangular, bull's horn, pointed, finger shaped or other irregular shapes [1,3]. The direction of protrusion also varies

It may protrude parallel to the sides only or upward and laterally. The degree of protrusion also varies and can be long or short.

Normally, the clavicle and the 1 rib cartilage are directly connected to the sternal styloid, and there is almost no distance between them. When the true sternal angle appears between them, the 1 rib cartilage will be squeezed downward due to the appearance of the bony protrusion, and thus all the other rib cartilages will be moved downward accordingly. This will undoubtedly compromise the intrinsic structure of the thorax. However, the appearance of the thorax does not depend on the shape of the local structures. In other words, the appearance of the thorax is not necessarily altered and does not necessarily result in a deformity of the thorax. This characteristic makes the true sternal angle highly invisible. In the absence of localized symptoms, it is difficult to detect, and most lesions are found on physical examination.

The symptoms of a true sternal horn depend on the effect of the bony prominence on the surrounding structures. If there is compression on the surrounding structures, there will be obvious symptoms [1,6]. If there is no compression, there will be no symptoms. Physical examination reveals a shallow supraclavicular fossa unilaterally or bilaterally, and a bony prominence palpable below the sternoclavicular joint, which is attached to

the sternal styloid in a fixed position and may have no tenderness. X-ray examination reveals an additional bony prominence on the lateral aspect of the sternal styloid, which is peripherally free and has no relationship to other bony structures, and is attached to the sternal styloid at the base, with trabeculae and a continuous bony cortex. CT examination reveals an abnormal bony prominence, which has no relationship to other bony structures, and has a continuous bony cortex and a continuous cortex. CT examination can reveal the abnormal bony protuberance. Three-dimensional reconstruction can clearly show the shape and structure of the bony prominence and its relationship to the sternal styloid.

The diagnosis of true sternal horn is relatively easy, but needs to be differentiated from some specific lesions [1,3]. The first one to be differentiated is osteochondroma. True sternal angle is a localized structural variant or deformity of the sternal stalk, which is a benign lesion with no distal calcification foci, which is the most significant difference from osteochondroma. The second thing to differentiate is lesions of the mediastinum. Upper mediastinal lesions sometimes appear as a mass in the plane of the sternal pedicle on X-ray, which is similar to the shape of a true sternal horn. It is difficult to distinguish between the two on X-ray, but the diagnosis can be easily made on CT.

When true sternal angle occurs, it may be combined with other rib shape abnormalities, such as cervical rib and rib bifurcation, etc[5]. Therefore, when making a diagnosis of true sternal angle, it is not only necessary to pay attention to the differentiation of other diseases, but also to clarify the presence of these combined deformities.

A true sternal angle hardly affects the overall appearance of the thorax, so localized symptoms become the only basis for deciding whether to operate or not. If there is no significant discomfort, surgery may not be considered. If symptoms are evident, surgery is indicated. The basic principle of surgery is to remove the bony prominence. This can be done by open surgery, where an incision is made directly on the surface of the protuberance and the protuberance is revealed and then removed. This method is simpler but has a visible surgical scar. Another option is thoracoscopic excision, which allows for a more subtle incision as it is made in the lateral chest wall.

Surgery for true sternal angles is simpler and usually not too difficult. However, sometimes there are special localized structures, such as the vascular nerves under the clavicle, the internal thoracic artery, and the structures of the superior mediastinum, which can pose a risk to the surgery, and therefore extra care is needed during the operation, or else associated complications may occur.

2. Sternal Deformities

Sternal deformities are often part of other deformities. In general thoracic deformities, the emphasis is usually on the abnormal shape of the thoracic cage as a whole, so the deformity of the sternum itself does not receive individual attention. However, deformities of the sternum alone are not uncommon and include many types.

Specific deformities. The more common deformity is the sternal cleft, which refers to a hole or fissure that occurs in the body of the sternum (Fig. 2-24-2). The mechanism of this deformity is unknown, and it has been suggested that it is similar to a sternal fissure, which is primarily the result of an impaired fusion of the centers of ossification of the sternum [7]. When the fusion disorder is more severe a sternal fissure is formed, which can be a partial or complete split of the sternum and is the most severe sternal deformity. If the fusion disorder is only localized to the center of ossification, a sternal cleft is formed. Sternocleidomalacia can exist alone or in complex thoracic deformities (Fig. 2-24-2). Simple sternal clefts are most often found during physical examination or surgical exploration, do not pose a specific risk in themselves, and are almost never clinically symptomatic. The other type of sternal deformity is characterized by a localized defect or absence, which may exist independently or in combination with other thoracic deformities (Figure 2-24-4). Another group of sternal deformities is more complex, with extremely complex localized shape variations

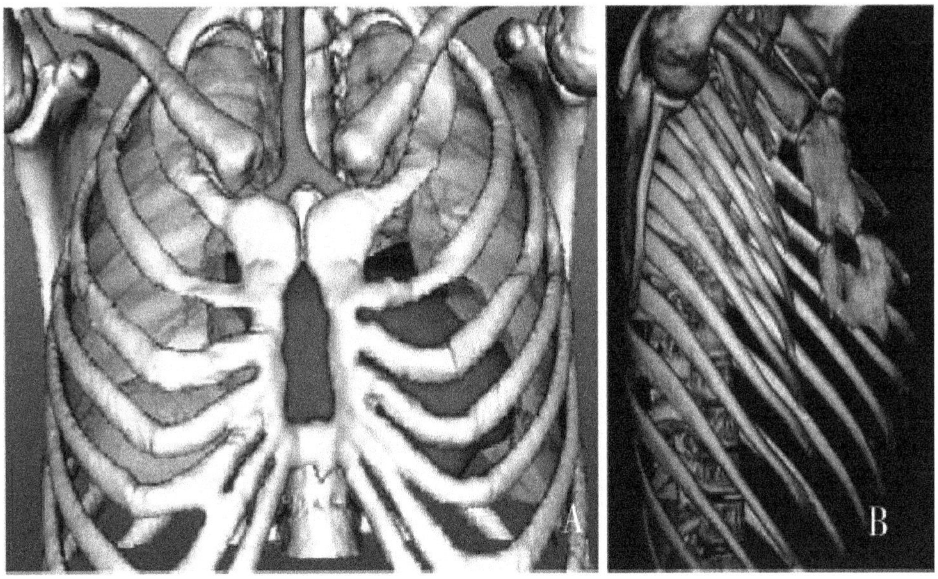

Figure 2-24-2 Sternal cleft (A. Cleft located median to the body of the sternum; B. Abnormal position of the sternum itself, median to the cleft)

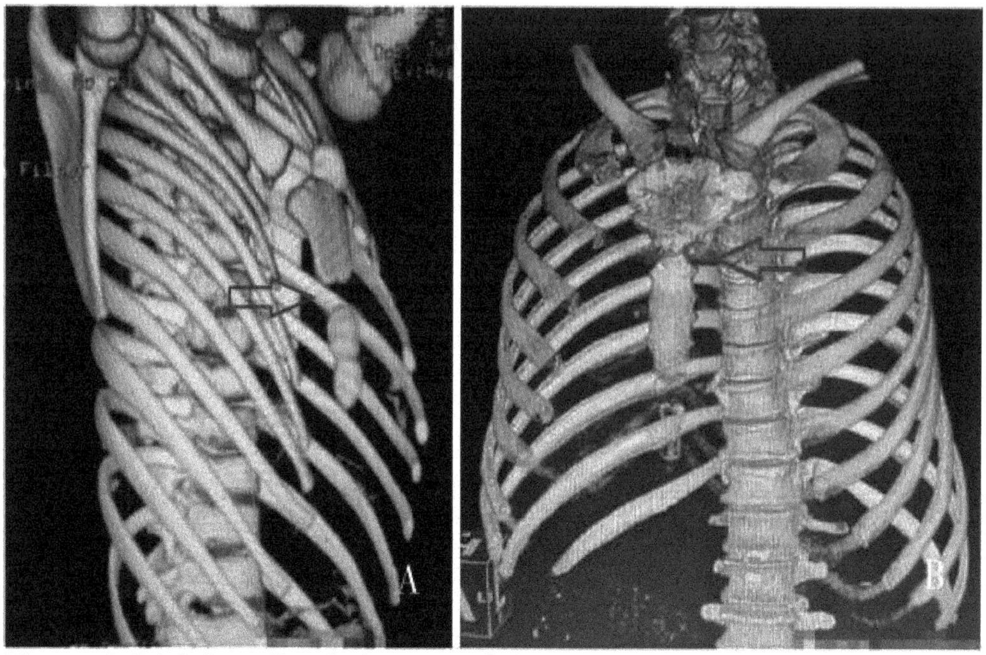

Figure 2-24-3 Localized absence of the sternum (A. Localized absence of the body of the sternum combined with asymmetric funnel chest; B. Localized absence of the sternum near the corner of the sternum).

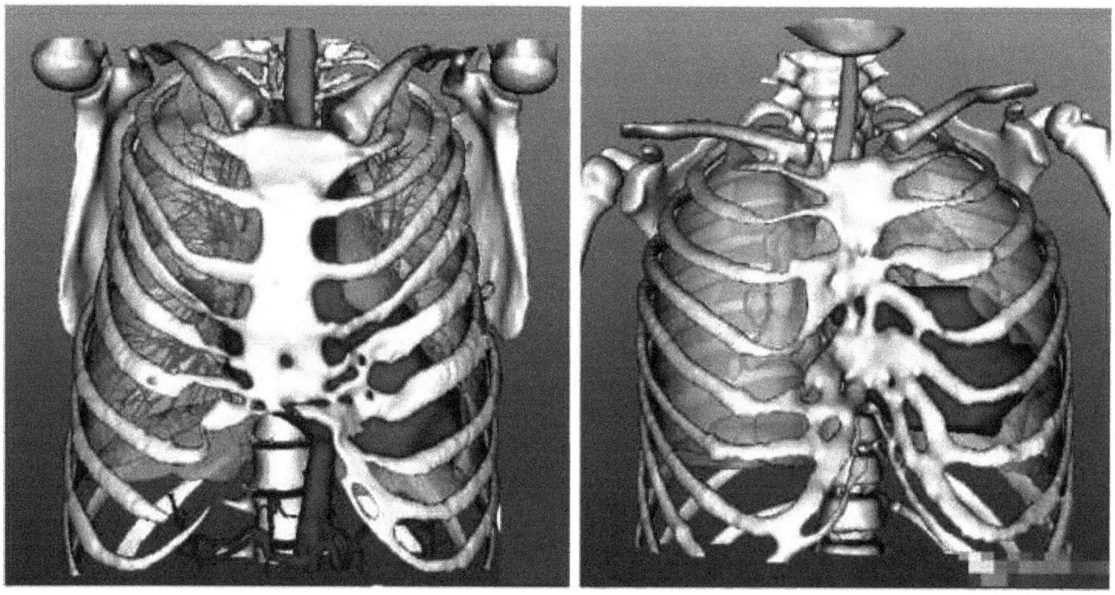

Figure 2-24-4 Complex localized deformity of the sternum (irregular shape, irregular changes, combined with localized extensive thoracic deformity)

3. Variation of the raphe

The raphe is a direct continuation of the lower end of the sternum, which is

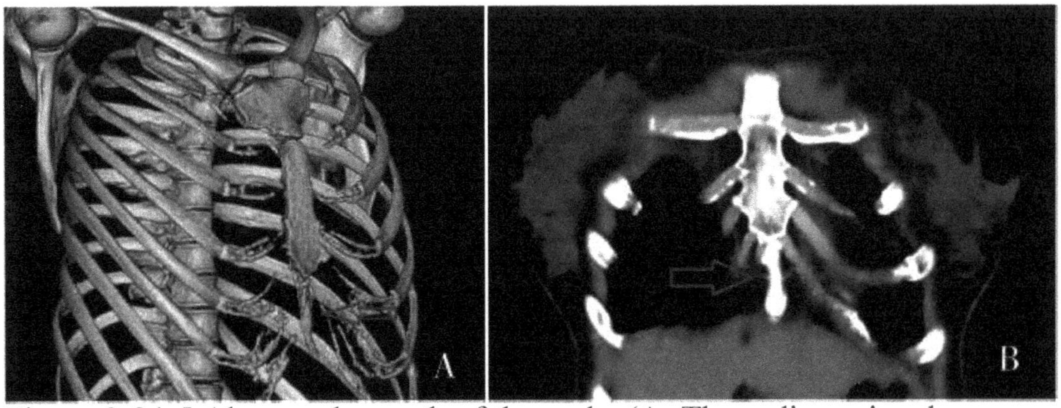

Figure 2-24-5 Abnormal growth of the raphe (A. Three-dimensional reconstruction showing the shape of the growing raphe; B. CT section showing the growing raphe)

often neglected because of its small size and hidden position. However, in some special cases, the raphe may change its shape or become deformed, which may even lead to special clinical symptoms and must be taken seriously.

Usually, the description of the raphe is taken from textbooks, and it is considered to be a straight bony structure with a neat terminal edge, no bifurcation, and no fissure. With the development of imaging, it has become possible to study the raphe by advanced means (Fig. 2-24-5). Recent studies have found that the size, location, and shape of the raphe are not fixed, and there are significant differences between individuals [8]. The first difference is the size of the raphe, which can be negligible in some cases and very long in others, with the longest raphe approaching 10 cm (Figure 2-24-6) [9]. The shape of the raphe also varies, with the most common shapes being concave and straight, and the less common shapes being convex and reverse S. The overall appearance of the raphe also varies. The overall appearance of the raphe also varies, in most cases appearing as a regular inverted triangle, but it can also be bifurcated into bifurcated and trifurcated patterns [10,11]. In the majority of cases, they are wide at the top and narrow at the bottom, and in a few cases, they may be narrow at the top and wide at the bottom. In addition,

Some raphe may have a fissure in the middle of the raphe (Fig. 2-24-5).

The shape of the raphe is varied and complex in its variability, and when small in size, it is generally of no clinical significance and does not require attention. Larger volumes of raphe are clinically significant in two ways: one is a matter of differential diagnosis. Some types of raphe may bulge at the end and form a distinct mass in the upper abdomen, which needs to be differentiated from a true abdominal mass; the second is the question of treatment. When the raphe is too long or the end of the raphe presses on the abdominal organs, the patient will have obvious symptoms, which can form the so-called raphe syndrome. At this time, targeted treatment is needed. If conservative treatment does not work, the raphe may need to be completely removed. This is an effective treatment for this condition

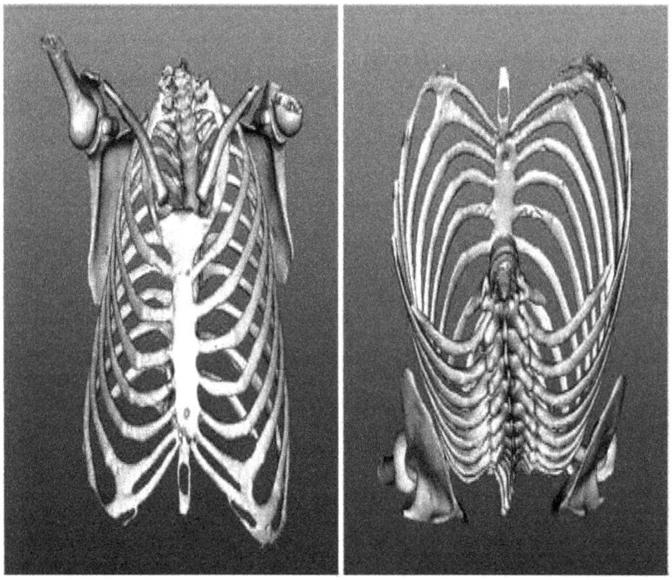

Figure 2-24-6 3-D reconstruction of the thorax showing an abnormality of the raphe, with the presence of an obvious cleft in the raphe.

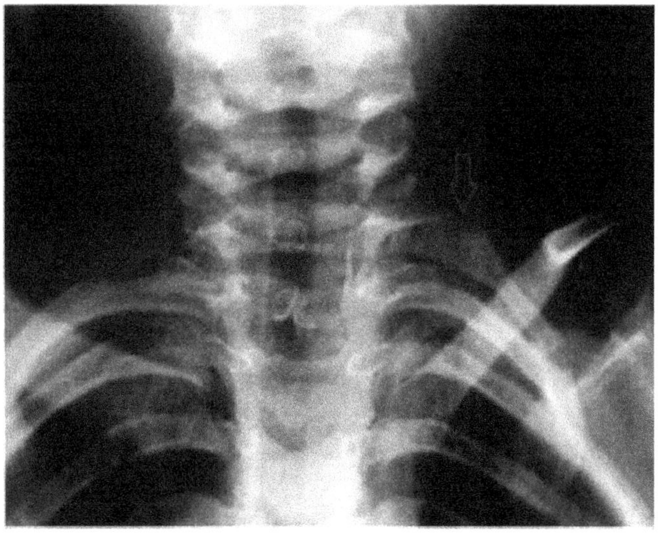

Figure 2-24-7 Cervical Ribs (Ribs attached to Cervical Vertebrae)

4. Cervical Ribs

With the deep lumbar back, it is of little clinical significance and is rarely of concern. Thoracic cervical ribs are a variant or deformity caused by an abnormality in the position of the ribs. Commonly found in fish and reptiles, cervical ribs normally do not exist in humans because the ribs attached to the cervical vertebrae have degenerated with the evolution of the species. If they are still present, they form a cervical rib (Figure 2-24-7). The presence of a cervical rib can be considered a rejuvenation phenomenon [12]. The incidence of this condition is low and has been documented to be approximately 0.5% ~ 1.0% [13]. In most cases, the cervical ribs appear in a low position, in relation to the 7th cervical vertebra and may occasionally be attached to the 6th cervical vertebra. The cervical ribs may be present on one side of the neck or on both sides at the same time, and may be accompanied by overgrowth of the transverse process of the 7th cervical vertebra.

Depending on the shape of the cervical ribs, they can be broadly categorized into four basic types [14]: (1) complete, (2) semi complete, (3) incomplete, and (4) residual. In most cases, the cervical rib is asymptomatic, and only 10% of patients have symptoms. The appearance of symptoms is mainly related to the compression of surrounding structures by the tip of the cervical rib. The most commonly involved structures are the brachial plexus and peripheral blood vessels. When these structures are compressed, they can cause conditions such as pain, numbness, impaired blood flow, or muscle atrophy in the upper extremities, resulting in the so-called thoracic outlet syndrome. Compression of the cervical ribs is the most common cause of this syndrome.

Asymptomatic cervical ribs can go unnoticed, and many patients are found on physical examination. Physical examination reveals a distinct mass in the supraclavicular fossa, which is fixed in position and firm, with roots attached to the cervical spine. Thoracic outlet syndrome presents with a positive compression test, abduction test, exercise test, and oblique muscle test [12,15]. Imaging can clarify the shape of the cervical rib.

The cervical rib does not usually require treatment when no symptoms are present, and mild symptoms can be treated conservatively. If symptoms are severe, surgical treatment is considered. The principle of surgery is to remove the cervical rib and the overgrown transverse process, and to release the surrounding fibrous bundles and the periosteum of the cervical rib. In cases of hypertrophy or spasm of the anterior oblique muscles, they need to be removed as well.

In the past, cervical rib surgery was usually performed by a plastic surgeon or hand surgeon, not by a thoracic surgeon. This is related to the special location of the cervical ribs[12,15] . Based on the anatomical location alone, the cervical rib is beyond the chest or chest wall. However, it still requires the attention of the chest wall surgeon because the surgical manoeuvre involves the apical structures of the chest wall.

5. The 12th rib variant

With the deep lumbar back, it is of little clinical significance and is rarely of concern to thoracic surgeons. However, variations in the shape of this rib may occur. The variation of the 12th rib occurs along with the vertebral body variation, which belongs to one kind of migration abnormality during spinal development, and can be manifested as unilateral rib dysplasia, bilateral rib dysplasia, and lumbarization of transverse processes on one side combined with short ribs on the other side, etc. (Fig. 2-24-8) [16]. X-ray frontal and lateral radiographs can accurately show the variation, and three-dimensional reconstruction examination can clarify the relationship between the variation and the surrounding structures more clearly. Since the 12th rib often serves as a marker for the localization of some specific structures, when a variant occurs in this rib, the localization of these structures may be affected. This is its only clinical significance. Since there are usually no clinical symptoms, no treatment is required.

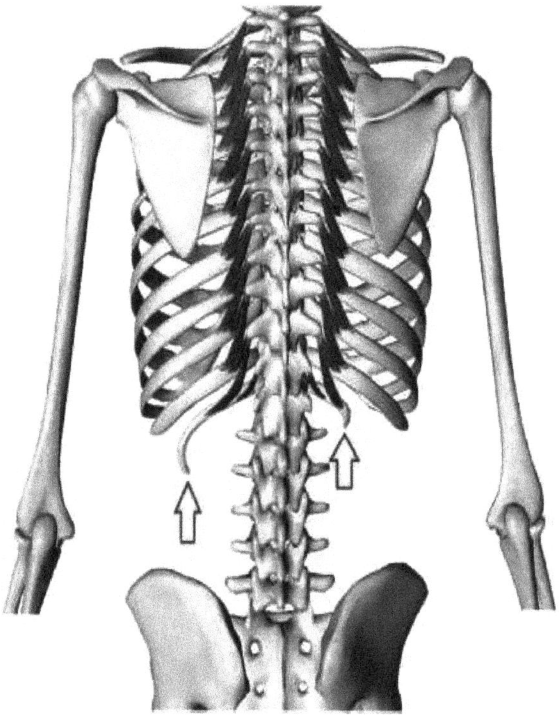

Figure 2-24-8 12th rib variant (left side rudimentary, right side abnormally shaped)

6. Lumbar Rib

A lumbar rib is a rare rib variation in which a rib is connected to a lumbar vertebra, forming this anomaly (Figure 2-24-9) [17]. The pathogenesis of lumbar ribs is unclear. They are generally asymptomatic and often go unnoticed, typically being discovered incidentally during physical examinations. They have little clinical significance and rarely attract attention. In the event of trauma, a lumbar rib should be differentiated from a transverse process fracture [17,18]. Lumbar ribs are usually bilateral and symmetrical, whereas transverse process fractures are mostly unilateral. Even when the variation is unilateral, the lumbar rib has an intact cortex and cancellous bone, whereas a fracture will show disruption of the cortical bone. Since lumbar ribs usually cause no symptoms and do not compress surrounding structures, no treatment is necessary.

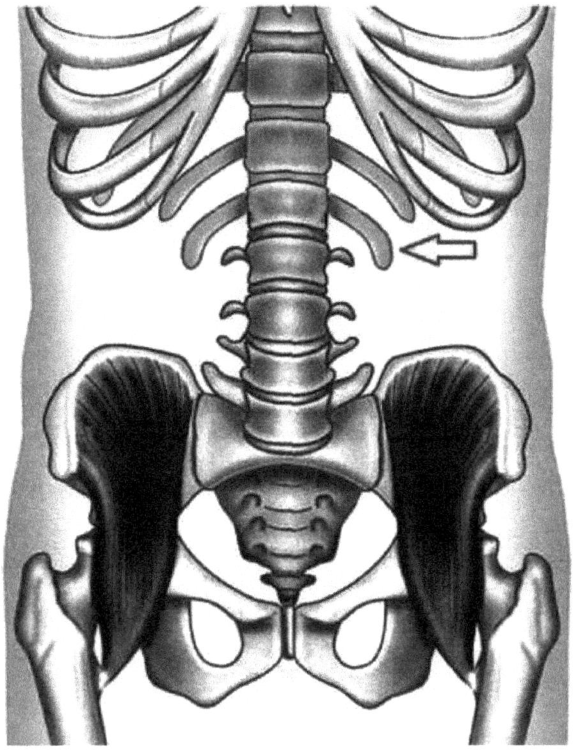

Figure 2-24-9 Lumbar ribs (ribs connected to lumbar vertebrae)

7. Variation with Thirteen Pairs of Ribs

Thirteen Pairs of Rib Variation A variation with thirteen pairs of ribs is an extremely rare rib anomaly (Figure 2-24-10). As the name suggests, it involves the presence of thirteen pairs of ribs. Since the ribs correspond to the thoracic vertebrae, patients with this variation also have thirteen pairs of thoracic vertebrae, which is the defining feature of this anomaly [19]. This differs from lumbar ribs, where the number of thoracic vertebrae remains normal. A thirteen pair rib variation generally does not cause clinical symptoms and therefore has little clinical significance and does not require treatment

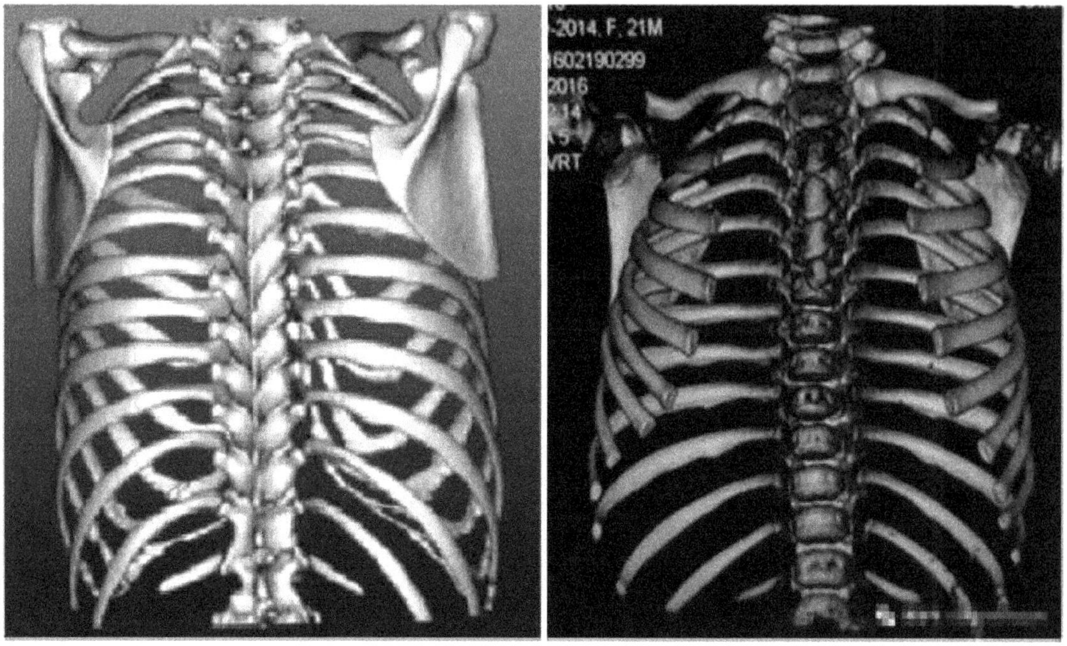

Figure 2-24-10 13 pairs of rib variations

8. Bifid Rib Deformity

Bifid rib deformity, also known as forked rib, is a structural anomaly that occurs in the rib itself (Figure 2-24-11). A study of 40,000 adult chest X-rays found 257 cases of bifid ribs, accounting for 0.6% of the population, indicating that this is a relatively common rib anomaly [20,21]. It is generally slightly more 3,4 common in males than females, with the third and fourth ribs being the most frequently affected. The specific manifestation is that the rib splits in the middle, forming a hole-like or forked structure. A bifid rib can exist independently or be associated with other deformities. When isolated, a bifid rib does not affect the appearance of the chest wall and produces no symptoms; it is most often discovered incidentally during routine examinations. Such isolated deformities generally have no clinical significance and do not require special treatment. However, if a bifid rib is present in conjunction with other anomalies, it should be managed according to the specific surgical requirements

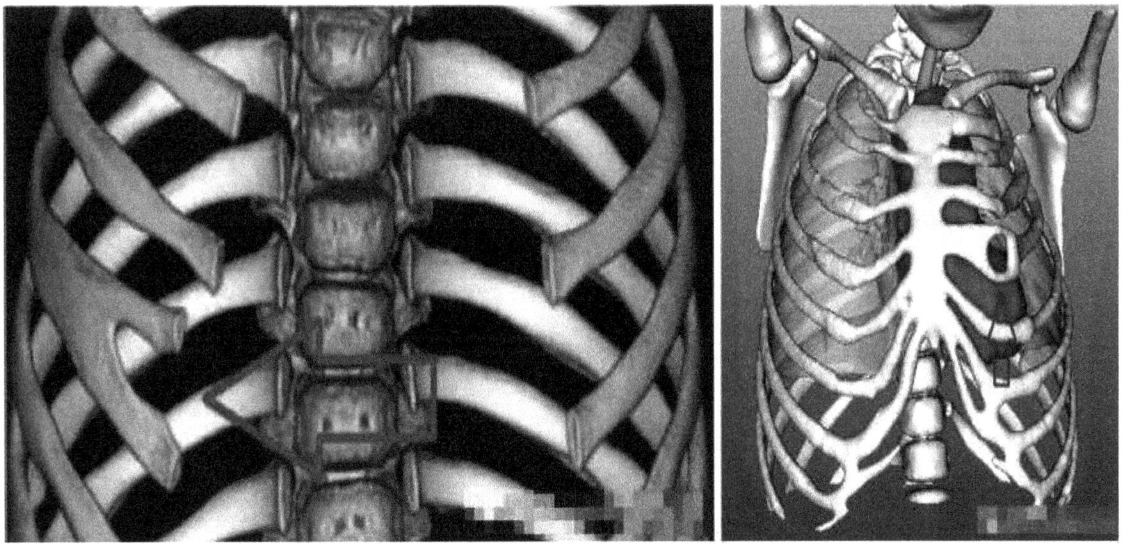

Figure 2-24-11. Bifid Rib Deformity

9. Rib Fusion Deformity

Rib fusion deformity refers to a condition in which adjacent ribs fuse together, forming a broad abnormal structure (Figure 2-24-12) [22]. It can exist independently or can be a local feature of other thoracic deformities. For example, localized rib fusion may occur in thoracic insufficiency syndrome [23] and Poland syndrome [24]. The pathogenesis of rib fusion deformity is not well understood. When rib fusion occurs independently, it usually causes no obvious symptoms and does not affect the external shape of the chest wall; it is often discovered incidentally during physical examinations. An isolated rib fusion deformity has no clinical significance and does not require special treatment. However, if it is associated with other deformities, it should be managed according to the specific clinical situation

10. Rib Absence

Rib absence refers to a deformity in which part or all of a specific rib is missing (Figure 2-24-13) [25]. This can present in two basic forms: partial absence of the rib and costal cartilage, or complete absence of both the rib and costal cartilage. The absence may be limited to a single rib or involve multiple adjacent ribs. In addition, rib absence may coexist with rib fusion, resulting in a more complex deformity (Figure 2-24-14). If rib absence leads to a local defect in the chest wall, it will constitute a chest wall defect, which will be discussed in detail in the relevant section

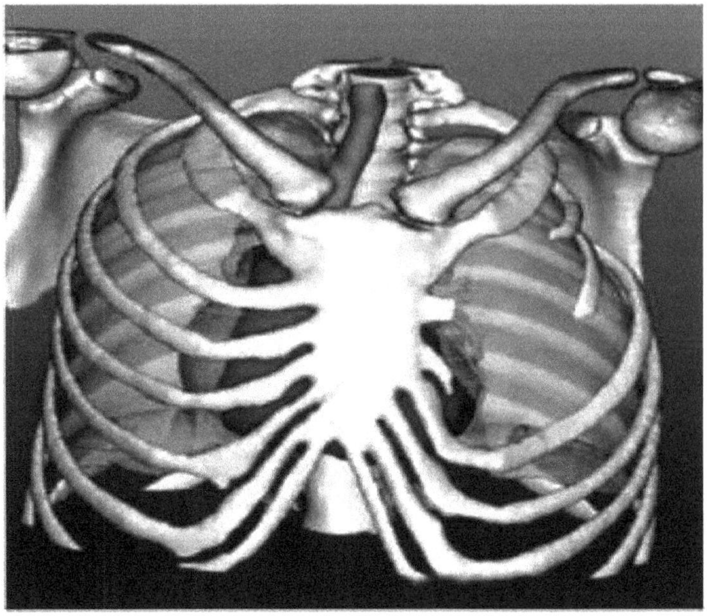

Figure 2-24-14 Rib loss and fusion

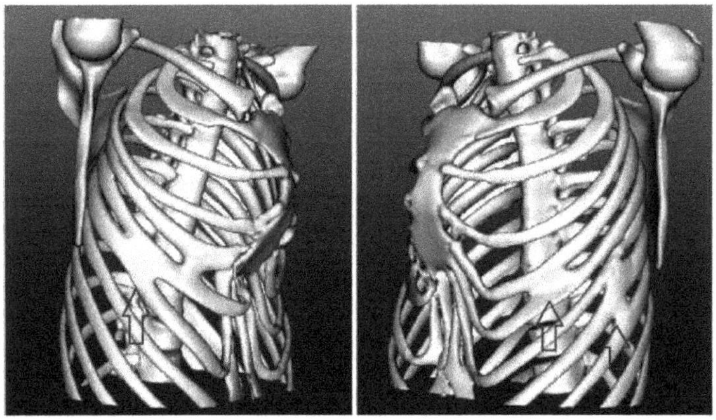

Figure 2-24-12 Rib Fusion Deformity

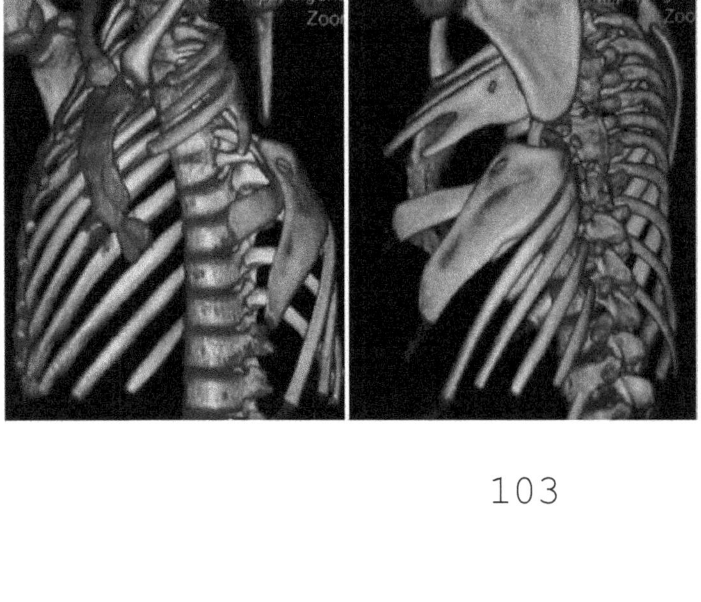

Figure 2-24-13. Rib Absence

The above has provided an overview of local structural anomalies of the sternum and ribs. Although many variations have been described, it is in fact impossible to cover every possible structural anomaly. From the perspective of isolated morphological research or other basic studies, these subtle structural variations may have particular significance. However, from a clinical perspective, if they neither affect the appearance of the chest wall nor cause any specific symptoms, they hold no clinical significance and therefore do not warrant further investigation.

REFERENCES

[1] Zhou, Yaping. 2021. "Clinical Analysis of 11 Cases of True Sternal Angle." *Chinese Journal of Drugs and Clinical Practice* 12 (6): 819–820.
[2] Chen, Xiaoqi. 2007. "A Case Report of Bilateral True Sternal Angle with Cervical Rib Variation." *Journal of Practical Radiology* 23 (4): 507.
[3] Lü, Zhengfei, Yuning Sun, Weiqing Han, et al. 2017. "Analysis of Digitized X-Ray Signs of Suprasternal Process Variation." *Contemporary Clinical Medicine* 30 (4): 3282–3283.
[4] Cao, Yongjie. 2005. "A Case of Bilateral True Sternal Angle Variation." *Journal of Clinical Radiology* 24 (1): 52.
[5] Lü, Zhengfei, Baolin Yu, Dongshi Jiang, et al. 2008. "A Case of Bilateral True Sternal Angle with Cervical Rib and Bifid Rib Variation." *Chinese Journal of Medical Imaging Technology* 24 (7): 1047.
[6] Sun, Qingju, Linxiang Liu, Huabin Yin, et al. 2002. "Multiple Bony Variations of the Thoracic Inlet: Five Cases." *Journal of Medical Imaging* 12 (1): 15, 32.
[7] Xie, Lunli, Peifeng Yang, Cheng Luo, et al. 2013. "A Case of Congenital Sternal Foramen with Variation and Deformity." *Anatomy and Clinics* 18 (6): 533.
[8] Xu, Yanyan, Hongliang Sun, Wu Wang, et al. 2012. "Evaluation of Xiphoid Process Anomalies in the Chinese Population Using 256-Slice Spiral CT." *Chinese Journal of Interventional Imaging and Therapy* 9 (4): 278–281.
[9] Zhong, Xinghua, Mingxi Chen, Shijun Liu, et al. 2003. "A Case of Elongated Xiphoid Process Variation." *Chinese Journal of Misdiagnosis* 3 (9): 1284.
[10] Vatzia, K., M. Fanariotis, K. G. Makridis, et al. 2021. "Frequency of Sternal Variations and Anomalies in Living Individuals Evaluated by MDCT." *European Journal of Radiology* 142: 109828.
[11] Akin, K., D. Kosehan, A. Topcu, et al. 2011. "Anatomic Evaluation of the Xiphoid Process with 64-Row Multidetector Computed Tomography." *Skeletal Radiology* 40 (4): 447–452.
[12] Song, Zhifei, Jie Ren, Hui Chen, et al. 2007. "Analysis of 13 Cases of Cervical Rib Syndrome." *Journal of Practical Hand Surgery* 21 (1): 9–11.
[13] Tan, Xiaoyi, Yuanli Du, Jin Cai, et al. 2011. "Surgical Treatment of Cervical Rib Syndrome." *Journal of Practical Medicine* 27 (2): 346–347.
[14] Zhang, Yaping, Zhaohui Wang, and Kanghua Li. 2004. "A Case Report of Bilateral Complete Cervical Ribs." *Chinese Journal of Modern Medicine* 14 (15): 159–160.
[15] Song, Zhifei, Hui Chen, Dongshan Luo, et al. 2004. "Brachial Plexus Function Analysis and Treatment Strategies in Patients with Cervical Rib Syndrome." *Chinese*

Journal of Clinical Rehabilitation 8 (35): 7978–7979, 8155.
[16] Shen, Zhe. 2011. "Analysis of Misdiagnosis Caused by 12th Rib Variation." In *Proceedings of the 2011 Sanya Summit Forum and Radiology Academic Conference*, 73.
[17] Liang, Shuzeng, and Hui Cheng. 2014. "The Significance of Congenital Lumbar Rib Deformity in Thoracic Trauma: Report of Two Cases." *Journal of Traumatic Surgery* 16 (3): 243.
[18] Song, Jiuhong, Fuxue Liu, Shikuan Ji, et al. 2004. "A Rare Case of Lumbar Rib Deformity." *Chinese Journal of Metallurgical Industry Medicine* 21 (5): 387.
[19] Guo, Jing, and Zuguo. 2014. "A Case of 13 Thoracic Vertebrae with 13 Pairs of Ribs Variation." *Journal of Dalian Medical University* (2): 202, 204.
[20] Ning, Jinbo, and Yimin Xie. 2018. "Advances in Research on Bifid Rib Deformity in Children." *Journal of Clinical Pediatric Surgery* 17 (5): 394–397.
[21] Gao, Daiping, Guanqiu Chen, and Changzhuo Tu. 2003. "A Case of Rib Deformity." *Imaging Diagnosis and Interventional Radiology* 12 (4): 214.
[22] Maonang, Yonghua Li, Wei Wang, et al. 2012. "A Case of Hemivertebra Combined with Three Fused Rib Deformity." *Chinese General Practice* 15 (33): 3894, 3896.
[23] Campbell, R. M. 2013. "VEPTR: Past Experience and the Future of VEPTR Principles." *European Spine Journal* 22 (Suppl 2): 106–117.
[24] Ashim, E. A. A., B. H. Quek, and S. Chandran. 2021. "A Narrative Review of Poland's Syndrome: Theories of Its Genesis, Evolution, Diagnosis and Treatment." *Translational Pediatrics* 10 (4): 1008–1019.
[25] Sun, Kai, Jianjun Ma, Tongsun Zhang, et al. 2014. "A Case of Symmetrical Free Variation of the Ninth and Tenth Ribs." *Journal of Anatomy* 37 (6): 843.

Straight Back Syndrome is a very distinct condition that was first reported by Rawlings in 1960 and has since gradually attracted increasing attention [1,2]. The main feature of Straight Back Syndrome is the loss of the normal physiological curvature of the thoracic spine, which is the fundamental cause of a series of related disorders. Under normal circumstances, the thoracic spine is slightly curved toward the dorsal side. This curvature provides sufficient space between the anterior chest wall and the thoracic spine to accommodate the mediastinal structures. When Straight Back Syndrome occurs, the normal thoracic curvature disappears, the space between the thoracic spine and the anterior chest wall becomes smaller, and all structures within the mediastinum are compressed, leading to various related conditions (Figure 2-25-1) [3,4]. The underlying cause of Straight Back Syndrome lies in the spine, which is the focus of spinal surgery. In its physiological state, the spine has a fixed shape, and when this shape changes, it becomes what is known as a deformity. Just like thoracic deformities or deformities in other regions, once the spine develops a deformity, it is considered a disease. The root cause of Straight Back Syndrome is a change in the shape of the spine, a clear deformity which makes it unequivocally a condition within the scope of spinal surgery. However, since the main damage occurs within the mediastinum and can affect many related structures, its treatment often involves multiple specialties. These include thoracic surgery,

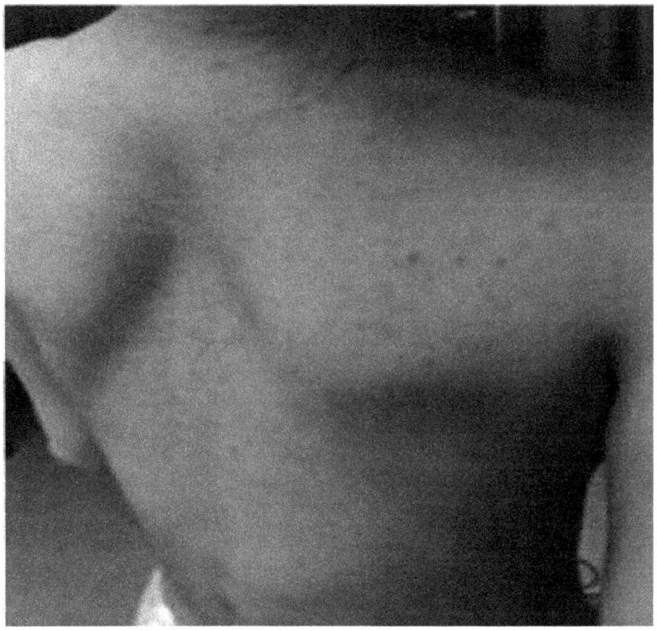

Figure-2-25-1. External Appearance of Straight Back Syndrome (Loss of Normal Thoracic Spinal Curvature

Syndrome is the loss of the normal physiological curvature of the thoracic spine, which is the fundamental cause of a series of related disorders. Under normal circumstances, the thoracic spine is slightly curved toward the dorsal side. This curvature provides sufficient space between the anterior chest wall and the thoracic spine to accommodate the mediastinal structures. When Straight Back Syndrome occurs, the normal thoracic curvature disappears, the space between the thoracic spine and the anterior chest wall becomes smaller, and all structures within the mediastinum are compressed, leading to various related conditions (Figure 2-25-1) [3,4]. The underlying cause of Straight Back Syndrome lies in the spine, which is the focus of spinal surgery. In its physiological state, the spine has a fixed shape, and when this shape changes, it becomes what is known as a deformity. Just like thoracic deformities or deformities in other regions, once the spine develops a deformity, it is considered a disease. The root cause of Straight Back Syndrome is a change in the shape of the spine, a clear deformity which makes it unequivocally a condition within the scope of spinal surgery. However, since the main damage occurs within the mediastinum and can affect many related structures, its treatment often involves multiple specialties. These include thoracic surgery, pulmonology, cardiology, and of course, chest wall surgery. Different specialties bring different perspectives to the study and treatment of this condition. Thoracic surgeons focus on mediastinal issues as a whole, pulmonologists focus on the trachea, cardiologists concentrate on the heart and great vessels, and chest wall surgeons focus not only on the chest wall but also on the overall mediastinum. Because each specialty focuses on different aspects, the treatment principles and methods also vary. In the pathogenic process of Straight Back Syndrome, although the chest wall is not the primary site of the lesion, its presence prevents the forward compression of the spine from being relieved outward, thereby causing various problems. From this perspective, the chest wall should be considered an indirect pathogenic factor and thus also warrants focused study

1.Etiology and Pathogenesis

The exact cause of Straight Back Syndrome is unknown. Some researchers believe it is an autosomal dominant hereditary condition, and there is some evidence to support this view, but the inheritance pattern is not fixed. Given that most patients develop the condition congenitally, some believe it is related to abnormal development of the thoracic vertebrae during the embryonic period. The development of the thoracic spine follows a specific program and sequence, and any stimulus during this time may cause changes in the shape of the spine. In fact, various spinal deformities may be linked to embryonic development. Unfortunately, the exact mechanism that leads to the loss of the spine's normal physiological curvature remains unclear.

From the perspective of the thoracic cage's integrity, the spine is an important structural component, closely connected to each rib. Therefore, spinal lesions may originate within the spine itself or arise from other structures of the thoracic cage. If there are structural abnormalities in the anterior chest wall, they may also lead to changes in the shape of the spine. Clinically, certain anterior chest wall deformities are often associated with straight back syndrome. For example, pectus excavatum and flat chest are frequently found together with this syndrome [5]. The mechanism of pectus excavatum combined with straight back syndrome may be related to direct traction by the ribs. When there is a depression in the anterior chest wall, the ribs on both sides of the depression may extend forward due to the depression, and because the posterior ends of the ribs are directly connected to the midline of the thoracic spine, they may pull the thoracic vertebrae forward. This forward movement results in the loss of the normal physiological curvature, forming straight back syndrome. The mechanism by which flat chest leads to straight back syndrome is roughly the same. However, in clinical practice, the vast majority of patients with straight back syndrome do not have clear anterior chest wall deformities, so the precise mechanism still requires further research.

The direct harm caused by straight back syndrome is a reduction in the mediastinal space, leading to compression of the heart and other mediastinal structures. When structures are compressed, their shapes may change (Figure 2-25-2) [2,6]. for hollow structures such as the heart, great vessels, trachea, and esophagus, the degree of shape change due to compression depends on three factors: first, the magnitude of the compressive force; second, their own mechanical strength; and third, their structural mobility

The mediastinum can be regarded as a relatively enclosed space. When pressure is exerted from the front and back, it is distributed relatively evenly. This means that all structures within the mediastinum are subjected to approximately the same compressive force. When the compressive force is the same, the impact on each structure largely depends on the structure's own characteristics. The first characteristic is the mechanical strength of each structure. The greater the strength, the stronger its resistance to compression and the lower the likelihood of deformation. Mechanical strength is a comprehensive concept that includes both the strength of surface structures and that of internal structures. Take the heart as an example: because the heart contains blood at different pressures within its chambers, different parts of the heart have completely different strengths. The left ventricle and the aorta have the greatest strength, followed by the right ventricle, while the atria and the veins have the least strength. From this, it can be inferred that the left ventricle is the least likely to be deformed by compression, whereas the right atrium and the superior and inferior vena cava are much more susceptible to shape changes due to compression. Aside from the heart, the trachea, supported by cartilage, has relatively high mechanical strength and is not easily deformed by compression. The esophagus, lacking any structural support, is therefore the most likely structure to be flattened. In addition to mechanical strength, structural change is related to another property, namely, the mobility of the structure. Structural mobility can be seen as the ability to avoid compression. When the mobility of a structure is poor, it is difficult to avoid compression and it will be subjected to direct compression, which will have a greater impact on the structure; on the other hand, if the mobility of a structure is high, the structure will avoid compression, and the pressure it is subjected to will decrease, and the impact on the structure will be reduced accordingly. Among the structures of the mediastinum, the esophagus is located on the left side of the spine for most of its travel and has a high degree of mobility. Although the aortic arch crosses its midsection anteriorly, the mobility of the esophagus is not affected by the fact that it is also located on the left side of the spine and not directly anteriorly. When the esophagus is compressed, it can be moved to the left side. Such movement can effectively defuse the compression and prevent obstruction from occurring. The trachea is located directly in front of the spine throughout its entire travel, and its two main left and right bronchioles extend into the thoracic cavity on each side and are directly connected to the lung tissue on both sides. The pulling of the main bronchi to the sides causes the trachea to become fixed and unable to deviate from the anterior aspect of the spine to the sides. Such a position is extremely unfavorable to the trachea. When the normal physiologic curvature of the spine disappears, the spine moves forward, causing direct compression of the trachea. As the trachea is fixed in position, it is impossible to avoid the compression, which may directly lead to the narrowing or even occlusion of the trachea, which will have a direct impact on breathing. Normally, due to the large caliber of the trachea, mild compression does not lead to abnormal respiratory function. However, if the compression is particularly severe, the trachea may collapse, with serious consequences. The heart and great vessels are the main structures in the mediastinum. The location of the large vessels entering and exiting the heart is relatively fixed, and the heart itself is relatively fixed and does not move much. In addition, because the heart occupies most of the space in the mediastinum, it is not completely free from compression, even with some movement, making it the structure most affected by compression.

The presence or absence of symptoms in patients with straight back syndrome is mainly related to the change in shape of the mediastinal structures after compression. As can be seen from the above analysis, the esophagus has a difficult time showing symptoms, and the trachea requires a more powerful compression to show symptoms. Although most parts of the heart are resistant to compression, there are also many parts that are susceptible to compression and deformation. Since the heart is an organically integrated whole, an abnormality in any one part may cause an abnormality in the functioning of the whole heart, and therefore, the heart is the structure in the mediastinum that is most likely to become symptomatic as a result of compression.

The front part of the heart is the right ventricle, which is close to the anterior chest wall. Because it is not mechanically strong and its position is relatively fixed, it is most susceptible to deformation due to compression, which may be manifested clinically as compression or narrowing of the right ventricular outflow tract. If the compression is severe, it can lead to problems in other areas, such as abnormal opening and closing of the pulmonary and tricuspid valves, and abnormal venous return in the upper and lower cavities. When these abnormalities occur, heart function will be impaired. In patients with straight back syndrome, there is usually no significant pathologic change in the spine itself, and the main harm comes from compression of the structures of the mediastinum. As mentioned above, of the many mediastinal structures that are compromised, the most important one is the heart, which is compromised by external forces and has no primary disease of its own, hence the term pseudocardiac disease [6]. This is not appropriate. Cardiac lesions can be categorized into structural and functional lesions. Structural lesions mainly refer to abnormalities in the internal structure of the heart, such as common congenital heart disease, rheumatic heart disease, coronary heart disease, and macrovascular disease, which are the more common structural diseases in clinical practice. However, in addition to structural lesions, a large number of functional lesions also exist in clinical practice. Among the various types of sunken thoracic deformities, the sunken front chest wall compresses the heart, causing various heart diseases, the main manifestation of which is that the shape of the heart changes first, followed by changes in the function of the heart. These changes may include abnormalities in the opening and closing of valves or changes in the channels for blood flow, but they do not involve changes in the inner structure of the heart, which, if the heart is treated as an organic whole, would be considered structural changes. However, since such changes are not the same as the traditional pathologic changes, they are not the same as the traditional pathologic changes, and they are not the same as the traditional pathologic

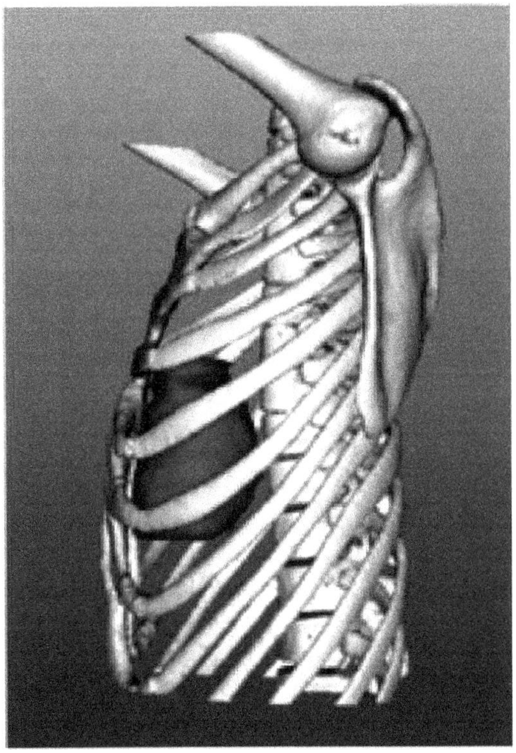

Figure 2-25-2. 3D Reconstruction of the Thorax in Straight Back Syndrome (Loss of Normal Thoracic Spinal Curvature and Compression of Mediastinal Structures)

changes. Because the compression can be relieved and the structure can return to normal, this condition is regarded as a functional disorder rather than a structural one. Although such diseases do not originate primarily within the heart itself, they are nevertheless classified as heart diseases, as they manifest through various definite clinical signs involving the heart. Therefore, they are real heart diseases, not pseudocardiac conditions. In patients with straight back syndrome, the heart also suffers significant compression, which constitutes the main pathological aspect of this syndrome. Thus, it falls within the category of functional heart disease it is indeed a genuine cardiac condition and not a pseudocardiac disorder

2.Clinical Presentation

Although the root cause of Straight Back Syndrome lies in the spine, the main harm it causes is concentrated in the mediastinum. Due to compression of mediastinal structures, a series of related clinical symptoms appears. When the heart is compressed, various associated lesions may occur, which can affect cardiac rhythm or directly impair cardiac function, ultimately manifesting through various symptoms. Many patients are misdiagnosed with different types of structural heart diseases [6]. In addition to cardiac manifestations, patients may also exhibit respiratory symptoms—particularly when the trachea is severely compressed—resulting in symptoms of significant airway obstruction [7,8].

The main physical signs of Straight Back Syndrome include abnormal spinal shape and heart-related signs. The physiological curvature of the spine disappears and may be accompanied by chest wall deformities. The heart may show various physical signs, mostly caused by functional changes rather than structural abnormalities.

3. Examinations

Physical examination can reveal the most important sign in patients with straight back syndrome, the loss of the normal thoracic spinal curvature. Imaging studies can demonstrate the abnormal shape of the spine and directly show the narrowing of the space between the thoracic vertebrae and the anterior chest wall. Cardiac-related examinations can directly exclude structural heart lesions。

4. Diagnosis and Differential Diagnosis

The diagnosis of straight back syndrome mainly involves three key points [3,4,6]: (1) Loss of the normal thoracic spinal curvature and narrowing of the space between the thoracic vertebrae and the anterior chest wall; (2) Clinical manifestations of compression of mediastinal structures; (3) Exclusion of structural heart disease. These three criteria show that obtaining the necessary diagnostic information is not difficult; however, misdiagnosis often occurs in clinical practice, with the condition being mistaken for purely structural heart disease. The main reason for misdiagnosis is related to the patient's presenting complaint at the first visit. Once an adult patient presents with heart-related complaints, cardiac disease is naturally considered first, and cardiologists typically do not pay attention to spinal issues, leading to inevitable misdiagnosis. Among chest wall disorders, pectus excavatum and flat chest can be associated with straight back syndrome [5]. Because chest wall deformities themselves can cause various compressive symptoms, coexisting straight back syndrome may easily be overlooked. In such cases, the straight back syndrome is not the primary cause. Compression symptoms are not solely caused by the straight back syndrome itself, but the condition can significantly aggravate compressive symptoms, so it must always be diagnosed simultaneously. The differential diagnosis of straight back syndrome mainly includes structural heart disease, which should be ruled out through appropriate diagnostic tests. Another condition that needs to be differentiated is airway disease. If the patient presents with significant dyspnea, airway evaluation is necessary to exclude other causes of obstruction.

5.Treatment

(1) Treatment of isolated straight back syndrome

Once straight back syndrome is clearly diagnosed, symptomatic treatment should be considered first. If symptomatic treatment is ineffective, intervention should target the narrowing of the mediastinum. There are two main approaches to relieve this narrowing:

Directly address the thoracic spine to restore its normal curvature; Reshape the anterior chest wall.

To change the shape of the thoracic spine, there are two possible methods: surgical treatment or conservative treatment. Because the thoracic spine is extremely robust, surgically altering its shape is extremely difficult, highly invasive, and the results are not guaranteed. Consequently, no doctor has ever attempted this approach. Clinically, some have tried conservative methods to modify the spinal curvature. This involves using special traction devices [1]. Such methods are minimally invasive and relatively easy to perform but may not yield satisfactory results.

The method of treating through the anterior chest wall is a more invasive surgical approach. Its principle is to remodel and reconstruct the anterior chest wall to expand the mediastinal space and relieve compression of the surrounding structures. This surgery can be performed using various techniques. The method we developed uses digitally designed material to reconstruct the anterior chest wall [7,8]. The specific procedure is as follows:

The patient is placed in a supine position, and a midline sternotomy is performed. Soft tissue is separated along the anterior surface of the sternum to expose the sternum and costal cartilages. The upper half of the sternum along with the attached costal cartilages on both sides, is respected. A slightly forward curved digital implant is then placed over the bony structures surrounding the defect in the upper chest wall and securely fixed to these bony structures. Finally, the incision is closed to complete the procedure.

This method alleviates compression through two mechanisms:

Resection of the upper half of the sternum and placement of the implant on the outer surface of the original sternum site effectively increases the anteroposterior diameter of the mediastinum by the thickness of the removed sternum.

The implant itself arches forward, further enlarging the mediastinal space.

Both mechanisms significantly increase the mediastinal space, achieving a definitive therapeutic effect. However, this method has inherent limitations, mainly in three aspects:

Significant surgical trauma: The procedure requires the removal of the sternum and multiple costal cartilages on both sides, with entry into both pleural cavities. The surgical field is extensive, resulting in considerable trauma; this is the biggest drawback of this approach.Prominent incision scar: The scar is located along the midline of the anterior chest wall, in an upper position, making it long, visible, and cosmetically undesirable. Presence of a foreign implant: The reconstructed chest wall must use artificial materials rather than autologous tissue. Once implanted, these artificial materials remain in the body permanently, which may cause discomfort for the patient and could lead to related complications.

These drawbacks are inherent to this procedure and cannot be completely avoided; therefore, it should not be used as a routine surgical option. It is reserved only for patients whose symptoms cannot be relieved by any other means.When discussing surgical treatment for straight back syndrome, some authors have mentioned the possibility of using minimally invasive surgery, that is, the so-called. The Nuss procedure aims to elevate the anterior chest wall to relieve mediastinal compression. Although this concept may seem reasonable in theory, it is actually impractical. Under normal circumstances, the anterior chest wall in straight back syndrome is structurally normal, that is, it is flat or slightly convex. The Nuss procedure is specifically designed to treat pectus excavatum (a depressed chest wall). Therefore, for a normal chest wall without any depression, the procedure is clearly ineffective. As a result, minimally invasive surgery alone cannot successfully treat isolated straight back syndrome. However, if straight back syndrome is accompanied by pectus excavatum or a flattened chest, minimally invasive surgery may be considered for correction.

(2) Surgery for Straight Back Syndrome Combined with Pectus Excavatum

In patients with straight back syndrome, the mediastinal space is already narrowed. If pectus excavatum is also present, the depression of the anterior chest wall further reduces the mediastinal space, resulting in various pronounced compression symptoms [5]. This is an absolute indication for surgical intervention. In such cases, the procedure is essentially the standard surgical correction for pectus excavatum. However, given the loss of normal spinal curvature, slight overcorrection should be considered during the repair; in other words, the anterior chest wall should be made to protrude slightly forward. This approach can achieve a better therapeutic outcome.

(3) Surgery for Straight Back Syndrome Combined with Flat Chest

Patients with straight back syndrome frequently also have a flat chest [5]. Although a flat chest does not show obvious anterior chest wall depression, it must be noted that the anteroposterior diameter of the thorax is already reduced, meaning the distance from the anterior chest wall to the spine is shorter than normal. If the natural thoracic kyphosis is completely lost, the resulting compression symptoms will be even more pronounced than in typical patients. Therefore, such patients also require surgical treatment. When surgery is performed, the specific procedure targets the correction of the flat chest. The operative technique is not significantly different from that used for isolated flat chest correction. The goal of flat chest surgery is to create anterior protrusion in the midline of the chest wall, restoring the normal curved contour of the entire anterior chest wall. This shape can significantly increase the mediastinal space, completely eliminate the compression of mediastinal organs, and ultimately achieve the intended therapeutic effect (see Figure 2-25-3).

6. Prognosis

Straight back syndrome is a condition caused by an abnormal shape of the spine. If obvious symptoms are present, symptomatic treatment should be considered first, as it can often yield good results without the need for further intervention. Only when symptomatic treatment is ineffective should treatment targeting the thoracic spine or anterior chest wall be considered. Spinal traction is a conservative approach and should be actively attempted if effective. If traction fails and symptoms persist, reconstruction surgery of the anterior chest wall may be necessary. Anterior chest wall reconstruction can reliably relieve mediastinal compression and produce immediate results. However, due to its inherent risks and limitations, this surgery must be approached with great

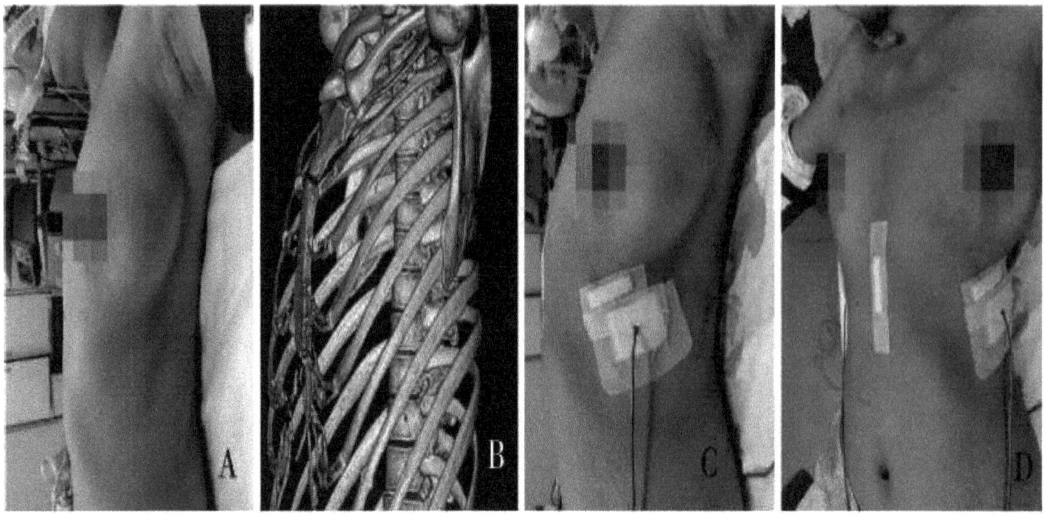

Figure 2-25-3 — Surgical treatment of straight back syndrome combined with flat chest, corrected using the Wung procedure. (A) External view of the chest wall showing typical features of a flat chest. (B) 3D reconstruction of the thorax demonstrating loss of normal thoracic kyphosis and a flattened chest wall. (C) Postoperative lateral view showing a significant increase in the anteroposterior diameter of the chest wall. (D) Postoperative external view of the chest wall showing restoration of normal shape and curvature.

caution and should not be treated as a routine procedure. for patients with straight back syndrome combined with pectus excavatum or flat chest, minimally invasive surgery can be used to reshape the anterior chest wall and generally achieves good results. These patients usually do not require full chest wall reconstruction. We once treated a female patient with straight back syndrome who had been diagnosed at another hospital with tracheal obstruction (see Figure 2-25-4). To resolve the obstruction, local doctors attempted tracheal stent implantation, but the procedure failed due to severe tracheal blockage. An ascending aortic aneurysm was suspected as the cause of the obstruction, but relevant examinations ruled this out. The final diagnosis was straight back syndrome. The patient was transferred to our hospital for surgical treatment. We performed anterior chest wall reconstruction using digitally designed materials [7,8]. Intraoperatively, in addition to the reconstruction, we used a special strap to lift the ascending aorta and fix it onto the digital implant to further relieve tracheal compression (see Figure 2-25-5). The surgical outcome was highly successful.

Once the procedure was completed, the tracheal compression was immediately resolved, the airway returned to normal caliber, and the patient's symptoms completely disappeared. Postoperative follow up confirmed that tracheal narrowing did not recur. This patient was an extremely severe case of straight back syndrome and the first in the world to receive this type of surgical treatment. Our experience suggests that when mediastinal compression in straight back syndrome cannot be resolved by other means, anterior chest wall reconstruction is the only reasonable option.By 2022, we had performed two chest wall reconstruction surgeries for straight back syndrome. The first case used customized digital material; the second used Matrix RIB. These two surgeries are the only such operations performed worldwide to date, and both were successful[9].

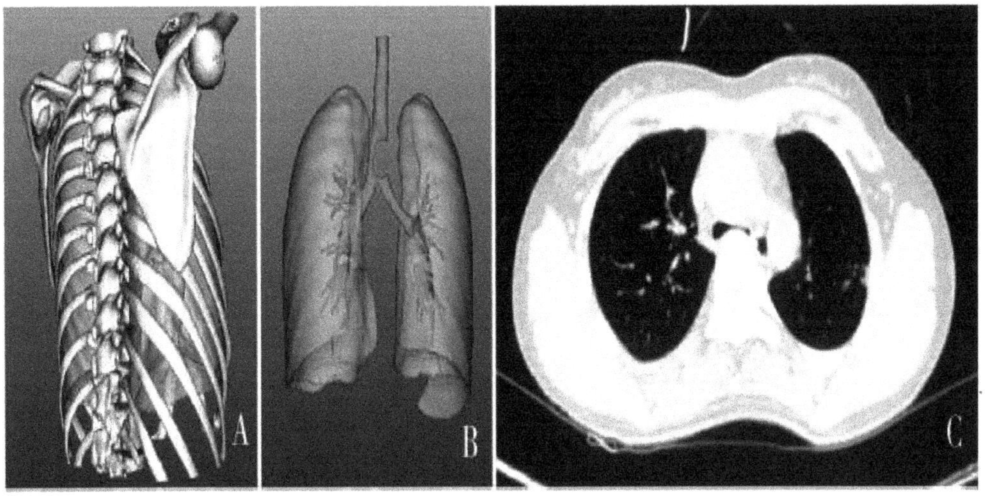

Figure 2-25-4 Imaging studies of a patient with straight back syndrome (A) 3D reconstruction of the chest showing loss of the physiological thoracic spinal curvature; (B) 3D reconstruction image showing severe compression of the main trachea with segmental imaging defect; (C) CT axial view showing severe tracheal compression with local occlusion.

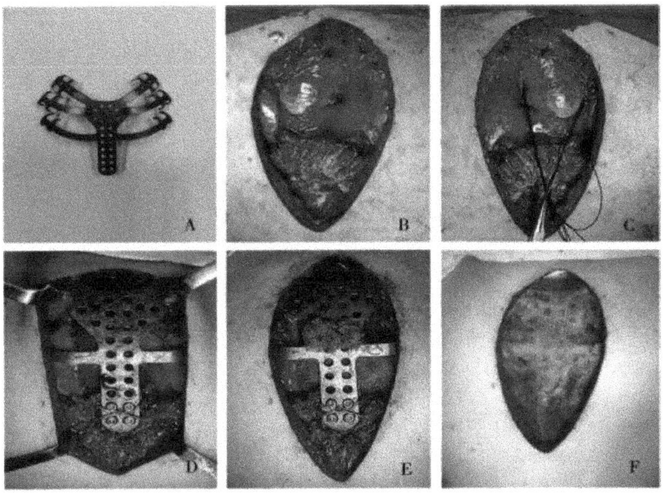

Figure 2-25-5 Chest wall reconstruction for a patient with straight back syndrome combined with tracheal obstruction using customized digital material. (A. Digitally designed material customized to the patient's anterior chest wall structure; B. Resection of the upper half of the sternum and the connected costal cartilages on both sides, with thymus tissue removed to expose the ascending aorta; C. Placement of traction

sutures around the ascending aorta; D. Insertion and secure fixation of the digital material into the anterior chest wall defect; E. The ascending aorta traction sutures pull and lift the supporting band to wrap around the ascending aorta, then the aorta is lifted and fixed to the digital implant; F. The digital material is covered with fibrous membrane and the incision is closed, completing the surgery.)

REFERENCES

[1] Rawlings, M. S. 1960. "The 'Straight Back' Syndrome: A New Cause of Pseudo Heart Disease." *American Journal of Cardiology* 5: 333–338.

[2] Betz, J. W., P. A. Oakley, and D. E. Harrison. 2018. "Relief of Exertional Dyspnea and Spinal Pain by Increasing Thoracic Kyphosis in Straight Back Syndrome (Thoracic Hypokyphosis) Using CBP® Methods: A Case Report with Long-Term Follow-Up." *Journal of Physical Therapy Science* 30 (1): 185–189.

[3] Wang, W. L. 2021a. "Why Is Straight Back Syndrome Easily Misdiagnosed as Heart Disease?" *Chest Wall Deformity Surgery Expert*, January 7.

[4] Wang, W. L. 2021b. "Straight Back Syndrome and Heart Disease." *Chest Wall Deformity Surgery Expert*, January 5.

[5] Wang, W. L. 2021c. "The Harm of Straight Back Syndrome Combined with Flat Chest or Pectus Excavatum." *Chest Wall Deformity Surgery Expert*, January 4.

[6] Wright, C. D. 2017. "Straight Back Syndrome." *Thoracic Surgery Clinics* 27 (2): 133–137.

[7] Wang, W. L. 2020. "World's First: Straight Back Syndrome with Severe Tracheal Stenosis Repaired Using Digitally Designed Material." *Chest Wall Deformity Surgery Expert*, December 29.

[8] Liu, Y., W. Wang, W. Long, et al. 2021. "Chest Wall Reconstruction with Digitally Designed Materials for Straight Back Syndrome with Tracheal Stenosis: A Case Report." *Annals of Translational Medicine* 9 (16): 1357.

[9] Wang, W. L. 2022. "World's Second: Chest Wall Reconstruction for Straight Back Syndrome (MatrixRIB Reconstruction Surgery)." *Chest Wall Deformity Surgery Expert*, April 18.

CHAPTER 3

CHEST WALL TUMORS

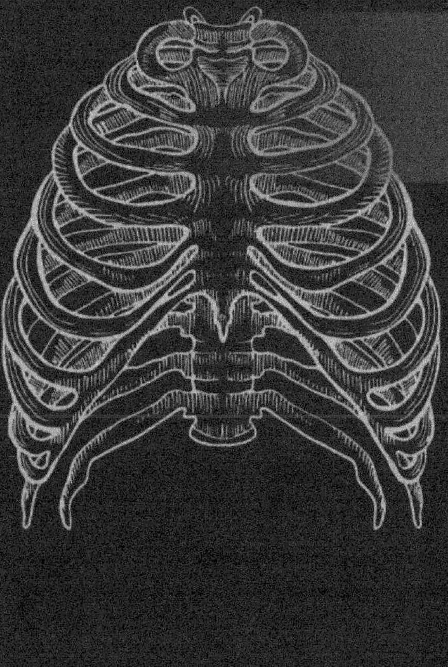

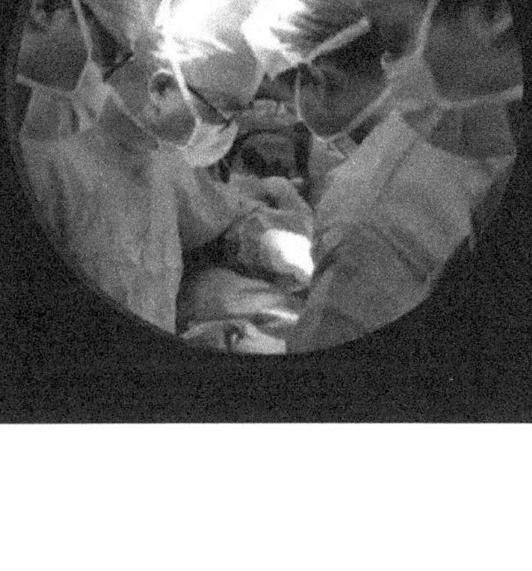

Chest wall tumors are relatively common and are also a frequently encountered condition in traditional thoracic Surgery. In earlier years, there were quite a few studies on chest wall tumors, with numerous related reports in the medical literature. From the perspective of thoracic Surgery, the literature mainly focused on treatment, particularly Surgical intervention. Topics related to Surgery and operative procedures can be readily found in those reports. However, over time, the number of publications on this subject has gradually declined, and fewer people are paying attention to this disease. In reality, patients with chest wall tumors are still frequently seen in clinical practice. This declining attention can generally be attributed to two main factors: ① Technical Bottlenecks: Thoracic Surgeons have primarily focused on the Surgical treatment of chest wall tumors, which mainly involves two basic components: first, the resection of the tumor itself; and second, the reconstruction of the chest wall [1-3]. Tumor resection is generally performed through open Surgery. From a technical standpoint, these procedures are not particularly difficult. Simple resection Surgeries have been well standardized, and there are no new techniques worth sharing. Chest wall reconstruction involves repairing the defect left after tumor resection using various materials. Technically speaking, reconstruction is also not very complex as long as appropriate materials are available, nearly all thoracic Surgeons can perform such procedures with ease [4,5]. This illustrates that Surgery for chest wall tumors is not considered a highly challenging procedure. According to past literature, the Surgical techniques have already become highly mature, having essentially reached their peak, making further breakthroughs difficult. As a result, the lack of technical advancement has become a bottleneck in the field of chest wall tumor treatment. Without overcoming this bottleneck, it is hard to make new progress, and without progress, there is little attention drawn to the condition. ② The Mainstream Focus in Thoracic Surgery. Traditional thoracic Surgery techniques are based on open procedures. However, with continuous advancements in technology, minimally invasive Surgery has gained increasing attention. In recent years, minimally invasive techniques have become prevalent across almost all thoracic Surgeries, primarily utilizing thoracoscopic (VATS) approaches. Thoracoscopic Surgery has, in fact, become synonymous with modern thoracic Surgery. Since thoracoscopy is used for procedures inside the chest cavity, when many thoracic Surgeons focus exclusively on thoracoscopic Surgery, the treatment of intrathoracic diseases becomes the mainstream of clinical thoracic Surgery. Leading hospitals and well-known specialists promote thoracoscopic procedures, and other Surgeons often follow suit without much critical thinking. Consequently, thoracic Surgery has essentially evolved into "thoracoscopic Surgery" or "Surgery for intrathoracic conditions," while chest wall procedures have been neglected. As a result, fewer Surgeons pay attention to diseases like chest wall tumors.

The development of treatment for any disease is closely tied to the level of attention it receives. When a condition lacks attention, related research diminishes, and progress becomes limited. This is precisely the dilemma faced by chest wall tumors. So, how can this dilemma be overcome? It is nearly impossible to forcibly redirect thoracic Surgeons' focus back to the treatment of chest wall tumors. The only viable path forward is to break through the existing technical bottlenecks. However, under the traditional concepts of thoracic Surgery, achieving such breakthroughs is nearly impossible. Fortunately, the emergence of the concept of chest wall Surgery has significantly changed the outlook for chest wall tumor treatment. With this new perspective, the bottlenecks are gradually being overcome, and substantial technological advances have been made. This has laid a strong foundation for the comprehensive development of treatment for chest wall tumors. The treatment of tumors can lead to entirely different outcomes when approached from a new perspective, which creates opportunities to break through existing bottlenecks.

The treatment outcomes of tumors can vary dramatically depending on the approach taken; this opens the possibility of breaking through existing bottlenecks. Chest wall Surgery, while originating from traditional thoracic Surgery, embraces a philosophy that differs significantly in its scope and focus. It not only includes the foundational principles of thoracic Surgery but also incorporates key interdisciplinary elements. Among these, two fields are particularly crucial: Orthopaedics, and Plastic and reconstructive Surgery. It can be said that chest wall Surgery represents a fusion of chest wall orthopaedics and chest wall plastic Surgery into a specialized discipline. With this understanding, when we revisit the treatment of chest wall tumors, we find numerous new opportunities in areas of practice that were previously unexplored. This change in perspective has led to a sudden and complete breakthrough of the previous bottleneck, enabling significant technical advancement. In other words, by integrating orthopaedic and plastic Surgical techniques into chest wall tumor treatment, it becomes possible to develop entirely new approaches methods that traditional thoracic Surgery alone could never have achieved. Thus, with the establishment of the core principles of chest wall Surgery, the Surgical treatment of chest wall tumors has truly entered a new era of development and renewal.

1. General Concept

Chest wall tumors refer collectively to all neoplastic growths that arise within the chest wall. These tumors may be primary, originating from structures within the chest wall itself, or secondary, resulting from metastases from other parts of the body. Primary tumors can develop in any of the tissues or structures that make up the chest wall, whereas metastatic tumors most commonly involve the bony components. Although metastases may also affect other areas of the chest wall, such occurrences are relatively rare. Reports on the incidence of chest wall tumors vary widely in the literature. However, due to the inconsistent and often imprecise nature of these data, most figures are of limited scientific value. From a histological perspective, chest wall tumors differ significantly from tumors of internal organs. Organ-based tumors typically originate in a single, isolated organ, with localized lesions and a relatively homogeneous tissue origin. As such, their effects are usually confined to the function of that specific organ. In contrast, the chest wall is not a single, uniform structure, but rather a composite anatomical region composed of various elements including bone, muscle, fascia, cartilage, and skin each of which has the potential to develop tumors. Consequently, chest wall tumors exhibit marked diversity in their tissue origins. This heterogeneity is one of the most distinctive features of chest wall tumors [6-9].

Structurally, the chest wall can be roughly divided into three main components: Bony structures, Soft tissues, and Skin. Correspondingly, chest wall tumors can also be broadly classified into three categories: Bony tumors, Soft tissue tumors, and Cutaneous tumors[10]. However, due to the integrated and overlapping nature of the chest wall's anatomical components, tumors in this region rarely remain confined to a single structure. The close interrelationship among tissues often leads to cross-involvement. Therefore, isolated chest wall tumors are uncommon, and once a tumor arises, it tends to affect multiple types of tissues and structures.

2. Hazards

The harmful effects of tumors are multifaceted and can be broadly divided into systemic and local complications [11]. Systemic hazards include the adverse effects caused by tumor-specific secretions, the metabolic burden placed on the body, and if present the consequences of distant metastases, which also fall under this category. Local hazards typically involve three main aspects [12,13]: Destruction of organ function due to the tumor itself, Compression of surrounding structures, and Infiltrative damage to adjacent tissues caused by the tumor.

In the case of chest wall tumors, if the lesion is localized and grows slowly, systemic symptoms are generally minimal or absent. However, if the tumor becomes more extensive or aggressive. If the tumor grows extensively, has a rapid growth rate, or presents with endocrine abnormalities, it can result in obvious systemic hazards. These systemic effects may manifest as a variety of general symptoms throughout the body. If distant metastasis occurs, it will lead to clinical symptoms corresponding to the affected sites.

The local hazards of chest wall tumors are the most prominent and also the most significant among all their effects. The first and foremost impact is the tumor's disruption of chest wall function. Although the chest wall is not an independent organ, it functions as an integrated structure with specific physiological roles. When a tumor arises in a particular area of the chest wall, the destruction of normal anatomical structures inevitably leads to functional impairment [14,15]. The normal physiological functions of the chest wall can be summarized as follows [10]: ① Maintaining the normal appearance of the thorax, thereby ensuring a healthy and aesthetically pleasing body image. The chest is located in the upper part of the torso, and the appearance of the chest wall directly influences a person's physique, posture, and gait. If the chest wall becomes deformed or abnormal in appearance, the patient's overall image will be significantly affected. ②Maintaining negative intra-thoracic pressure to ensure proper respiratory function. The chest wall must have sufficient rigidity, which primarily comes from its bony structures. Under the support of these bones, a stable negative pressure is maintained within the thoracic cavity. This negative pressure is fundamental for normal breathing mechanics. If the structural integrity of the chest wall is compromised, its function is also affected, potentially leading to the loss of negative pressure within the chest cavity, thereby causing serious impairment of pulmonary ventilation. ③Providing attachment points for various muscles and participating in chest wall movements. In general, bodily movements are carried out by muscles acting on bones. Although the bones of the chest wall are not as mobile as those of the limbs, they do play a role in specific movements. These movements are achieved through the actions of the muscles on the surface of the chest wall, and though the range is limited, they hold significant physiological importance. If this mobility is lost, a range of complications may arise. ④Protecting vital thoracic organs and creating a secure environment for them. The thoracic cavity contains multiple vital organs, among which the lungs and heart are particularly sensitive to external pressure. The chest wall serves as a protective barrier for these organs. Without this structural protection, the heart and lungs could be easily compressed, which would severely impair their function.

From the above analysis, it is evident that although the chest wall is located on the body surface, it plays a very important physiological role. When chest wall tumors occur, under the destructive effects of the tumor, the four aforementioned functions are almost inevitably affected. First is the impact on appearance. Chest wall tumors can not only protrude on the body surface themselves but may also alter the overall shape of the thorax, causing deformities in appearance. This will have a significant effect on the patient's overall image. Second is the impact on respiration. Once a chest wall tumor develops, it may grow not only outwardly towards the body surface but also inwardly into the thoracic cavity. The volume within the thoracic cavity is limited. Tumor growth inward means a reduction in thoracic cavity volume, which will change the pressure within the chest. This undoubtedly directly affects the negative intrathoracic pressure and subsequently impairs respiratory function. Additionally, the tumor may compress lung tissue, directly impacting its physiological function. Third is the impact on movement. Chest wall tumors can directly affect the attachment of various chest wall muscles, and may even invade these muscles. When muscles are affected, their related movements will inevitably be impaired. Fourth is the impact on the protective function. Chest wall tumors can directly destroy the chest wall, causing it to lose its basic structure and function. At this point, the chest wall will no longer be able to protect the organs within the thoracic cavity. Once this protective function is lost, the functions of the thoracic organs will be adversely affected.

The second type of local harm caused by chest wall tumors comes from the tumor's compression of surrounding structures. This compression can be either longitudinal or transverse. Transverse compression mainly affects the internal structures of the chest wall, such as the ribs, costal cartilages, sternum, muscles, mammary glands, and the spine. Longitudinal compression primarily impacts the organs within the thoracic cavity, with the lungs being the most susceptible to compression, followed by the heart and major blood vessels. Under normal circumstances, each structure of the chest wall has its unique function. When the surrounding structures are compressed by the tumor, their anatomy is altered and their function impaired, leading to various complications.

The third type of local harm caused by chest wall tumors comes from the infiltrative destruction of surrounding structures by the tumor. This type of damage is mostly caused by malignant tumors, although some benign tumors can also exhibit infiltrative growth, eventually damage the surrounding structures and cause loss of their normal anatomy and function. Malignant tumors of the sternum can cause extensive destruction, not only damage the adjacent costal cartilages and ribs but also invade outward to the skin and inward to the thoracic cavity organs. As the tumor continues to invade surrounding tissues, it may affect the clavicle, scapula, spine, and other structures. The higher the malignancy of the tumor, the more severe and extensive the local invasion. Malignant rib tumors can also infiltrate adjacent structures, leading to corresponding damage.

3. Clinical Manifestations

The clinical symptoms of chest wall tumors are a direct reflection of the various types of damage they cause [16–18]. The most common symptom is pain, which is generally well-localized and corresponds closely to the site of the lesion, representing a direct manifestation of the tumor's local effects. The pain is often described as dull, though in some cases it may be severe. However, not all patients experience pain; some may remain pain-free throughout the entire course of the disease. If the tumor invades the pleura or directly affects the lung, the patient may present with notable respiratory symptoms, such as coughing or even dyspnea (difficulty breathing). When the tumor compresses the heart or major blood vessels, symptoms related to the cardiovascular system may also appear.

Since the chest wall is located on the body surface, tumors that occur there are often easily detected externally. Therefore, the most direct physical sign of a chest wall tumor is the presence of a localized mass. The characteristics of this mass vary depending on whether the tumor is benign or malignant. For benign tumors, the overlying skin typically appears normal, the mass has well-defined borders, grows slowly, and, if originating from superficial soft tissue, may have some degree of mobility. In contrast, malignant tumors may cause infiltration of the overlying skin, and in severe cases, even ulceration. The mass usually has poorly defined borders, may be fixed to surrounding structures, grows rapidly, and is highly destructive. Additionally, the origin of the mass influences its characteristics. Tumors arising from bony structures tend to be firm in texture, while those originating from soft tissues are generally softer. Recognizing these features helps in understanding the basic nature of the tumor.

4. Examination

In addition to local signs, chest wall tumors may also present with other physical signs if they affect intra-thoracic structures. However, these signs are generally non-specific; they can indicate the severity of the tumor, but not its nature. Theoretically, tumors involving bony structures can lead to pathological fractures. Since the sternum is rarely subjected to external force, pathological fractures of the sternum are uncommon. In contrast, the ribs are more fragile, and when the tumor causes bone destruction, a sufficiently strong external force may result in a pathological rib fracture. In some cases, this fracture may be the first clinical manifestation of a chest wall tumor.

For further examination of chest wall tumors, the following information needs to be understood [11]: ①Information about the tumor itself, including the tumor's location, size, internal structure, and nature. This is key information for understanding the tumor. ② Relationship with surrounding structures: including whether there is adhesion, infiltration, or compression. This information is crucial for determining treatment. ③ Information about important surrounding structures: including whether there are accompanying lesions, damage, or involvement of special structures nearby. This is also critical for treatment decisions. ④ Overall systemic condition: including all other information related to tumor diagnosis and treatment. This is essential clinical information.

Imaging examinations are the basic methods for evaluating chest wall tumors [16,17]. X-ray examination is the most elementary imaging method and can clarify the approximate location of the tumor, its relationship with surrounding structures, as well as the general condition of the heart, lungs, and thorax. However, it is difficult to obtain detailed information about the tumor itself through X-rays, so it is not the primary examination method. CT scanning is the most fundamental and useful diagnostic tool for chest wall tumors, capable of providing nearly all necessary diagnostic information. Whole-body radionuclide scans and PET-CT can clarify the overall systemic condition, but these examinations are not always necessary [15]. If the local tumor mass is clear, even when distant metastases exist, Surgery may not be contraindicated, so the value of such examinations is limited. Three- dimensional reconstruction imaging is an advanced and valuable examination. Besides providing various details about the tumor itself, it can also finely display the entire chest wall structure [17,19]. This type of imaging is valuable not only for tumor diagnosis but also for Surgical planning. Especially for the increasingly popular digital material reconstruction surgeries, this examination is essential. However, the results of three-dimensional reconstruction cannot be directly obtained from ordinary CT scans and require special software processing. Due to the complexity and high cost of the procedure, it has not yet become widespread.

The determination of the nature of chest wall tumors requires pathological examination, while preoperative qualitative assessment can be done through cytological examination. Since chest wall tumors are mostly located on the body surface, except for some special locations, performing these examinations is not very difficult. Cytological examination has some significance in guiding treatment but its role is limited. Considering that methods of obtaining cells cause a certain degree of trauma, cytological examination should not be regarded as a mandatory preoperative test.

5. Diagnosis and Differential Diagnosis

The diagnosis of chest wall tumors is relatively straightforward; a basic diagnosis can be made based on clinical manifestations and various examinations. If cytological examination results are available, a definitive diagnosis can be obtained. However, the confirmation should be made after Surgery, and pathological examination is not mandatory before Surgery. The differential diagnosis of chest wall tumors mainly involves distinguishing them from benign masses, such as chest wall abscesses, tuberculosis, and certain deformities. This differentiation helps in Surgical decision-making. However, from the perspective of performing Surgery, differential diagnosis is not decisive because Surgery is necessary for any mass. Sometimes it is difficult to determine the nature of the mass preoperatively. Even negative results may be false negatives; therefore, regardless of the results, Surgery should be actively pursued without overemphasizing the nature of the lesion before Surgery [11]. Especially when the nature is suspicious or very difficult to define, Surgery should be performed as soon as possible.

6. Indications for Surgery

Once a chest wall tumor is detected, Surgery is an absolute indication regardless of the nature of the tumor. Even if nature cannot be clearly identified, the chest wall. Even the presence of a mass itself requires early removal. Some people believe that certain pathological types of masses are not suitable for Surgical treatment. This viewpoint is worth questioning. As mentioned above, besides their own harm, masses may also affect the function of important organs. For example, when a chest wall tumor severely invades the thoracic cavity, the tumor mass may directly compress the heart and lungs, leading to severe impairment of cardiopulmonary function. Such lesions, whether benign or malignant, should not be considered contraindications for Surgery. If not removed in time, the patient may quickly lose their life, without any chance for further rescue or treatment. However, when considering Surgery, some objective contraindications must not be forgotten. If the patient's overall condition is extremely poor, or the local invasion is too extensive, and the expected Surgical outcome is very poor, Surgery should not be forcibly performed.

7. Surgical Principles

Chest wall tumors are one of the most fundamental diseases treated by chest wall Surgery. Therefore, Surgical treatment must follow the general principles of chest wall Surgery, which include both therapeutic and reconstructive purposes [8,9,14]. These two aspects coexist but may be emphasized differently depending on the situation. For patients with severe tumor invasion, the therapeutic aspect is absolutely the primary concern, with the goal of eliminating the lesion and prolonging life. However, for lesions with less severe harm, in addition to thorough removal of the lesion, the reconstructive aspect should also be emphasized. During the specific procedure, all relevant factors must be fully considered, and the Surgery should be carried out based on the priorities.

The therapeutic nature of chest wall tumor Surgery is reflected in the removal of the lesion, while the reconstructive aspect is achieved through the reconstruction of the chest wall. The most basic procedure in chest wall tumor Surgery is lesion excision. If the resection area is extensive, reconstruction must be performed. If a soft tissue tumor does not involve the bony structures and can be completely removed without large defects in the soft tissue and skin, chest wall reconstruction may not be necessary. However, the vast majority of chest wall tumors may invade bony structures. To completely remove the tumor, the bony structures must also be excised. The removal of bony structures results in defects in the chest wall's bony framework, which affects the integrity of the thorax. To maintain the chest wall's function, reconstruction must be performed. This is another important aspect of chest wall tumor Surgery [16–21].

8. Basic Characteristics of Chest Wall Surgery in Managing Chest Wall Tumors

Chest wall tumors are not a new disease; they have long been recognized in traditional thoracic Surgery. The knowledge related to chest wall tumors in thoracic Surgery has become quite mature. However, as stated at the beginning of this book, chest wall Surgery is a new discipline. When chest wall tumors are viewed from the perspective of chest wall Surgery, their meaning changes significantly; this is precisely what this specialty needs to focus on.

Compared with traditional thoracic Surgery, the perspective of chest wall Surgery incorporates elements from orthopaedics and plastic Surgery [11]. Viewing the clinical management of chest wall tumors from an orthopaedic perspective adds two dimensions: first, the breadth of the disease; second, the depth of the disease. The breadth refers mainly to content related to the traditional chest wall structures but previously not considered part of the chest wall, such as tumors of the clavicle, scapula, and vertebral bodies. These tumors were not traditionally managed under thoracic Surgery. However, in chest wall Surgery. Aspects require the attention of chest wall Surgery. The "depth" aspect mainly refers to applying orthopaedic concepts and techniques in managing chest wall tumors. For example, when treating tumors in the upper sternum that involve the sternoclavicular joint and clavicle, traditional orthopaedic techniques can assist chest wall Surgeons in handling very challenging issues.

Viewing chest wall tumors from the perspective of plastic Surgery broadens the field of vision and improves many aspects of care. For instance, the techniques for chest wall reconstruction are very limited if relying solely on thoracic Surgery. Once plastic Surgery techniques are incorporated, chest wall tumor Surgery no longer follows the traditional thoracic Surgery approach but takes on a completely new form. This breakthrough represents overcoming the Surgical bottleneck in chest wall tumor treatment. Chest wall Surgery has brought new life to the management of chest wall tumors.

REFERENCES

[1] Harati, K., J. Kolbenschlag, B. Behr, et al. "Thoracic Wall Reconstruction after Tumor Resection." Frontiers in Oncology 5 (2015): 247.

[2] Sandler, G., and A. Hayes-Jordan. "Chest Wall Reconstruction after Tumor Resection." Seminars in Pediatric Surgery 27, no. 3 (2018): 200–206.

[3] Sanna, S., J. Brandolini, A. Pardolesi, et al. "Materials and Techniques in Chest Wall Reconstruction: A Review." Journal of Visualized Surgery 3 (2017): 95.

[4] Sandri, A., G. Donati, C. D. Blanc, et al. "Anterior Chest Wall Resection and Sternal Body Wedge for Primary Chest Wall Tumour: Reconstruction Technique with Biological Meshes and Titanium Plates." Journal of Thoracic Disease 12, no. 1 (2020): 17–21.

[5] Tamburini, N., W. Grossi, S. Sanna, et al. "Chest Wall Reconstruction Using a New Titanium Mesh: A Multicenter Experience." Journal of Thoracic Disease 11, no. 8 (2019): 3459–3466.

[6] Bagheri, R., S. Z. Haghi, M. Kalantari, et al. "Primary Malignant Chest Wall Tumors: Analysis of 40 Patients." Journal of Cardiothoracic Surgery 9 (2014): 106.
[7] Friesenbichler, J., A. Leithner, W. Maurer-Ertl, et al. "Surgical Therapy of Primary Malignant Bone Tumours and Soft Tissue Sarcomas of the Chest Wall: A Two-Institutional Experience." International Orthopaedics 38 (2014): 1235–1240.
[8] Wang, Wenlin. "MatrixRIB Surgery: Resection and Reconstruction of Large Chest Wall Tumors." Thoracic Deformity Surgery Expert, October 22, 2021.
[9] Wang, Wenlin. "Fourth Surgery for Chest Wall Tumor: Tumor Resection + MatrixRIB Chest Wall Reconstruction." Thoracic Deformity Surgery Expert, October 20, 2021.
[10] Wang, Wenlin. "Chest Wall Surgery: Basic Structure and Function of the Chest Wall." Jinri Toutiao, October 31, 2021.
[11] Wang, Wenlin. "Related Issues of Chest Wall Tumors." Jinri Toutiao, October 31, 2021.
[12] Scarnecchia, E., V. Liparulo, R. Capozzi, et al. "Chest Wall Resection and Reconstruction for Tumors: Analysis of Oncological and Functional Outcomes." Journal of Thoracic Disease 10 (Suppl 16) (2018): S1855–S1863.
[13] Sørensen, T. R., M. Raedkjaer, P. H. Jørgensen, et al. "Soft Tissue Sarcomas of the Thoracic Wall: Higher Mortality and Local Recurrence—A Single-Institution Long-Term Follow-Up Study." International Journal of Surgical Oncology (2019): 2350157.
[14] Zhang, Jianhua, Li Bin, Gou Yunjou, et al. "Reconstruction of Bony Chest Wall Defects Using Artificial Composite Materials: Report of 23 Cases." Chinese Journal of Modern Medicine 22, no. 12 (2012): 41–43.
[15] Zhang, Y., Li J. Z., Hao Y. J., et al. "Sternal Tumor Resection and Reconstruction with Titanium Mesh: A Preliminary Study." Orthopaedic Surgery 7, no. 2 (2015): 155–160.
[16] Xu, Qiming, Zhou Naikang, Liu Ying, et al. "Diagnosis and Surgical Treatment of 105 Cases of Chest Wall Tumors." Chinese Journal of Clinical Oncology 34, no. 13 (2007): 750–753.
[17] Xu, Qinzi, Sun Wei, Ai Bo, et al. "Sternal Tumor Resection and Thoracic Reconstruction with Autologous Rib and Pedicled Omental Flap Transplantation." Chinese Journal of Physician Continuing Education 33, no. 35 (2010): 12–14.
[18] Kirklin, J. W., and T. T. Myre. "Resection of Tumors of the Sternum." Annals of Surgery 144, no. 6 (1956): 1023–1028.
[19] Wang, Wenlin. "Next-Generation Chest Wall Reconstruction Techniques: Digital Material Chest Wall Reconstruction." Thoracic Deformity Surgery Expert, September 7, 2020.
[20] Foroulis, C. N., A. D. Kleontas, G. Tagarakis, et al. "Massive Chest Wall Resection and Reconstruction for Malignant Disease." OncoTargets and Therapy 9 (2016): 2349–2358.
[21] Wang, Wenlin. "MatrixRIB Surgery: Upper Sternal Tumor Resection and Reconstruction." Thoracic Deformity Surgery Expert, October 19, 2021.

The chest wall is a complex structure composed of multiple components and various tissues, each of which can develop tumors. These tumors all fall under the category of chest wall tumors. Therefore, the origins of chest wall tumors are quite complex, much more so than tumors of isolated organs. To thoroughly study these tumors, it is necessary to analyze them from multiple levels and perspectives. Only in this way can the essential nature of chest wall tumors be understood.

1. Benign and Malignant Tumors

Like tumors in all other parts of the body, chest wall tumors can be classified as benign or malignant. Common benign chest wall tumors include [1-10]: fibrous dysplasia, chondroma, eosinophilic granuloma, osteochondroma, giant cell tumor of bone, aneurysmal bone cyst, osteoblastoma, desmoplastic fibroma, haemangioma, myofibroma, myolipoma, fibro lipoma, myxoid lipoma, neurofibroma, and schwannoma. Common malignant chest wall tumors include [1-10]: chondrosarcoma of the ribs, plasma cell myeloma, Hodgkin's lymphoma of the sternum, fibrosarcoma, rhabdomyosarcoma, primitive neuroectodermal tumor, malignant peripheral nerve sheath tumor, leiomyosarcoma, Angio leiomyosarcoma, and various malignant metastatic tumors.

The distinction between benign and malignant tumors is one of the most important concerns for both doctors and patients. Not only do their pathological characteristics differ completely, but their Surgical methods and prognoses also vary [1]. Benign tumors can originate from various tissues, and their common features include slow growth, localized position, and clear boundaries with surrounding tissues. Malignant tumors can also originate from various tissues but generally grow rapidly, exhibit infiltrative growth, have unclear boundaries with surrounding tissues, can invade nearby structures, and may even metastasize to distant sites. The primary harm caused by benign tumors comes from local mass effect and compression, but they can also undergo malignant transformation and become malignant tumors. The harm caused by malignant tumors is multifaceted; in addition to local mass effect and compression, they can directly destroy primary and surrounding structures and may even cause systemic damage. Differentiating between benign and malignant tumors is a crucial clinical task that not only determines the entire treatment plan but also ultimately decides the patient's outcome.

2. Tumor Structural Origin

The chest wall is a composite structure composed of various differently shaped components, which can essentially be divided into three main categories. Corresponding to these structures, three types of tumors are clinically observed: tumors of the bony chest wall structures [1-4], soft tissue tumors [11-14], and skin tumors [15]. Tumors originating from different structures generally retain some characteristics of their tissue of origin. For example, bone tumors have distinct gross morphology and structure compared to soft tissue tumors.

The morphology and structure of bone tumors differ significantly from those of soft tissue tumors. Distinguishing the structural origin of the tumor is mainly important for guiding treatment. Since the Surgical approaches for the three types of tumors are fundamentally different, it is crucial to differentiate their structures before Surgery.

3. Tumor Location

The structural origin of a tumor only provides a general idea of where it may occur, which is rather vague and does not accurately reflect the tumor's exact location. To gain a more precise understanding of a tumor, it is essential to clearly identify its location. Based on different locations, chest wall tumors can be classified as sternal tumors, rib tumors, pectoralis major tumors, pectoralis minor tumors, and so on. For even greater precision, more detailed descriptions can be used for example, a tumor of the 10th left rib, or a tumor in the midsection of the sternum. The more specific the location, the more accurate the description, and such detailed descriptions hold greater clinical significance. When describing the location of a tumor, another concept closely related to location is the area of invasion. Some tumors may initially arise in a specific site, but as they grow, they may extend beyond that original location. This information is also extremely important, as it directly determines the overall Surgical strategy and specific details of the operation. For example, in the case of a sternal tumor, whether there is invasion into surrounding structures and the extent of that invasion are major factors that affect the success or failure of the Surgery. Therefore, thorough understanding is essential before the operation.

4. Tissue Origin of Tumors

The chest wall is composed of various structures, which, when further subdivided, consist of different tissues. Each type of tissue within these structures has its own unique characteristics. When a tumor originates from a specific tissue, it tends to inherit the distinctive properties of that tissue. This is what contributes to the diverse nature of chest wall tumors.

5. Cellular Origin of Tumors

There is extensive documentation regarding the cellular origins of chest wall tumors. We have summarized the commonly used terms found in the literature and identified the following specific classifications [1–4]:

Malignant mesothelioma, malignant lymphoma, malignant fibrous histiocytoma, malignant plasmacytic lymphoma of the sternum, osteosarcoma, bone cyst, myeloma, osteochondroma, bone lymphoma, osteoblastoma, giant cell tumor of bone, chondrosarcoma, fibrous dysplasia of bone (fibro- osseous dysplasia), rib hemangioma, rib lipoma, rib giant cell tumor, benign mesenchymal tumor of the rib, costal chondroblastoma, periosteal osteosarcoma of the rib, intravascular proliferation of the rib, ossifying fibroma of the rib, costal chondroblastoma, differentiated osteosarcoma of the rib, non-ossifying fibroma of the rib, mesenchymal chondrosarcoma of the rib, differentiated chondrosarcoma of the rib, serous chondrosarcoma of the rib, rib hemangioma with cartilaginous metaplasia, costal chondromyxoid fibroma, primary aneurysmal bone cyst of the rib, enchondroma, dermoid cyst, malignant fibrous histiocytoma, aggressive fibromatosis, cavernous hemangioma, rhabdomyosarcoma, cavernous hemangioma, plasmacytoma, mesenchymal hamartoma, eosinophilic granuloma, phosphaturic mesenchymal tumor, Askin tumor, epidermoid cyst, aneurysmal bone cyst, liposarcoma, lipoma, synovial sarcoma, myofibroma, alveolar soft part sarcoma, squamous cell carcinoma, solitary fibrous tumor of the pleura, primitive neuroectodermal tumor, primary neuroendocrine carcinoma, dermatofibrosarcoma, spindle cell sarcoma, schwannoma, malignant peripheral nerve sheath tumor, neuroblastoma, neurofibroma, elastofibroma, neurofibrosarcoma, chondroma, chondrosarcoma, soft tissue sarcoma, angioleiomyoma, angiolipoma, hemangioma, hemangioendothelioma, angiofibrolipoma, fibroma, xanthofibroma, histiocytoma, fibrosarcoma, fibrous dysplasia, giant cell tumor of the sternum, pleural mesothelioma, small round cell malignant tumor.
The names listed above reveal the cellular origins of chest wall tumors and represent their most fundamental pathological characteristics. For thoracic Surgeons treating chest wall tumors, it is essential to have a deep understanding of these pathological attributes. However, one critical issue must be clarified: the accuracy of these tumor names. Due to the varying expertise levels of the physicians who assigned these names, there may be discrepancies in both their accuracy and appropriateness. Therefore, when studying these tumor types, it is crucial to remain clear-headed and not be misled by irresponsible or inaccurate pathological terminology.

6.Some Special Chest Wall Tumors

(1) Fibrous Dysplasia of the Rib

Fibrous dysplasia of the rib is a benign tumor, also known as rib fibrous dysplasia, and was first reported by Lichtenstein in 1938. The fundamental lesion involves the destruction and resorption of normal bone and bone marrow, which are gradually replaced by pathologically proliferative fibrous tissue [16–18]. This lesion can occur in any part of the skeletal system, but it is most

commonly found in the craniofacial bones, femur, and tibia, with the ribs also being a relatively common site. Fibrous dysplasia of the rib is a relatively rare benign rib tumor.
Some scholars believe its occurrence is related to developmental defects, others suggest it may be associated with local infections or repair responses following injury, while some attribute it to genetic mutations. The pathogenesis of the disease remains controversial, and no explanation has gained universal acceptance. Pathologically, the condition is generally classified into three types: Monostotic type the lesion is confined to a single rib. Polyostotic type the lesion involves multiple ribs. Albright's syndrome characterized by skin and mucosal pigmentation, precocious puberty, and often endocrine hyperfunction. Rib fibrous dysplasia is most commonly seen in adolescents, affecting both males and females, though it is more frequent in females. In the early stages, it may not show any specific symptoms. Most patients seek medical attention due to localized pain, deformity, or even pathological fractures. Imaging features vary depending on the maturity and proportion of fibrous tissue, osteoid tissue, and newly formed bone trabeculae within the lesion (see Figure 3-2-1). There are four classic imaging patterns: ① Cystic expansile change primarily due to fibrous tissue proliferation, appearing as solitary or multiple cystic expansile radiolucent areas, often surrounded by a sclerotic margin. ② Ground-glass appearance a significant feature marked by newly formed bone trabeculae, often superimposed on cystic expansile lesions, showing as diffusely increased density within the radiolucent areas. ③ Loofah-like change characterized by thickened bone trabeculae distributed along the longitudinal axis, repeatedly twisted and interspersed with a small amount of proliferative fibrous tissue. ④ Moth-eaten bone destruction the main feature is scattered areas of bone resorption, resembling the pattern of bone being eaten away. It may contain mature bone trabeculae and may exhibit cortical bone continuity disruption; in severe cases, osteolytic changes may be present. Fibrous dysplasia of the rib has the potential for malignant transformation, possibly developing into chondrosarcoma, osteosarcoma, or fibrosarcoma, with a malignant transformation rate of approximately 2% - 3% [17, 18].

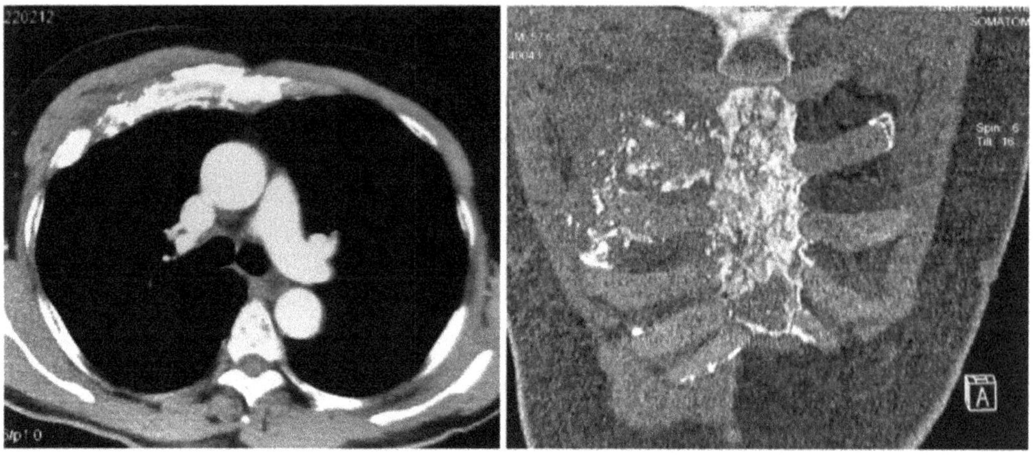

Figure 3-2-1 CT Imaging Features of Rib Fibrous Dysplasia

(2) Chondroma

Chondroma is a common benign tumor that can be classified into extraosseous chondroma and enchondroma [19–22]. Extraosseous chondroma occurs outside the skeletal system, located within soft tissues and unrelated to any bony structure. Chondromas associated with bone include synovial chondroma and enchondroma: Synovial chondroma originates from synovial membranes found in joint cavities, tendon sheaths, or bursae. These give rise to multiple cartilaginous nodules within the joint space, forming synovial chondromas. Enchondroma, by contrast, occurs within the medullary cavity of bones. It is one of the most common benign bone tumors, accounting for 12%-24% of all benign bone tumors and 3%-10% of all bone tumors. It is composed of mature cartilage tissue and typically arises in the diaphysis or metaphysis of bones. Because the tumor is centrally located within the bone, it is sometimes referred to as a central chondroma. Enchondromas commonly occur in patients aged 30–40 years. Most patients are asymptomatic, though some may seek medical attention for painless swelling. The most frequent locations are the small tubular bones of the hands and feet, especially the proximal and middle phalanges. X-rays features of enchondromas include: Cystic or irregular low-density areas, sometimes appearing ground-glass or fluffy, Well-defined borders, occasionally with chondroid

calcification, the lesion may cause expansile growth, thinning the cortical bone, in flat or irregular bones, imaging findings may be atypical, Radiolucent defects are often seen on X-rays, clearly demarcated from surrounding bone, usually without periosteal reaction or reactive new bone formation, The lesion is typically central, with thinned and expanded cortex, Reactive sclerosis may be seen around the tumor, scattered granular calcified spots may be present. Chondromas of the chest wall can occur in the ribs, sternum, or soft tissues: Rib chondromas are rare, Sternal chondromas most often affect the body of the sternum, though they can also occur at the xiphoid process, which is extremely rare, There are also reports of primary osteochondromas within chest wall soft tissues, unrelated to the skeletal system, occurring solely in soft tissue, Although chondromas are benign, they do carry a risk of malignant transformation.

(3) Osteochondroma

Osteochondroma is also a relatively common benign bone tumor. It is characterized by the growth of a bony outgrowth capped with cartilage, which arises from the external surface of the bone [23, 24]. Among all benign bone tumors, osteochondromas account for approximately 38.5%, and they make up about 12% of all bone tumors. This tumor can appear as solitary or multiple lesions. A solitary osteochondroma is also known as an exostosis, and it is the most common type of osteochondroma. Osteochondromas most frequently occur at the metaphysis of long bones, with the distal femur and proximal tibia being the most commonly affected sites accounting for around 50% of cases. The condition typically arises in children and adolescents, and is most often seen in patients under the age of 20, with a higher incidence in males than females. Rib osteochondromas are extremely rare, and when they do occur, they are most commonly found near the costochondral junction. Tumors in other parts of the rib are even rarer (Figure 3-2-2). Complications may include: Damage to intercostal nerves and vessels, Hemothorax due to vessel rupture, Compression of the lungs or other intrathoracic structures if the tumor becomes large, Spinal cord compression if the tumor arises from a rib adjacent to the thoracic spine. Osteochondroma must be differentiated from rib tuberculosis and other benign rib lesions. Although osteochondromas are benign, they carry a risk of malignant transformation, most commonly into chondrosarcoma.

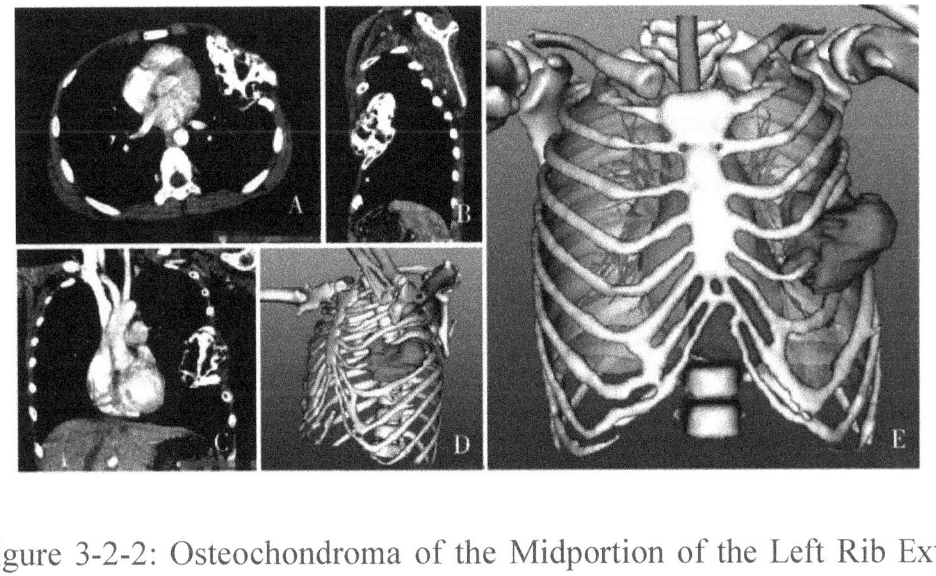

Figure 3-2-2: Osteochondroma of the Midportion of the Left Rib Extremely Rare (A, B, C: CT imaging features of the tumor; D, E: Three-dimensional reconstruction images of the tumor)

(4) Giant Cell Tumor of Bone

Giant cell tumor of bone (GCTB) is a relatively common bone tumor, second only to osteochondroma, accounting for 18.2%-20.0% of benign bone tumors (Figure 3-2-3). Most cases are benign, but a small number exhibit locally aggressive behaviour [25,26]. GCTB most commonly occurs in adults between the ages of 20 and 40,

with females more frequently affected than males. It typically arises in the epiphyseal regions of long bones, especially the distal femur and proximal tibia. GCTBs occurring in the ribs are rare. Some studies report that rib giant cell tumors account for only about 0.6% of all GCTB cases. Histologically, giant cell tumors are composed mainly of multinucleated giant cells and mononuclear stromal cells, and may also exhibit changes such as: Cystic degeneration, Fibrosis, Hemorrhage, Hemosiderin deposition. Typical Radiographic Features: Eccentric expansile bone destruction, the cortical shell may be intact or disrupted, no ossification or calcification, the lesion typically shows well-defined margins, and no surrounding bone sclerosis. Pathological fractures may occur, and when they do, periosteal reaction and adjacent soft tissue masses can be observed. These features may indicate potential malignant transformation. CT imaging can demonstrate: Cortical bone disruption, surrounding soft tissue involvement. Internal structure of the lesion, aiding in differential diagnosis and Surgical planning.

The pathological grading of giant cell tumor of bone (GCTB) was initially divided into three grades: Grade I & II: Benign, Grade III: Malignant. Later, a more detailed three-stage clinical classification was developed, integrating clinical presentation, X-ray imaging, and pathological features: Stage I: No clinical symptoms, Lesion visible on X-ray, Pathology shows benign features. Stage II: Clinical symptoms present, X-ray shows an expansile lesion, but no cortical destruction, Pathology remains benign. Stage III: Clinical symptoms present, X-ray shows aggressive growth, with cortical bone destruction or defect, Possible soft tissue mass, Pathology may show benign or malignant characteristics. This classification helps guide treatment strategy and assess prognosis for patients with giant cell tumors.

Campanacci and colleagues proposed a grading system for giant cell tumors of bone (GCTB) based on X-ray findings, particularly the extent of bone lysis and cortical destruction. This system divides GCTB into three grades [27]: Grade I: Lesion has well-defined margins, Sclerotic rim present, no periosteal reaction, no soft tissue mass (or, if present, it has well-defined edges), This is the most common grade, accounting for 70%-80% of cases. Grade II: Partially ill-defined margins, may show signs of outward (extraosseous) extension, Cortical breakthrough and soft tissue mass may be present, Mass edges are often poorly defined, frequently associated with pathological fractures. This accounts for approximately 20% of cases. Grade III: Lesion has ill-defined boundaries, typically shows aggressive, outward-growing destruction, often accompanied by pathological fractures, Also accounts for around 20% of cases. Campanacci grading system reflects the biological behaviour of the tumor and is considered a scientific and practical classification method. Data show a strong correlation between the Campanacci grade and the recurrence rate of GCTB Higher grade = more extensive destruction of local normal bone structure = higher likelihood of recurrence.

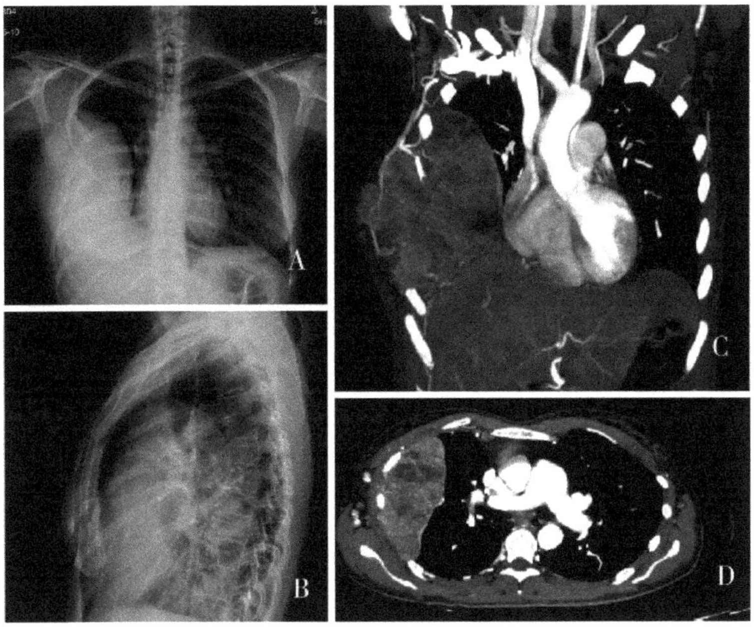

Figure 3-2-3: Giant Cell Tumor of Bone, (A, B: Radiographic (X-ray) features of the tumor; C, D: CT imaging features of the tumor)

(5) Aneurysmal Bone Cyst (ABC)

Aneurysmal bone cyst is a rare, tumor-like bone lesion, accounting for approximately 1.3% of all bone tumors [28–30]. It occurs most frequently in individuals under 20 years old, typically affecting the epiphyseal regions of long bones and the spine. Rib involvement is rare, and no cases in the sternum have been reported. Etiology and Pathogenesis: The exact cause remains unclear. Some researchers believe it is related to elevated local venous pressure. When venous outflow is obstructed for various reasons, vascular beds expand, leading to bone resorption and the formation of these lesions. Radiological Features: Cystic, expansile, lytic bone destruction, resembles an aneurysm, hence the name. The cortical bone becomes extremely thin due to expansion. Bony septations may be present; in some cases, cortical discontinuity can be seen. The lesion is typically filled with homogeneous fluid without calcification. Fluid–fluid levels may be observed on imaging. These fluid–fluid levels are not specific and must be differentiated from similar features seen in: Telangiectatic osteosarcoma, Chondroblastoma, Giant cell tumor. While often referred to as a "cyst," ABC is not a true cyst because the cavity does not contain only fluid. Pathology: Histological examination reveals: A spongy, trabecular internal structure, Numerous large vascular channels, Fibrous septa separating blood- filled spaces. This vascular and cystic nature is what gives ABC its name and unique imaging appearance.

(6) Eosinophilic Granuloma

Eosinophilic granuloma is a lesion that occurs in isolated histiocytic tissue, characterized by abnormal differentiation of a non-neoplastic nature. It is considered a proliferative disease of the reticuloendothelial system involving the bone [31,32]. It is more commonly seen in young males, with frequent involvement of the skull, ribs, and vertebrae, followed by the long bones. Although the sternum can also be affected, it is less common. The disease typically presents as a solitary lesion, but multiple lesions can occasionally occur, especially in children under the age of 5. As for its pathogenesis, some believe it is related to trauma and originates from hematoma within the tissue, although the exact mechanism remains unclear. The most typical sign of this bone disease is an increase in eosinophils in the peripheral blood, with the eosinophil level correlating with the activity of the lesion. Eosinophil levels are lower during the quiescent phase and higher during the active phase, and they return to normal after the lesion is removed. Eosinophilic granuloma involving the sternum and ribs can be complex and diverse, making diagnosis difficult and prone to misdiagnosis, often being mistaken for bone tumors or chronic osteomyelitis. The lesions usually present with significant changes on X-ray imaging, though clinical symptoms are often mild or absent. X-ray examination may show the lesion as a unilocular, multilocular, or irregular-shaped area, possibly with mild to moderate expansion, thinning of the bone cortex, and clearly defined margins. In a few patients, extensive osteolytic changes may be observed.

(7) Multiple Myeloma

Multiple myeloma is generally classified into multiple myeloma and solitary plasmacytoma. Multiple myeloma is the most common type of malignant plasma cell disease and is also known as plasma cell myeloma or Kahler disease [33,34]. A key characteristic of multiple myeloma is osteolytic bone lesions, where trabecular bone is destroyed and the bone marrow cavity is filled with tumor tissue. The tumor tissue appears gray-white in color. The cortical bone becomes thinned and may be invaded and destroyed. Due to the resulting fragility of the bone, pathological fractures can occur. Common sites of involvement include the clavicle, sternum, ribs, sacroiliac bones, skull, and other areas. Lesions often appear at multiple locations throughout the body simultaneously, so Surgical intervention should be approached with caution. Radiotherapy is generally not suitable; chemotherapy is considered the ideal treatment. Solitary plasmacytoma originates from neoplastic plasma cells and arises within the bone marrow cavity. It is also referred to as solitary plasma cell myeloma [35,36], and falls under the category of malignant plasma cell tumors. It accounts for approximately 2% of all myelomas, though some sources suggest it may represent up to 8%. These tumors are most commonly found in the spinal column and other axial bones, but may also occur in long bones and flat bones rich in cancellous (spongy) bone such as the femur, tibia, pelvic bones, and zygomatic bones. The patella and ribs are rarely affected (Fig. 3-2-4).

The diagnostic criteria for this tumor are: ① Cytological examination confirms a plasma cell bone tumor; ② Urine Bence-Jones protein test is negative; ③ Multiple bone marrow biopsies from sites other than the lesion are negative. ④ X-ray examinations of bones outside the lesion show no abnormalities; ⑤ No systemic symptoms and no obvious physical signs; ⑥ No progression of the lesion during 2–3 years of follow-up. Some experts propose a simplified set of diagnostic criteria, stating that the diagnosis can be confirmed if any one of the following conditions is met: ① Local bony structure is confirmed to be plasma cell myeloma, and bone marrow examinations from other sites are all negative; ② All skeletal examinations outside the lesion show no abnormalities; ③ Urine Bence-Jones protein test is negative, and there are no systemic symptoms. Solitary plasmacytoma is rarely found in the chest wall, but once diagnosed, treatment usually targets the isolated nature of the lesion. Radiotherapy is often the first choice, although Surgery can also be considered as a primary treatment option. The final treatment plan should be tailored to the specific circumstances of the patient.

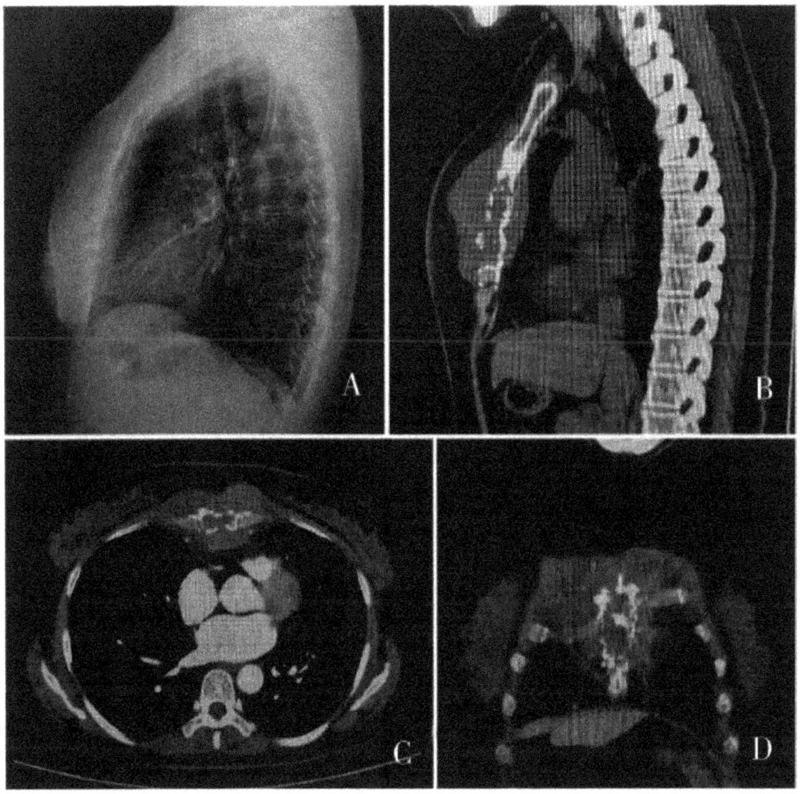

Figure 3-2-4: Solitary Plasmacytoma of the Sternum (A. X-ray findings; B, C, D. CT findings)

(8) Rhabdomyosarcoma

Rhabdomyosarcoma is a malignant tumor that arises from mesenchymal tissue differentiating toward striated muscle [37–39]. It accounts for 4.5% of all childhood malignant tumors, and 50% of all soft tissue sarcomas. The two peak incidence periods are between ages 2-6 and 10-18, with males more frequently affected than females. The vast majority of patients are under the age of 11. The younger the patient, the poorer the prognosis. Historically, the pathological classification of rhabdomyosarcoma included three types: Embryonal, Alveolar, and Pleomorphic types. With advances in understanding, a sclerosing type has recently been added. Additionally, spindle cell subtype, originally part of the embryonal type, has now been reclassified and combined with the sclerosing type to form a new category: spindle cell and/or sclerosing rhabdomyosarcoma. Among all histological types: The embryonal type is the most common, accounting for approximately 60% of cases; The alveolar type is less common, at about 20%; The remaining 20% comprises other subtypes.

Embryonal type typically occurs in younger children, and commonly affects the genitourinary tract, head and neck, and retroperitoneum; Alveolar type is more frequently seen in adolescents and adults, often affecting the limbs; Pleomorphic type is rare, mainly occurring in deep muscles of middle-aged and elderly men; Spindle cell and/or sclerosing types often occur in the paratesticular region and retroperitoneum.

Rhabdomyosarcoma of the chest wall is extremely rare. The site of onset has no obvious specificity and can occur in various parts of the chest wall. The tumor may arise in the superficial muscle layer or in the deep muscle layer. Tumors in the deep muscle layer are more likely to invade adjacent organs and are prone to causing destruction of bony structures. Imaging examinations may reveal the following features: ① The tumor is relatively large, located in the outer layer of the chest wall, and appears as a soft tissue mass. It may involve inner chest wall structures. ② The lesion is oval or round in shape, with small lobulations. It infiltrates surrounding tissues and has an unclear boundary with muscle tissue. ③ The tumor typically shows no signs of calcification or fatty tissue. ④ After contrast- enhanced scanning, the lesion shows uneven enhancement, with the most obvious enhancement at the periphery. Tumor blood vessels may be seen within the lesion. Areas of cystic degeneration and necrosis generally do not enhance.⑤ It often invades adjacent soft tissues, with bone structures being less commonly affected. If bone invasion occurs, it is usually mild.⑥ Distant metastasis from the lesion may occur, most commonly to the lungs. Surrounding lymph nodes may also be involved.

(9) Osteosarcoma

Osteosarcoma is the most common malignant bone tumor. It originates from poorly differentiated primitive cells specifically from osteoblastic-type cells within primitive mesenchymal cells and is therefore sometimes referred to as osteogenic sarcoma [40, 41]. This tumor accounts for 44.6% of all malignant bone tumors and 15.5% of all primary bone tumors. It is more common in young individuals, with a higher incidence in males than in females. The most frequently affected sites are areas where the epiphyseal (growth plate) activity is most active, namely the metaphysis of long bones. The most common sites include: Distal, femur,Proximal tibia, Followed by the proximal humerus. These three sites together account for approximately 85% of all osteosarcomas. Osteosarcomas of the sternum and ribs are relatively rare. The causes of osteosarcoma are complex, and multiple factors can lead to its development. Most osteosarcomas are primary tumors, but some may occur secondarily from the malignant transformation of other bone tumors, or may develop after radiation therapy for various other tumors.

Imaging examinations play an important role in the diagnosis of osteosarcoma. The typical imaging features include [42, 43]: ① Bone destruction, ②Tumor bone formation, ③Periosteal reaction, ④Soft tissue mass. The most characteristic findings are bone destruction and tumor bone formation, which are key criteria for diagnosing osteosarcoma. In addition, osteosarcoma often presents with a typical "Codman triangle" appearance.

In X-ray examinations, osteosarcoma is classified into three types based on the degree of bone destruction and the amount of tumor bone formation [43]: ①Sclerotic Type: This type is primarily characterized by tumor bone formation. There are large amounts of patchy or cloud-like tumor bone within the tumor. The density is high and may show ivory-like appearance. Bone destruction is not obvious. A significant amount of tumor bone may also be present in the surrounding soft tissues, accompanied by obvious periosteal proliferation. ②Osteolytic Type: This type is mainly marked by bone destruction. There is extensive osteolytic destruction. Pathological fractures are commonly seen. There may be a small amount of periosteal reaction and tumor bone. ③Mixed Type: This type is a combination of sclerotic and osteolytic types. Both types of X-ray features may appear simultaneously.

CT scanning is a commonly used examination for patients with osteosarcoma. It can detect tumor masses with heterogeneous density both inside and outside the bone. Within the tumor, the following may be observed: Newly formed tumor bone, Ring-shaped calcified tumor cartilage, and signs of necrotic cystic degeneration [42]. Compared to X-ray examination, CT is more sensitive and can more clearly display various features of the tumor.

Based on the site of occurrence, osteosarcoma can be classified into central type and peripheral type. Central Type: The central type includes: Conventional central osteosarcoma, Telangiectatic osteosarcoma, Small cell (cellular) osteosarcoma, low-grade central osteosarcoma. The conventional central osteosarcoma is further subdivided into: Osteoblastic type, Chondroblastic type, Fibroblastic type. Peripheral Type The peripheral type of osteosarcoma includes: Paraosseous osteosarcoma, periosteal osteosarcoma, and surface high-grade malignant osteosarcoma. This classification system is relatively complex but can accurately reflect the clinicopathological characteristics of osteosarcoma, directly affecting treatment outcomes and prognosis.

The ribs themselves are relatively thin, and this characteristic affects the presentation of osteosarcoma. In the early stages of rib osteosarcoma, the tumor bone mostly appears as spotty, striped calcification shadows, which are difficult to distinguish from general calcification. The typical 'Codman triangle' is rarely seen (Figure 3-2-5). Due to the atypical pathological features, it is necessary to differentiate it from chondrosarcoma, Ewing's sarcoma, suppurative osteomyelitis, and rib cartilage tuberculosis.

(10) Chondrosarcoma

Chondrosarcoma is a malignant bone tumor originating from cartilage tissue and is considered one of the three most common malignant bone tumors [44-47]. The incidence of chondrosarcoma accounts for 20% of all bone tumors, second only to osteosarcoma and multiple myeloma. Chondrosarcoma is more commonly seen in adults, with the onset age ranging from 40 - 60 years, and occurs significantly more often in males than in females. The femur and tibia are the most frequent sites of occurrence, followed by the pelvis. The bones of the chest wall can also develop chondrosarcoma, but the incidence there is low and it is not commonly encountered clinically. Chondrosarcoma is primarily a primary tumor but can also result from the malignant transformation of certain benign tumors, such as osteochondroma and enchondroma. Pathologically, chondrosarcoma is generally classified into six types: conventional medullary type, mesenchymal type, clear cell type, periosteal type, myxoid type, and dedifferentiated type. Besides this classification method, there are other systems that directly classify it into conventional, dedifferentiated, mesenchymal, and clear cell types. According to the tumor's origin site, it can also be divided into central and peripheral types. Central tumors originate from the medullary cavity and grow concentrically, while peripheral tumors arise from the cortex or periosteum and grow outward.

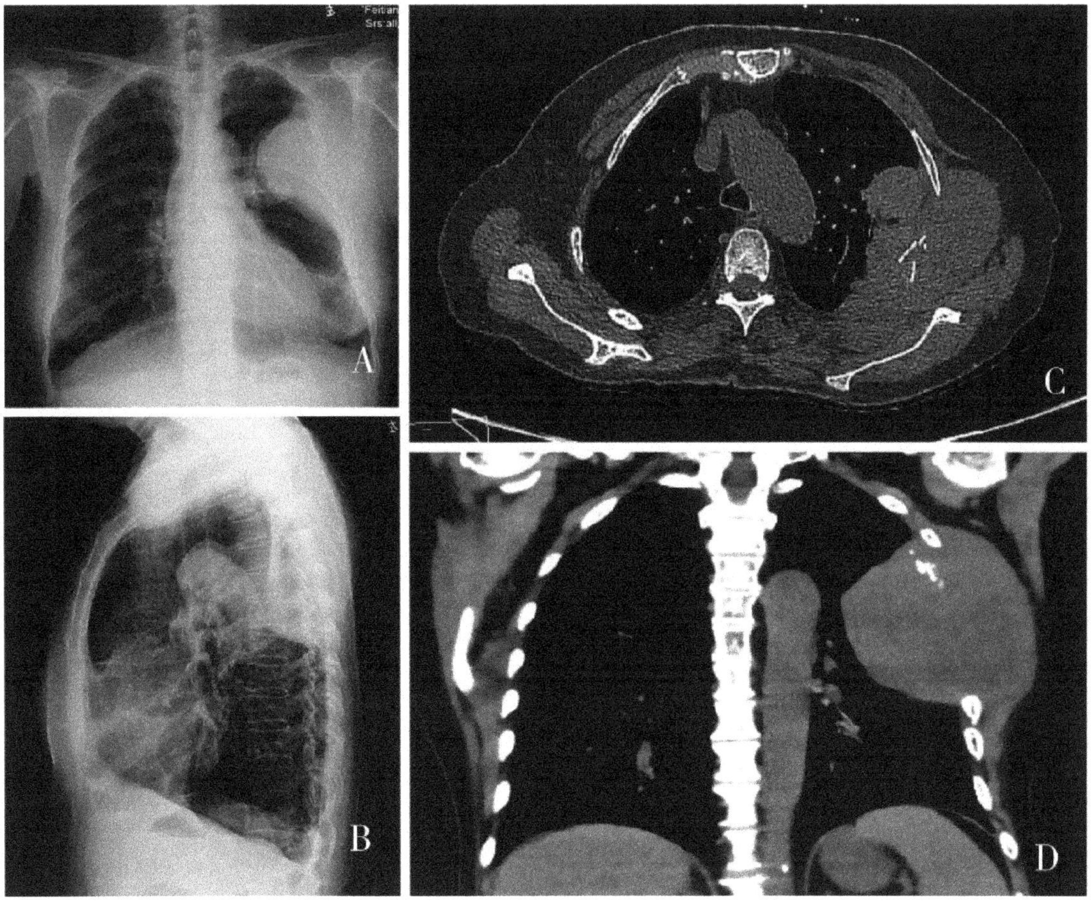

Figure 3-2-5 Rib Osteosarcoma (A, B. X-ray signs of the tumor; C, D. CT signs of the tumor)

The WHO classifies chondrosarcoma into three grades: Grade I [47,48]: low-grade malignancy, highly differentiated, and mild atypia; Grade III: highly malignant, with nuclear changes including binucleation and multinucleation; Grade II: intermediate between Grade I and Grade III.
Chondrosarcoma grows slowly and may infiltrate either along the chest wall or into the thoracic cavity. Rib chondrosarcoma originates from the rib cartilage, while sternum chondrosarcoma can develop from any part of the sternum, with lesions typically located centrally within the bone. Imaging studies often reveal characteristic features of chondrosarcoma (Figure 3-2-6) [48], including: ①Osteolytic bone destruction; ②Cartilage calcification; ③Periosteal reaction; ④Formation of tumor bone. Differentiating chondrosarcoma from osteosarcoma primarily hinges on the nature of the calcification. In osteosarcoma, calcification arises directly from primitive bone cells, representing primary calcification. Conversely, in chondrosarcoma, calcification is secondary, resulting from the malignant transformation of cartilage cells. Generally, chondrosarcoma is less aggressive, and Surgical

treatment tends to have favorable outcomes. Osteosarcoma, on the other hand, is typically more malignant and associated with a poorer prognosis.

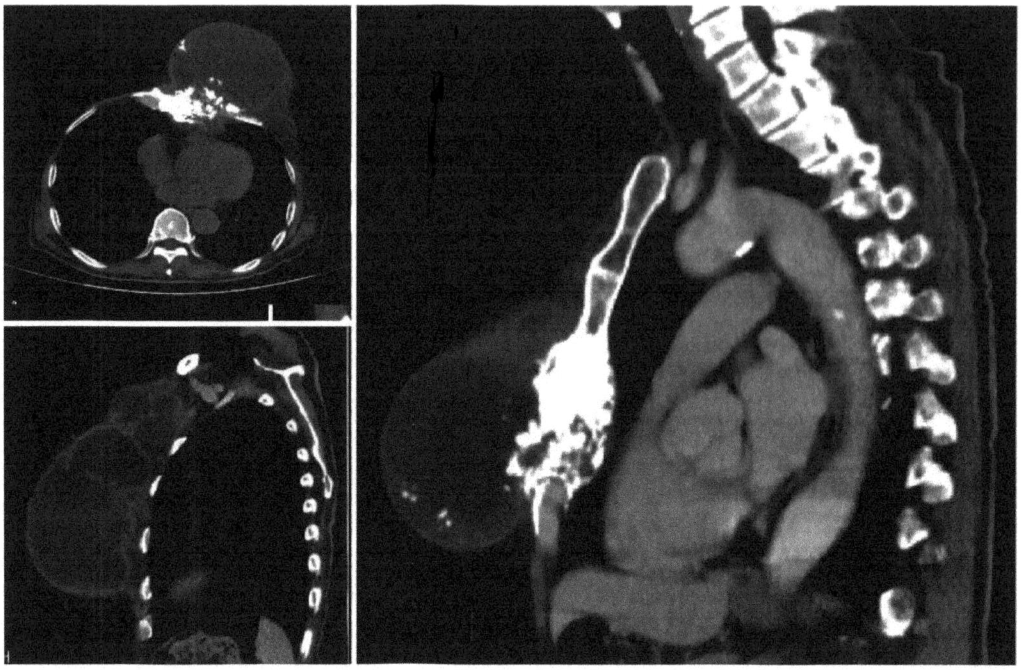

Figure 3-2-6 CT Features of Sternum Chondrosarcoma

(11) Chest Wall Metastases

Chest wall tumors can be broadly categorized into two types: primary tumors and metastatic tumors. The incidence of metastatic tumors is significantly higher than that of primary tumors. Since metastatic tumors are almost always malignant, they represent the most common type of malignant chest wall tumor [49–52]. Metastases to the chest wall primarily originate from cancers such as breast cancer, lung cancer, prostate cancer, Hodgkin's lymphoma, thyroid cancer, nasopharyngeal carcinoma, malignant tumors of the superior mediastinum, esophageal cancer, liver cancer, and gastric cancer. The metastatic sites are mostly bony structures, mainly the sternum and ribs, but other parts of the chest wall can also be affected (Figure 3-2-7). Bone metastases can present in three different forms [49]: ① Osteolytic metastases: This is the most common type, characterized by bone destruction. The bone damage can appear as irregular, moth-eaten areas or patchy destruction. Both the bone marrow and cortex may be involved. Cortical destruction may have either clear or blurred margins. Generally, there is no periosteal reaction, but soft tissue masses may form around the lesion. ② Osteoblastic metastases: This type is less common. It manifests as spotty, nodular, or densely sclerotic areas within the bone. The proliferative areas are evenly distributed, with normal trabeculae disappearing and blending into the bone cortex. There may be localized sclerosis and expansion, but usually no periosteal reaction or surrounding soft tissue masses.③ Mixed metastases: This less common type exhibits feature of both osteolytic and osteoblastic metastases. Typical imaging shows small patchy areas of bone destruction alongside small spots of high-density sclerotic proliferation.

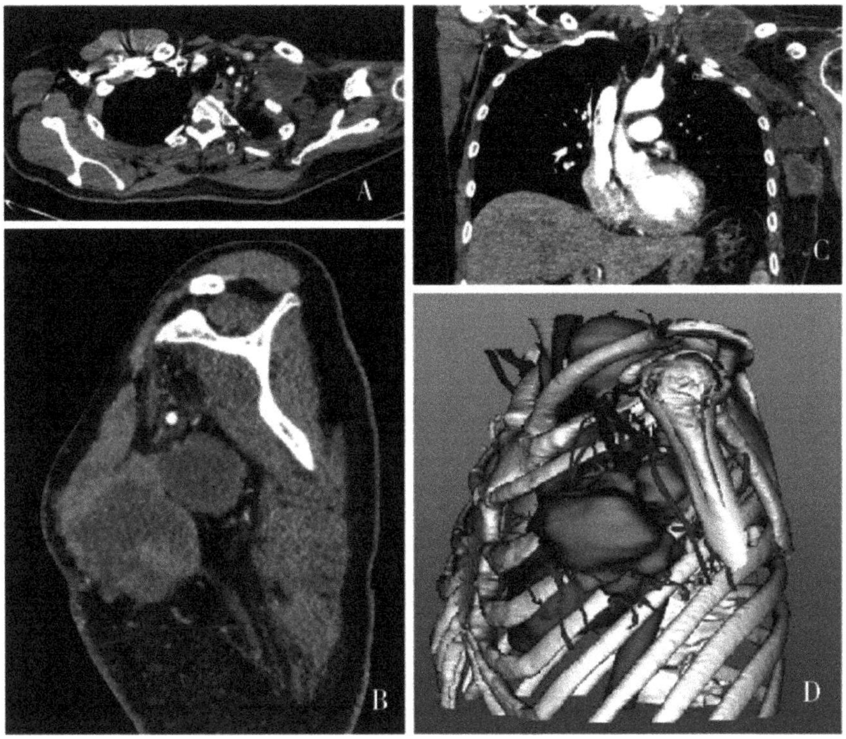

Figure 3-2-7 Chest Wall Metastatic Tumor. The tumor originates from skin cancer and is a squamous cell carcinoma. (A, B, C. CT signs of the tumor; D. 3D reconstruction image of the tumor)

Rib metastases tend to have a distinct distribution pattern, most commonly affecting the anterior ends of the lower ribs. Sternal metastases can occur at various locations, but are most frequently found in the body and manubrium of the sternum, with the xiphoid process rarely involved. The primary route of bone metastasis is hematogenous spread (via the bloodstream), although tumor cells may also enter the circulatory system indirectly through lymphatic channels, ultimately leading to metastatic spread.

When a primary tumor in another part of the body metastasizes to the chest wall, it is often accompanied by metastases to other regions. In such cases, the chest wall lesion represents only one part of a systemic metastatic process. Therefore, once a chest wall metastasis is confirmed, it is crucial to clarify two key points: The location of the primary tumor, and The presence of metastases elsewhere in the body. Only after both of these questions are answered can an optimal treatment strategy be developed. This approach highlights the most significant difference between the diagnosis and treatment of metastatic tumors and primary chest wall tumors.

(12) Invasive Tumors of the Chest Wall

Chest wall metastases are tumors that have spread from distant primary sites to the chest wall via various pathways. In these cases, there is no direct anatomical connection between the primary tumor and the chest wall metastasis meaning, spatially, the primary and metastatic lesions are not contiguous. However, in clinical practice, there is another category of chest wall tumor that results from direct invasion by adjacent malignancies. These tumors may originate in the lungs, mediastinum, pleura, breast, or even the retroperitoneum [53–56]. As these tumors expand and grow destructively, they may eventually involve the chest wall, forming a special type of chest wall tumor (Figure 3-2-8). In such cases, the invading lesion and the chest wall involvement are anatomically continuous, forming a single, uninterrupted mass clearly different from a metastasis. It's important to note that while these invasive tumors may also form metastatic lesions in the chest wall through distant spread, metastases lack direct spatial continuity with the primary tumor. Cytologically, metastatic and invasive tumors may appear identical; however, their gross morphology can differ significantly. This distinction has direct implications for Surgical management. For invasive tumors, where the lesion is continuous with the primary site, resection (if indicated) must involve en bloc removal of the entire affected area as a single Surgical procedure. In contrast, metastases being anatomically separate from the primary tumor typically require independent resections of each lesion.

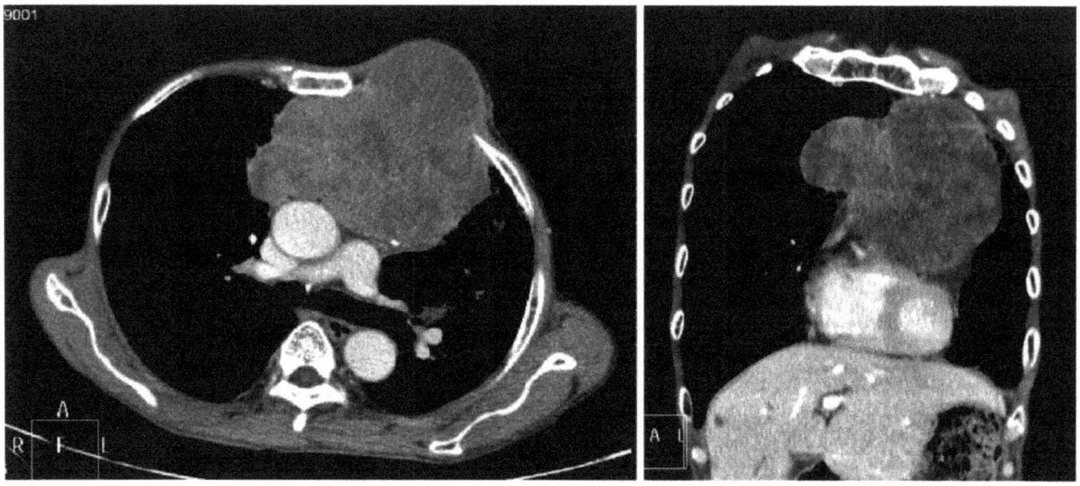

Figure 3-2-8: Tumor Originating from the Mediastinum

7. Significance of Understanding Tumor Pathology

Clinical management of chest wall tumors involves many aspects, primarily diagnosis and treatment. While these tasks may appear straightforward on the surface, they are in fact complex and demand a high level of clinical skill. Successfully managing such cases is a significant test of a physician's technical ability. At the core of all clinical efforts lies a fundamental requirement: understanding the nature of the tumor. Every tumor possesses a range of distinct characteristics, but its essential nature is revealed through its pathological features. The pathological characteristics of a tumor encompass a wide array of elements. These features directly influence the tumor's morphology, gross appearance, biological behavior, level of threat, progression, prognosis, and more. They determine the patient's symptoms and signs, influence the selection of diagnostic tests, guide the diagnostic process, shape the treatment plan, and ultimately affect the patient's outcome [1]. Therefore, when chest wall tumors are studied as a key area in thoracic Surgery, understanding their pathological characteristics becomes especially critical. For thoracic Surgeons aiming to achieve optimal clinical outcomes, a solid grasp of the pathological features of various tumors is essential it forms the foundation of all diagnostic and therapeutic work.

REFERENCES

[1] Wang, Wenlin. "Basic Characteristics of Chest Wall Tumors." Toutiao, October 31, 2021.
[2] Lü, Yongge, Luo Diling, Yang Maohong, et al. "Imaging Analysis of 65 Cases of Sternal Tumors." Journal of Jinan University (Natural Science and Medical Edition) 30, no. 2 (2009): 225–228.
[3] Zhang, Jianhua, Li Bin, Gou Yunjian, et al. "Reconstruction of Bony Chest Wall Defects with Artificial Composite Materials: A Report of 23 Cases." Chinese Journal of Modern Medicine 22, no. 12 (2012): 41–43.
[4] Shah, A. A., and T. A. D'Amico. "Primary Chest Wall Tumors." Journal of the American College of Surgeons 210, no. 3 (2010): 360–366.
[5] Xue, Liang, Jiang Ming, Yuan Yunfeng, et al. "Clinical Analysis of 12 Cases of Sternal Tumor Resection and Titanium Mesh Reconstruction." Journal of Fudan University (Medical Edition) 42, no. 3 (2015): 389–392.
[6] Xu, Qiming, Zhou Naikang, Liu Ying, et al. "Diagnosis and Surgical Treatment of 105 Cases of Chest Wall Tumors." Chinese Clinical Oncology 34, no. 13 (2007): 750–753.
[7] Lenze, U., A. Angelini, F. Pohlig, et al. "Chondrosarcoma of the Chest Wall: A Review of 53 Cases from Two Institutions." Anticancer Research 40, no. 3 (2020): 1519–1526.
[8] Han, Yulong. "Repair and Reconstruction of Chest Wall Defects After Tumor Resection." China Medicine 5, no. 10 (2010): 928–929.
[9] Scarnecchia, E., V. Liparulo, R. Capozzi, et al. "Chest Wall Resection and Reconstruction for Tumors: Analysis of Oncological and Functional Outcomes." Journal of Thoracic Disease 10, suppl. 16 (2018): S1855–S1863.
[10] Bagheri, R., S. Z. Haghi, M. Kalantari, et al. "Primary Malignant Chest Wall Tumors: Analysis of 40 Patients." Journal of Cardiothoracic Surgery 9 (2014): 106.

[11] Friesenbichler, J., A. Leithner, W. Maurer-Ertl, et al. "Surgical Therapy of Primary Malignant Bone Tumors and Soft Tissue Sarcomas of the Chest Wall: A Two-Institutional Experience." International Orthopaedics 38, no. 6 (2014): 1235–1240.
[12] Sorensen, T. R., M. Raedkjaer, P. H. Jørgensen, et al. "Soft Tissue Sarcomas of the Thoracic Wall: Higher Mortality and Local Recurrence—A Single-Institution Long-Term Follow-Up Study." International Journal of Surgical Oncology (2019): 2350157.
[13] Nakahashi, N., M. Emori, H. Tsuchie, et al. "Treatment Outcome of Chest Wall Soft Tissue Sarcomas: Analysis of Prognostic Factors." Journal of Surgical Oncology 120, no. 7 (2019): 1235–1240.
[14] Cipriano, A., and W. Burfeind. "Management of Primary Soft Tissue Tumors of the Chest Wall." Thoracic Surgery Clinics 27, no. 2 (2017): 139–147.
[15] Ma, Chaoyang, Guo Xiaolin, Ji Huifan, et al. "A Case Report of Primary Liver Cancer with Chest Wall Skin Metastasis." Journal of Clinical Hepatology 32, no. 4 (2016): 772–773.
[16] Vanderelst, A., G. Spiegel, and P. De Francquen. "Fibrous Dysplasia of the Rib." Journal Belge de Radiologie 71, no. 6 (1988): 742–743.
[17] Hoshi, M., S. Matsumoto, J. Manabe, et al. "Malignant Change Secondary to Fibrous Dysplasia." International Journal of Clinical Oncology 11, no. 3 (2006): 229–235.
[18] Van Rossem, C., P. Pauwels, J. Somville, et al. "Sarcomatous Degeneration in Fibrous Dysplasia of the Rib Cage." Annals of Thoracic Surgery 96, no. 4 (2013): E89–E90.
[19] Hughes, E. K., S. L. James, S. Butt, et al. "Benign Primary Tumours of the Ribs." Clinical Radiology 61, no. 4 (2006): 314–322.
[20] Karabakhtsian, R., D. Heller, M. Hameed, et al. "Periosteal Chondroma of the Rib: Report of a Case and Literature Review." Journal of Pediatric Surgery 40, no. 9 (2005): 1505–1507.
[21] Han, Min, Liu Entao, and Zhang Shengjian. "A Case of Extraskeletal Chondroma." Chinese Journal of Medical Imaging Technology 23, no. 1 (2007): 84.
[22] Gong, Lihua, Qian Zhanhua, Liu Baoyue, et al. "Clinicopathological Analysis of Enchondroma and Primary Chondrosarcoma of Long Bones." Journal of Diagnostic Pathology 19, no. 4 (2012): 248–251.
[23] Sharma, A. K., S. Patel, D. Meena, et al. "Large Sternal Exostoses Presenting as Stridor: A Surgical and Anesthetic Challenge." Journal of Cardiac Surgery 35, no. 9 (2020): 2388–2391.
[24] Zhao, T., and H. Zhao. "Computed Tomographic Image Processing and Reconstruction in the Diagnosis of Rare Osteochondroma." Computational and Mathematical Methods in Medicine (2021): 2827556.
[25] Du, H., H. Xu, and G. Che. "Malignant Giant Cell Tumor of the Rib with Lung Metastasis in a Man." Journal of Thoracic Disease 6, no. 9 (2014): 1307–1310.
[26] Sakanoue, I., H. Hamakawa, E. Onishi, et al. "Giant Cell Tumor of the Rib with Direct Invasion into the Thoracic Spine." General Thoracic and Cardiovascular Surgery 65, no. 5 (2017): 293–296.
[27] Zhang, Dianhong, Zhang Huaishuan, and Li Jiazhen. "Advances in the Treatment of Giant Cell Tumor of Bone." Chinese Journal of Practical Medicine 38, no. 7 (2011): 98–99.

[28] Kumar, V., R. S. Singh, S. Rawat, et al. "A Large Aneurysmal Bone Cyst of the Rib." Asian Cardiovascular and Thoracic Annals 27, no. 4 (2019): 313–315.
[29] Guo, J., and C. Liang. "A Giant Aneurysmal Bone Cyst of the Rib: Case Report." Oncology Letters 7, no. 1 (2014): 267–269.
[30] Medina, M., and S. Paul. "Aneurysmal Bone Cyst Arising from the First Rib: A Rare Cause of Thoracic Outlet Syndrome." Thoracic and Cardiovascular Surgeon Reports 5, no. 1 (2016): 74–76.
[31] Godfrey, G. C., J. M. Miller, and M. Ginsburg. "Eosinophilic Granuloma of the Rib." U.S. Armed Forces Medical Journal 11 (1960): 217–223.
[32] Pappas, C. A., H. F. Rheinlander, and M. J. Stadecker. "Pleural Effusion as a Complication of Solitary Eosinophilic Granuloma of the Rib." Human Pathology 11, no. 6 (1980): 675–677.
[33] Sharma, D., V. Rawat, and R. Yadav. "A Rare Case of Multiple Myeloma Presenting as Lytic Lesion of the Rib." Journal of Clinical and Diagnostic Research 10, no. 3 (2016): PD20–PD21.
[34] Goto, T., A. Maeshima, Y. Oyamada, et al. "Definitive Diagnosis of Multiple Myeloma from Rib Specimens Resected at Thoracotomy in a Patient with Lung Cancer." Interactive Cardiovascular and Thoracic Surgery 10, no. 6 (2010): 1051–1053.
[35] Tajima, K., N. Uchida, Y. Azuma, et al. "Surgical Resection of a Solitary Plasmacytoma Originating in a Rib." Annals of Thoracic and Cardiovascular Surgery 20 (Suppl) (2014): 609–612.
[36] Haser, G. C., H. K. Su, M. J. Pitman, et al. "Extramedullary Plasmacytoma of the Cricoid Cartilage with Solitary Plasmacytoma of the Rib." American Journal of Otolaryngology 36, no. 4 (2015): 598–600.
[37] Ruiz-Mesa, C., J. M. Goldberg, A. J. Coronado Muñoz, et al. "Rhabdomyosarcoma in Adults: New Perspectives on Therapy." Current Treatment Options in Oncology 16, no. 6 (2015): 27.
[38] Saenz, N. C., F. Ghavimi, W. Gerald, et al. "Chest Wall Rhabdomyosarcoma." Cancer 80, no. 8 (1997): 1513–1517.
[39] Siregar, K. B., and A. Azrah. "Pleomorphic Rhabdomyosarcoma of the Chest Wall with Intercostal Muscle Infiltration: A Case Report." International Journal of Surgery Case Reports 75 (2020): 380–384.
[40] Douglas, Y. L., K. J. Meuzelaar, B. van der Lei, et al. "Osteosarcoma of the Sternum." European Journal of Surgical Oncology 23, no. 1 (1997): 90–91.
[41] Rad, M. P., S. H. Fattahi-Masoum, P. Layegh, et al. "Primary Osteosarcoma of the Sternum: A Case Report and Review of the Literature." Archives of Bone and Joint Surgery 2, no. 4 (2014): 272–275.
[42] Zhang, X., and Z. Guan. "PET/CT in the Diagnosis and Prognosis of Osteosarcoma." Frontiers in Bioscience (Landmark Edition) 23 (2018): 2157–2165.
[43] Kundu, Z. S. "Classification, Imaging, Biopsy, and Staging of Osteosarcoma." Indian Journal of Orthopaedics 48, no. 3 (2014): 238–246.
[44] Brito, I. M., S. Teixeira, G. Paupério, et al. "Giant Chondrosarcoma of the Chest Wall: A Rare Surgical Challenge." Autopsy and Case Reports 10, no. 3 (2020): e2020166.
[45] Lenze, U., A. Angelini, F. Pohlig, et al. "Chondrosarcoma of the Chest Wall: A Review of 53 Cases from Two Institutions." Anticancer Research 40, no. 3 (2020): 1519–1526.

[46] Jiang, Zhiming, and Zhang Huizhen. "Differential Diagnosis and Special Histological Types of Chondrosarcoma." Clinical and Experimental Pathology 23, no. 5 (2007): 517–519.
[47] Zhang, Dongliang, Wu Dongqiang, and Zhang Zhihao. "Two Case Reports of Costal Chondrosarcoma and Literature Review." Zhejiang Clinical Medical Journal 21, no. 4 (2019): 570–571.
[48] Xue, Jinliang, Zhang Chao, Jin Chao, et al. "A Case of Well-Differentiated Chondrosarcoma of the Rib." Henan Medical Research 29, no. 5 (2020): 959–960.
[49] Tian, Peilin, Zhu Hongzhou, and Jiang Mingqiang. "CT and Clinical Analysis of Metastatic Tumors of the Sternum." Radiologic Practice 16, no. 6 (2001): 419–421.
[50] Porsok, S., M. Mego, D. Pind'ak, et al. "Chest Wall Tumor as a Rare Clinical Presentation of Hepatocellular Carcinoma Metastasis." Klinická Onkologie 30, no. 4 (2017): 299–301.
[51] Hyun, Y. S., H. S. Choi, J. H. Bae, et al. "Chest Wall Metastasis from Unknown Primary Site of Hepatocellular Carcinoma." World Journal of Gastroenterology 12, no. 13 (2006): 2139–2142.
[52] Dilek, O. N., E. O. Gur, T. Acar, et al. "Chest Wall Metastasis of Endometrial Cancer: Case Report and Review of the Literature." Acta Chirurgica Belgica 119, no. 4 (2019): 243–247.
[53] McCaughan, B. C., N. Martini, M. S. Bains, et al. "Chest Wall Invasion in Carcinoma of the Lung: Therapeutic and Prognostic Implications." Journal of Thoracic and Cardiovascular Surgery 89, no. 6 (1985): 836–841.
[54] Thomas-de-Montpreville, V., A. Chapelier, E. Fadel, et al. "Chest Wall Resection for Invasive Lung Carcinoma, Soft Tissue Sarcoma, and Other Malignancies: Pathologic Aspects in a Series of 107 Patients." Annals of Diagnostic Pathology 8, no. 4 (2004): 198–206.
[55] Sepesi, B. "Management of Breast Cancer Invading the Chest Wall." Thoracic Surgery Clinics 27, no. 2 (2017): 159–163.
[56] Ren, Anmin, and Zheng Weicai. "A Case of Chest Wall Metastasis after Surgery for Retroperitoneal Aggressive Fibromatosis." Hebei Medical Journal 33, no. 7 (2011): 1113–1115.

Chest wall tumors represent a fundamental category of diseases within chest wall Surgery. As such, their treatment should strictly follow the basic Surgical principles specific to this field. Chest wall Surgery is characterized by two essential and often competing objectives: oncologic resection (disease eradication) and reconstruction (restoration of form and function) [1,2]. Oncologic resection requires the complete removal of the tumor. To achieve this, Surgeons must exercise not only the tumor itself but also any surrounding tissues that may be at risk of harboring residual disease. Given that these tumors often originate from normal chest wall structures, the surrounding tissues typically include essential components of the chest wall. As a result, radical excision often leads to significant structural damage, compromising the integrity of the chest wall and making reconstruction more complex. In contrast, successful reconstruction aims to preserve or restore the anatomical and functional integrity of the chest wall. This goal necessitates minimizing tissue removal, which may conflict with the need for wide oncologic margins. Thus, there is an inherent tension between achieving oncologic control and maintaining structural integrity. These two goals, tumor eradication and reconstruction are interdependent yet contradictory. Optimal outcomes require a careful balance between the two. While this balance is relatively straightforward to achieve in routine Surgical cases, chest wall tumors pose a unique challenge due to their location and complexity. Striking the right compromise between thorough tumor resection and feasible reconstruction can be a difficult but critical aspect of Surgical decision-making in these cases.

In cases of benign tumors or extremely aggressive malignant tumors, balancing oncologic resection and reconstruction is relatively straightforward, as these represent two clinical extremes. For benign tumors, the risk to the patient is minimal, allowing greater emphasis to be placed on preserving or restoring chest wall structure and aesthetics. Conversely, in cases of highly aggressive malignancies, the priority is unequivocally on achieving complete tumor removal. In such situations, functional and cosmetic considerations must be willingly compromised to ensure oncologic control. When treatment clearly favors one objective, the other must often be sacrificed accordingly.

While balancing disease eradication and reconstruction is relatively straightforward in cases of either benign tumors or highly aggressive malignancies, managing this balance becomes more complex in typical, less clear-cut cases. In these situations, several factors must be considered, including the nature and behavior of the tumor, the Surgeon's technical capabilities, and the expectations or concerns of the patient and their family. Despite these external influences, the fundamental guiding principle must always be the nature of the disease itself. For instance, a patient may prioritize cosmetic outcomes after Surgery; however, if achieving complete tumor removal poses significant risk or necessitates sacrificing aesthetic results, oncologic safety must take priority. Even benign tumors though less aggressive are not to be underestimated, and effective treatment must remain the foremost concern.

1. Disease Treatment

For chest wall tumors, the primary method of treatment is tumor resection [3]. Ideally, once the lesion is clearly identified, complete excision should be performed. However, in clinical practice, Surgical removal is not always straightforward and requires careful consideration of various practical factors.

First, it is essential to distinguish the nature of the tumor, as different types require different Surgical approaches. For benign tumors, treatment can be achieved simply by removing the tumor itself. In contrast, malignant tumors demand a more rigorous excision; in addition to removing the tumor, a certain margin of healthy tissue around the lesion must also be excised. This margin removal is the minimum requirement for an adequate resection.

Second, the feasibility of complete tumor resection must be considered. For chest wall tumors, the ideal approach is the complete removal of all tumor tissue, also known as radical resection. However, in certain special circumstances, complete excision is not practical, and only partial resection can be performed. These situations include: ①Invasion of critical structures: When the tumor involves vital anatomical structures that cannot be removed. For example, tumors near the thoracic inlet may invade nerves or blood vessels beneath the clavicle. If these structures are involved, complete resection is not possible. ②Involvement of dangerous structures: Some tumors lie close to major blood vessels, or may directly invade them. Attempting radical excision in such cases may lead to intra operative complications. To ensure a safe procedure, partial resection may be necessary. ③Tumor obscured by important structures: When the tumor is located deep beneath structures that cannot be safely retracted or exposed, complete removal is difficult. For instance, tumors on the deep surface of the scapula may be challenging to fully expose, requiring partial resection. ④Extensive tumor invasion preventing reconstruction: When the tumor involves a very large area, especially if the skin or soft tissue is extensively affected, complete resection may leave a defect too large to repair. Without sufficient tissue for reconstruction, radical excision is not feasible. Incomplete tumor removal significantly reduces the effectiveness of Surgery. Such procedures are termed palliative Surgery. Although palliative Surgery is not curative, it may be necessary in certain cases. It can provide valuable time for further treatment and thus holds both clinical necessity and rational

justification.
Third, the risks associated with tumor resection must be carefully considered. The surrounding anatomical structures can significantly impact the safety of the Surgery, and certain characteristics of the tumor itself may also affect Surgical risk. For example, large vascular tumors, such as giant hemangiomas, may cause uncontrollable bleeding during removal. When performing Surgery on such tumors, it is essential to thoroughly evaluate the inherent risks and select the most appropriate Surgical approach to ensure the safest and most effective treatment plan.
Fourth, the functional implications of involved structures must be carefully considered. Both the tumor-invaded and adjacent normal tissues usually serve specific physiological functions. When removing the tumor or resecting surrounding tissues, the functional consequences of removing these structures must be taken into account to avoid serious complications. For example, in malignant tumors at the upper end of the sternum, standard Surgical guidelines often call for removal of the nearby sternoclavicular joint and part of the clavicle. However, considering the unique functions of the sternoclavicular joint, the extent of resection should be carefully reassessed. Similarly, for chest wall tumors invading the lung, if pulmonary function is not taken into account, maximal lung tissue removal might be pursued. Yet, if the patient already has compromised lung function, the extent of lung resection must be carefully limited to preserve respiratory capacity and prevent further deterioration.
In summary, although the curative aspect of chest wall tumor Surgery is fundamentally achieved through tumor resection, it is subject to many practical limitations. While tumor removal may seem straightforward in theory, the various constraints discussed make the procedure highly challenging in practice. Achieving complete tumor excision with an optimal balance of outcomes demands not only advanced Surgical skills but also careful judgment and planning.

2. Reconstruction

The essence of reconstructive Surgery is to alter the shape of a local area of the body. In a broad sense, reconstructive Surgery includes any procedure that changes shape, but clinically, meaningful reconstruction is defined by its ability to meet specific patient needs. In chest wall tumor Surgery, the tumor and certain surrounding structures must be removed. Since these structures often serve important functions, reconstruction is necessary to restore function. In this context, reconstruction refers specifically to the restoration of the chest wall [4]. Chest wall reconstruction has two fundamental goals: one is to restore the structural integrity of the chest wall, and the other is to optimize the appearance of the chest wall, making it as normal and aesthetically as pleasing as possible. These two objectives represent the core attributes of reconstructive Surgery. Achieving both ensures a successful and ideal reconstruction.

(1) Structural reconstruction

Reconstruction aims to restore the relevant anatomical structures. The closer the restored structure resembles the original, the better the outcome. The chest wall is a complex assembly of bones, soft tissues, and other specialized components. An ideal reconstruction should address two main aspects: restoring the components themselves and reestablishing their spatial relationships. Component restoration involves recovering as much of the original tissue as possible, while spatial reconstruction ensures that these components maintain their proper arrangement to function correctly. While the best outcome is achieved by replicating the chest wall's natural physiological structure, this level of precision is rarely achievable in practice. Clinically, reconstruction is often an approximate process. Typically, the bony framework is rebuilt first, with soft tissues and other structures restored as needed to preserve key physiological functions. As a result, what is commonly performed is partial rather than complete reconstruction of the chest wall.
Reconstruction procedures are generally categorized into three types: reconstruction of the bony structures, soft tissues, and skin.

(2) Reconstruction of Bony Structures

Most chest wall tumors invade the bony components of the chest wall, which must be removed during Surgery. This resection inevitably leaves defects in the bony framework. Therefore, reconstruction of the bony structures is a key part of most chest wall tumor Surgeries. The primary goal of this reconstruction is to restore the normal shape and stability of the thoracic cage. To achieve this, specialized materials are used to rebuild the bony framework.
Reconstruction of bony structures is not a new Surgical procedure and has been widely performed in the past [5,6]. The key challenge in these Surgeries is not the technique itself, which is relatively straightforward, but rather the choice of materials. When appropriate materials are used, the Surgery is simpler and the outcomes are significantly better; conversely, unsuitable materials can complicate the procedure and lead to suboptimal results. Historically, a variety of materials have been employed in clinical practice for chest wall reconstruction, including autologous tissue, allografts, devitalized xenografts, biological materials, synthetic polymers, and metals [3–10]. These materials differ widely in composition, shape, and effectiveness. Previous literature has outlined basic criteria for ideal reconstructive materials [8-10], such as adequate hardness, some degree of malleability, good tissue compatibility, absence of biological toxicity, and suitability for X-ray imaging. These requirements were reasonable and have generally been met by most materials used in the past. However, with ongoing advances in technology, some of these criteria such as the need for X-ray transparency are now considered less essential.
From the essence of reconstructive Surgery, an ideal reconstruction must

restore the structure as closely as possible to its original form; this is the fundamental requirement of any reconstructive procedure. Regarding the bony framework, achieving this goal requires that the reconstructed area closely approximates the physiological shape of the original bony structure [8–10].

For instance, after removing a rib, the reconstructed area should ideally replicate the rib's basic shape. The same principle applies to reconstructing the sternum. However, most previous reconstruction Surgeries have fallen short of this ideal. They often only restore certain chest wall functions, such as providing enough rigidity or preventing abnormal breathing patterns, but don't fully achieve the anatomical accuracy desired. In earlier clinical practice, these limited reconstructions became common partly because there was no solid scientific framework guiding the procedures, and partly because suitable materials were not available. Consequently, Surgeons had to work within these constraints, focusing on meeting only the minimum functional needs.

Working under the minimum functional requirements has been the norm in the past. However, a significant advancement in recent years in chest wall reconstruction has been the development of reconstruction materials designed according to the anatomical shape of the bony structures. There are three basic types of reconstruction materials: ①Traditional materials, such as various steel plates, meshes, and bone cement, which have been widely used clinically. These materials are convenient but were not originally designed specifically for reconstruction, so Surgical outcomes often fall short of expectations. ②Modular materials, which are newer and consist of components designed for different chest wall structures. ③These can be temporarily assembled during Surgery to best meet the specific needs of the procedure. A widely used example is MatrixRIB, which has proven effective in many chest wall reconstruction Surgeries (Figure 3-3-1). Customized, patient-specific materials that are manufactured based on detailed information about the patient's local defect. These require a special fabrication process and cannot be produced on demand during Surgery. Instead, they must be prepared preoperatively. Current personalized materials include digital materials, which come in two forms: 3D-printed implants [11] digitally customized implants [12]. In theory, these materials can replicate the original anatomy most closely, leading to more ideal reconstruction outcomes (Figure 3-3-2).

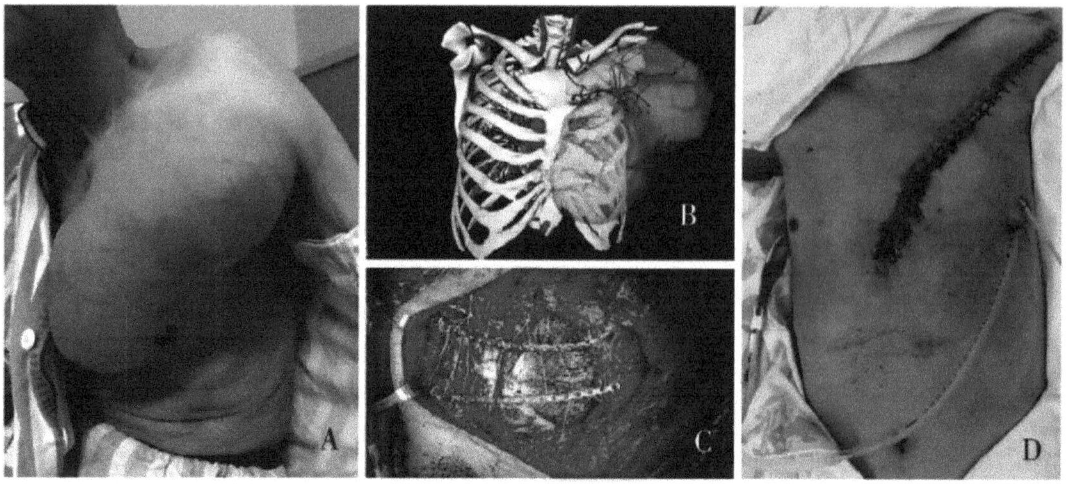

Figure 3-3-1 Modular material (MatrixRIB) chest wall reconstruction: (A. large anterior chest wall tumor;B. 3D reconstruction showing tumor location; C. tumor resection and reconstruction with MatrixRIB; D. postoperative chest wall appearance)

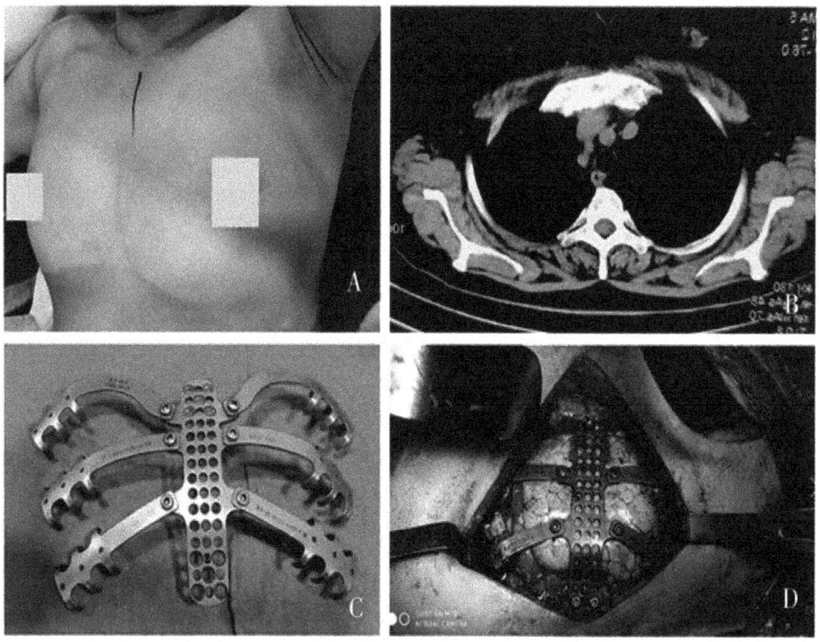

Figure 3-3-2 Chest wall reconstruction using digital materials: (A. patient with sternal tumor; B. CT image showing sternal tumor details; C. digital material designed based on local lesion data; D. digital material placed in chest wall defect after tumor resection for reconstruction)

Reconstructing the bony structure is usually straightforward. The primary task is to securely attach the reconstruction material to the surrounding bone around the defect. The material often requires precise shaping to fit the Surgical needs. Personalized design materials are theoretically the easiest to fix, as they are custom-made to match the patient's anatomy. However, this depends on achieving true customization. Successful design and fabrication of personalized materials require close collaboration and clear communication between Surgeons and engineers. Poor communication can result in materials that do not meet Surgical requirements, making the procedure more difficult.

(3) Soft Tissue reconstruction

Besides the bony framework, the chest wall contains abundant soft tissue, much of which often must be removed during chest wall tumor Surgery, leading to significant defects. To restore chest wall integrity, reconstruction of soft tissue is essential. Soft tissue reconstruction serves three key purposes: First, it fills the defect and maintains the normal physiological function of the chest wall. Although reconstructing the bones is fundamental after tumor removal, the chest wall is not solely made up of bone. Without soft tissue to fill the gaps between bones, complete reconstruction is impossible, and the basic airtight seal of the thoracic cavity cannot be preserved. Thus, soft tissue reconstruction is a vital supplement to bone reconstruction. Second, it corrects surface depressions and deformities, helping the chest wall maintain a more natural and aesthetically pleasing appearance. The goal of reconstruction Surgery is not only to restore chest wall integrity but also to achieve a normal or attractive external contour. No matter how precise the bone reconstruction, its appearance is limited to skeletal shape alone.

If left unrefined, the skeletal contours alone do not resemble a normal chest wall appearance. Therefore, soft tissue is essential to improve aesthetics. This is a critical part of every reconstruction procedure. The third function of soft tissue reconstruction is to cover the implanted materials and support proper postoperative healing. Achieving a good structural and cosmetic result depends first on the successful healing of the Surgical wound. If reconstruction materials are placed too close to the skin surface without sufficient soft tissue coverage, they can compromise wound healing and increase the risk of complications. To prevent this, adequate soft tissue must be used to wrap and cushion the artificial materials, an essential step in all reconstruction Surgeries.

The fundamental role of soft tissue reconstruction in chest wall tumor Surgery highlights the high demand for soft tissue. Since soft tissue cannot be replaced with artificial materials or transplanted from donors, the patient's own tissue is the only viable source. However, the quantity of autologous soft tissue is inherently limited, making it a valuable and finite resource. To ensure an adequate amount of soft tissue for reconstruction, it is essential to preserve as much tissue as possible within the Surgical field. If local soft tissue is insufficient, nearby regional tissue should be prioritized. Should that still prove inadequate, tissue must be harvested from other parts of the patient's body. This careful and stepwise approach is necessary to meet the demands of effective chest wall reconstruction.

Among the various tissues in the human body, the greater omentum is one of the most commonly used soft tissues in reconstruction [8]. It offers not only substantial volume but also strong anti-infective properties, making it a preferred choice for filling defects in other Surgical areas, especially when there is a risk of infection. However, in chest wall tumor Surgeries, the greater momentum is less frequently used due to its distance from the Surgical site and the generally low presence of infection in the operative field. When large soft tissue defects are present, muscle flaps of various types become the primary source for reconstruction, as they are more accessible and versatile in these cases.

In chest wall tumor surgeries, the most commonly used muscle flap is the pectoralis major flap, followed by the latissimus dorsi flap. For lesions located in the lower anterior chest wall, the rectus abdominis flap may be considered. These muscle flaps are often combined with skin flaps, forming a frequently used reconstructive option in sternal tumor resections. [8–10].

In soft tissue reconstruction, particular attention must be given to the reconstruction of the intercostal structures. Under normal conditions, the intercostal spaces are filled with intercostal muscles. However, during reconstruction Surgery, if no specific intervention is taken, these spaces may be covered loosely with soft tissue rather than securely reconstructed. This loose coverage does not anchor the soft tissue to the bony reconstruction materials, which may result in herniation of intrathoracic contents into the space between the reconstruction material, leading to a range of complications. Essentially, such an approach does not constitute true intercostal reconstruction. To address this issue, after reconstructing the bony structure, various types of synthetic mesh or fiber membranes are commonly used as internal linings, typically placed on the inner side of the reconstruction material. For added protection, an additional layer can be applied to the outer surface. Once properly lined, the reconstructed material is effectively separated from the thoracic organs, thereby achieving functional intercostal reconstruction and enhancing the overall Surgical outcome.

The above procedure primarily targets the reconstruction of intercostal structures. Although fiber membranes are not autologous tissue, their use can still be considered part of soft tissue reconstruction. Some refer to this as "pleural reconstruction," but this term is not entirely appropriate. The parietal pleura is an extremely thin anatomical layer, and reconstructing it in its original form is virtually impossible. Fiber membranes differ significantly from the pleura in both structure and function, and they are often used to cover the outer surface of reconstruction materials rather than replicate the pleura itself. Therefore, it is inaccurate to describe this procedure as pleural reconstruction.

(4) Skin reconstruction

Chest wall tumors can originate from various structures of the chest wall and may involve the skin. Some tumors even arise directly from the skin, causing direct damage. When the skin is affected, it must be removed along with the tumor during treatment. If the area of skin removal is small, direct suturing is possible; however, if the area is large, direct closure becomes very difficult. In such cases, various skin flaps are needed for reconstruction [8]. Skin flap reconstruction falls under the field of plastic Surgery. If the chest wall Surgeon is not skilled in this procedure, collaboration with a plastic Surgeon is necessary to complete the operation.

Similar to soft tissue reconstruction, the availability of skin from the patient's own body is extremely limited. Therefore, during skin reconstruction, it is essential to strictly follow relevant guidelines to maximize the effective use of the available skin.

(5) Aesthetic reconstruction

Aesthetic reconstruction focuses on restoring the appearance of the chest wall and involves three levels of requirements: ①Basic reconstruction: Ensures the Surgery is successfully completed without obvious symptoms or major complications postoperatively. ②Intermediate reconstruction: Aims to restore the chest wall's appearance as normally as possible, avoiding noticeable deformities. ③Advanced reconstruction: Not only ensures Surgical success but also strives to make the chest wall look as aesthetically pleasing as possible. Aesthetic reconstruction is not an independent procedure but is integrated into the reconstruction of various structures bone, soft tissue, and skin carried out simultaneously. To achieve satisfactory aesthetic results, it is essential to carefully consider the overall appearance of the chest wall, meticulously shape and structure the reconstructive materials, and thoughtfully plan the Surgical details. Only through this comprehensive approach can an ideal aesthetic outcome be achieved.

Achieving a perfect aesthetic reconstruction is not easy and requires attention at every step. First, during the reconstruction of the bony structure, a solid foundation must be laid to create a flawless chest contour. As the chest wall's skeletal framework, this is the basis for the entire reconstruction, so it must be completed satisfactorily. Second, during soft tissue reconstruction, the surface deformities of the chest wall must be carefully shaped to achieve a normal appearance. Third, in skin reconstruction, special attention must be given to the design and execution of incisions to minimize scarring and its impact on aesthetics.

Chest wall tumor Surgery is highly destructive, so achieving even a primary or intermediate level of reconstruction is already a significant accomplishment. To reach an advanced level of reconstruction, beyond standard reconstructive techniques, some cosmetic skills are also required. This raises the technical demands of the procedure and inevitably increases the cost for the patient. From a purely tumor treatment perspective, many may not support such elaborate procedures. However, if a more aesthetically pleasing outcome can be achieved at a relatively low additional cost, it would be widely welcomed. This trend places higher demands on chest wall Surgeons. Traditionally, the focus of chest wall tumor Surgery has been mainly on treating the disease, a reluctant choice due to the inability to simultaneously ensure both effective treatment and good appearance. It is easy to imagine that if patients could receive not only successful treatment but also an aesthetically pleasing chest wall, they would be much more willing to undergo Surgery. Therefore, placing greater emphasis on cosmetic elements in chest wall Surgery will be a key direction for Surgeons and one of the important paths for the discipline's future development.

REFERENCES

[1] Wang, W. 2021. "Basic Nature of Chest Wall Surgery." *Jinri Toutiao*, October 31, 2021.

[2] Wang, W. 2021. "Chest Wall Surgery: Shaping and Reconstruction." *Jinri Toutiao*, October 31, 2021.

[3] Foroulis, C. N., A. D. Kleontas, G. Tagarakis, et al. 2016. "Massive Chest Wall Resection and Reconstruction for Malignant Disease." *OncoTargets and Therapy* 9: 2349–2358.

[4] Sandler, G., and A. Hayes-Jordan. 2018. "Chest Wall Reconstruction After Tumor Resection." *Seminars in Pediatric Surgery* 27 (3): 200–206.

[5] Ferraro, P., S. Cugno, M. Liberman, et al. 2010. "Principles of Chest Wall Resection and Reconstruction." *Thoracic Surgery Clinics* 20 (4): 465–473.

[6] Rocco, G. 2011. "Chest Wall Resection and Reconstruction According to the Principles of Biomimesis." *Seminars in Thoracic and Cardiovascular Surgery* 23 (4): 307–313.

[7] Salo, J. T. K., and E. J. Tukiainen. 2018. "Oncologic Resection and Reconstruction of the Chest Wall: A 19-Year Single-Center Experience." *Plastic and Reconstructive Surgery* 142 (2): 536–547.

[8] Seder, C. W., and G. Rocco. 2016. "Chest Wall Reconstruction After Extended Resection." *Journal of Thoracic Disease* 8 (Suppl 11): S863–S871.

[9] Harati, K., J. Kolbenschlag, B. Behr, et al. 2015. "Thoracic Wall Reconstruction After Tumor Resection." *Frontiers in Oncology* 5: 247.

[10] Sanna, S., J. Brandolini, A. Pardolesi, et al. 2017. "Materials and Techniques in Chest Wall Reconstruction: A Review." *Journal of Visualized Surgery* 3: 95.

[11] Aragon, J., and I. P. Mendez. 2016. "Dynamic 3D-Printed Titanium Prosthesis: A Novel Design for Large Chest Wall Resection and Reconstruction." *Journal of Thoracic Disease* 8 (6): E385–E389.

[12] Wang, W. 2020. "Digital Materials for Chest Wall Reconstruction: Combined Surgery for Recurrent Breast Cancer with Superior Vena Cava and Chest Wall Reconstruction." *Thoracic Deformity Surgery Expert*, May 11, 2020.

The chest wall is an organic whole with specific functions, and its effective functioning depends on maintaining structural integrity. In the treatment of chest wall Surgical diseases, it is often necessary to remove part of the chest wall structure [1], and many chest wall diseases themselves involve structural defects [2]. These factors lead to the disruption of the chest wall's integrity and affect its normal function. Therefore, whenever there is a chest wall defect, whether primary or secondary, after lesion resection, reconstruction is required. The chest wall consists of three basic components: the bony structure, soft tissue, and skin. To restore the integrity of the chest wall, reconstruction must address all three. Due to the unique nature of these structures, soft tissue and skin reconstructions require the use of autologous tissue, while reconstruction of the bony structure is more complex and allows for a variety of material choices. These materials may include autologous tissue, allogeneic materials, xenogeneic materials, or even synthetic materials. Since the sources vary, their properties and characteristics differ as well. To ensure the success of the reconstruction Surgery, an in-depth understanding of these materials is essential.

1. Materials for reconstructing Skin and Soft Tissue

For simple skin defects, various types of skin flaps can be considered for reconstruction. These flaps may be sourced from the area surrounding the lesion or from other parts of the body. They can be pedicled flaps with a vascular supply or free flaps. Additionally, flaps can be purely skin-based or composite flaps that include soft tissue.

There are various options for soft tissue reconstruction materials. In terms of tissue source, these can include muscle tissue or adipose (fat) tissue. Generally, tissues located nearby are preferred. Muscle flaps or other soft tissues surrounding the lesion are commonly used for soft tissue reconstruction [3]. The momentum, a composite soft tissue, is particularly useful for certain soft tissue defects in the lower chest wall [4].

When simultaneous reconstruction of skin and soft tissue is needed, various types of musculocutaneous flaps can be used [5-9]. The pectoralis major flap and latissimus dorsi flap are the most commonly employed and can cover most areas of the upper and lateral chest wall. For the mid-lower chest wall, the rectus abdominis flap is highly effective. In cases of extensive defects or when the above flaps cannot be used such as when the internal thoracic artery is unavailable due to coronary artery bypass grafting, flaps from distant parts of the body may be considered. Various pedicled musculocutaneous flaps from remote sites then become valuable options for reconstruction.

Skin and soft tissue reconstruction materials are all derived from the patient's own body, which provides the major benefits of no immune rejection and excellent tissue compatibility. When well supplied with blood, these tissues also have strong resistance to infection. However, because they must be harvested from other areas of the body, there are inherent limitations: ① the amount of tissue available is limited and cannot be harvested indefinitely; ② harvesting causes additional trauma that may affect the function of the donor site; ③ the procedure requires incisions on the body surface, which can impact the appearance of the donor area; ④ the harvesting process adds complexity and length to the Surgery.

To minimize the drawbacks of harvesting skin and soft tissue for reconstruction, the following principles should be observed: ① Proximity priority: If the skin or soft tissue near the defect can meet the reconstruction needs, these should be chosen first. Harvesting nearby tissue avoids unnecessary damage to distant sites and simplifies the Surgery. ② Concealed area priority: When sufficient tissue is not available nearby and distant harvesting is required, donor sites located in less visible or concealed areas should be preferred to minimize cosmetic impact on the donor site. ③ Non-essential area priority: Tissue should not be taken from regions with

critical physiological functions, as harvesting there could impair those functions. Instead, tissues should be sourced from areas with less functional importance. ④ Rich blood supply priority: Adequate blood supply is essential for the tissue to survive and function properly after reconstruction. Therefore, donor tissue with good vascularization must be prioritized. ⑤ Minimization of harvested tissue: To reduce damage to the donor site, the smallest amount of tissue needed to achieve reconstruction should be harvested.

Skin and soft tissue are essential materials for chest wall reconstruction. Although it may not be necessary to deliberately harvest tissue from other parts of the body for small defects, the undeniable fact is that whenever there is a defect and soft tissue and incisions are sutured, reconstruction of soft tissue and skin is inevitably involved, often done unconsciously. This means that in many reconstruction Surgeries, the reconstruction of skin and soft tissue is overlooked. When the procedure is neglected, the importance of these materials is also undervalued. Conversely, if more attention is paid to these materials and procedures, the reconstruction outcomes will inevitably be more ideal.

2. Bone Structure reconstruction Materials

The target structures for bone reconstruction materials are the various bones of the chest wall, and their purpose is to fulfill the functions of the original bones. Therefore, all materials should possess properties similar to those of natural bone. Considering that these materials need to be permanently implanted in the human body, higher standards are required for their characteristics. The ideal materials should have the following fundamental properties [3-9]: ① Tissue Compatibility: Since the materials will remain permanently inside the body, they must be accepted by the human body and not be recognized as foreign objects that trigger a strong rejection response. Without good tissue compatibility, the material fails the basic requirement for implantation. ② Infection Resistance: After implantation, reconstruction materials need to integrate with surrounding structures and persist long-term. Ensuring wound healing is the first step for material survival. Materials with strong anti-infective properties help prevent infection of the incision and wound, laying a solid foundation for successful implantation. Without this property, pathogens can easily colonize and multiply on the material's surface, leading to infections and ultimately Surgical failure. ③ Adequate Mechanical Strength: Bone reconstruction materials are meant to replace bone, so they must possess sufficient mechanical strength. This is the minimum requirement for any bone substitute. Materials that do not meet strength requirements are unsuitable for reconstruction. ④ Necessary Plasticity: The ultimate purpose of reconstruction materials is to be used in Surgery. During the procedure, the material must be shaped to fit the defect precisely. To ensure successful reconstruction, adjustments to the material's shape and other physical parameters are necessary, requiring the material to have a certain degree of plasticity. This property is essential for smooth Surgical handling. Additionally, because the normal chest wall possesses some flexibility, the implanted material should also have a degree of flexibility and must not be overly rigid. ⑤ Non-toxicity: Synthetic materials may sometimes have inherent toxicity due to manufacturing processes. Prolonged exposure to such toxicity can cause harm to the body. Therefore, reconstruction materials must be non-toxic; otherwise, they cannot be used in Surgery. ⑥ No Carcinogenic Risk: Some materials may not exhibit general toxicity but could pose a carcinogenic risk. Such materials are even less suitable for use in reconstruction. Different authors may phrase the requirements for reconstruction materials differently, but the core criteria remain consistent. This consensus underscores the fundamental standards that materials must meet. Any material failing to satisfy these basic properties is deemed unsuitable for reconstructive surgery.

(1) Autologous Bone Materials

Autologous bone materials are primarily sourced from the patient's own skeletal structures [3]. The two most commonly used types are: autologous ribs and autologous iliac bone. Both of these can be utilized for reconstructing relatively large chest wall defects.

Ribs are part of the chest wall's bony structure, so using autologous ribs for chest wall reconstruction may seem contradictory, but it is justifiable when repairing more critical defects, such as those in the sternum, a key load-bearing and stabilizing structure. Sacrificing local ribs to restore thoracic stability can be necessary. Autologous ribs have advantages like easy accessibility, no rejection risk, and survival without vascular pedicles. However, they also have drawbacks: harvesting ribs creates new local defects, the available quantity is limited, and their fixed shape offers poor plasticity, which can affect aesthetic outcomes. While using autologous ribs can be a reasonable compromise when better options are unavailable, alternative materials are generally preferred due to these limitations.

Autologous iliac bone is also a commonly used material for chest wall reconstruction, particularly for repairing internal defects. Although it shares similar advantages with autologous ribs, such as biocompatibility and no rejection, it must be harvested from a more distant site, which brings comparable drawbacks. Therefore, if alternative materials are available, autologous iliac bone should generally be avoided.

(2) Allogeneic Bone Materials

Allogeneic bone materials are a special category of materials whose physical properties can closely match those of the target reconstruction site [3]. However, these materials have obvious drawbacks: ①there are restrictions on the source of the materials and they cannot be obtained in large quantities; ② there are problems with tissue compatibility and rejection may occur; ③ there are ethical restrictions. Because of these defects, it is difficult to use these materials on a large scale in clinical practice.

(3) Allogenic bone material

Xenograft bone materials are specially treated animal bone materials, which are easier to obtain than autologous or allogeneic materials, but have more problems, among which histocompatibility is the key problem that restricts their wide application, and it is extremely difficult to solve this problem.

(4) Xenogeneic Membranous Materials

Xenogeneic membranous materials mainly include specially processed bovine pericardium, porcine pericardium, and dura mater-like materials [10]. Theoretically, the repair of bony defects requires rigid materials for reconstruction. However, in clinical practice, doctors often use these membranous materials for reconstructive Surgeries. The fundamental reason is that these membranous structures possess sufficient mechanical strength. When firmly fixed to the bony structures surrounding the defect, they can fulfill part of the chest wall's functional requirements. Although these functions are not complete, they are generally sufficient to meet basic physiological needs. Clinically, such materials are occasionally used in reconstructive Surgeries and have yielded relatively satisfactory results.

Xenogeneic membranous materials have many advantages: they are relatively easy to obtain and are simple to handle. However, they also face issues such as biocompatibility. Additionally, as materials for reconstructing bony defects, membranous materials often struggle to meet all the necessary technical requirements.

(5) Artificial Materials

Based on different design approaches, artificial materials can be categorized into three types: ①General materials; ②Standardized materials; ③Custom-designed materials. General materials are not specifically designed for chest wall reconstruction and are mostly used temporarily during reconstruction Surgeries. Standardized materials are designed with modular components tailored to the needs of chest wall reconstruction, which can be assembled during the operation according to Surgical requirements. Custom-designed materials are specially created based on the individual Surgical needs of each patient and, in theory, can best meet Surgical demands.

(i) General Materials

1. Metal Materials.

Metal materials are among the most commonly used reconstructive materials in clinical practice. These include stainless steel, titanium alloys, and other types of metals [3]. Metal materials can be processed and designed according to reconstruction requirements to ensure that their physical properties meet Surgical needs as much as possible, which gives them certain advantages.

Currently, titanium alloys are the most widely used in clinical settings. They are available as plates or meshes, with titanium mesh being particularly common. Titanium alloys are lightweight, highly inert, and have good biocompatibility, making them the most frequently used reconstructive material today. Titanium mesh can be trimmed to fit the size of the defect and then fixed around the damaged area. It has sufficient hardness to effectively restore the integrity of the chest wall. However, this material lacks elasticity and cannot provide the chest wall with good physiological function. As a result, patients may experience various discomforts or even complications after Surgery. Therefore, it is not considered an ideal material.

Other metal materials include stainless steel, Kirschner wires, and medical-grade steel wires. These materials are not specifically designed for reconstructing the bony structure of the chest wall. While they may fulfill the requirements of certain reconstruction Surgeries, they often fail to achieve optimal results. The use of Kirschner wires is generally a last resort and reflects a lack of Surgical preparedness. Some practitioners use steel wires to weave a mesh back and forth across the defect. Clearly, such a mesh cannot be compared to a titanium mesh and is likewise an inappropriate approach.

MatrixRIB is a special type of metal material originally designed to stabilize fractured ribs. It is shaped similarly to a rib, and its length can be selected as needed, while the curvature can be adjusted during Surgery. In rib fracture Surgeries, this material is relatively easy to use. In recent years, it has gradually been applied to chest wall reconstruction Surgeries as well. It is now used not only for rib reconstruction but also for the reconstruction of other bony structures [11]. Since this material does not require intraoperative modification and can flexibly accommodate various Surgical needs, it is considered a relatively ideal reconstructive material.

2. Synthetic Materials

In clinical practice, many synthetic materials have been used for the reconstruction of bony structures. These materials are readily available, but due to various technical limitations, they often cannot fully meet Surgical requirements. Synthetic materials that have been used in clinical settings include plexiglass (acrylic), bone cement, various synthetic membranes, and other synthetic compounds.

Plexiglass has the advantages of being cuttable and moldable. With thorough preoperative preparation, it is possible to achieve a suitable shape that meets Surgical needs. However, many of its physical, chemical, and biological properties do not align with the ideal requirements for reconstructive materials. As a result, it is not considered an ideal material for reconstruction and has been rarely used in recent years [10].

Bone cement is a commonly used reconstructive material, but it is not used on its own. Instead, it is typically sandwiched between two layers of polypropylene mesh in what is referred to as a "sandwich" configuration [12,13]. Bone cement itself is not a single type of material; it can include polymethyl methacrylate (PMMA), calcium phosphate cement, and magnesium phosphate cement. Bone cement is relatively strong, easy to shape, simple to operate, and can be molded into a perfect form. However, bone cement also has several significant drawbacks: First, It is difficult to form a strong bony union with human bone and is prone to loosening; Second, It has poor tissue compatibility and always remains a foreign object in the body; Third, It carries risks of allergenicity and carcinogenicity, making long-term use unsafe; Fourth, It is too rigid and lacks elasticity, failing to meet physiological demands. Fifth, When used in reconstruction Surgeries, it is generally shaped into flat plates, which differ significantly from the natural curvature of the chest wall's bony structures. This mismatch can affect function and lead to postoperative discomfort.

In addition to the above-mentioned synthetic materials, synthetic membranous materials are also used in clinical chest wall reconstruction. Similar to xenogeneic membranes, these are also membranous in form. When used as materials for bony reconstruction, they inherently suffer from natural limitations. However, in situations where no other materials are available, the use of such membranes can be considered reasonable as a temporary substitute. Currently used synthetic membrane materials in clinical practice include polytetrafluoroethylene During the reconstruction of defects, when these materials are tightly fixed and stretched over the center of the defect, they provide basic mechanical strength, which helps eliminate paradoxical respiration in the defect area and partially restore the integrity of the thoracic cage. However, such materials still fall far short of meeting the requirements for reconstructing bony structures, and therefore, they are not considered ideal reconstructive materials.

All of the materials mentioned above are non-degradable synthetic materials. For a long time, there has been interest in using degradable materials to replace non-degradable ones. The basic idea is that, in the early postoperative period, these materials can provide essential support for reconstruction, and as the body's own tissues gradually regenerate, the materials will be absorbed and ultimately eliminated as foreign substances. This concept has a certain degree of rationality. However, for bony structures which are special and difficult to regenerate this idea seems unrealistic. Once the reconstruction material degrades, if the body's own bone structure has not regenerated, it can lead to problems with the shape and structure of the chest wall. Therefore, such materials are not suitable for use in the reconstruction of bony structures.

Currently, the most extensively studied degradable material is poly-p-dioxanone. This material has good degradability, and basic research has shown that it can be used for reconstruction of human structures. However, it is precisely because of its degradability that its application in chest wall bone structure reconstruction surgeries is limited [13].

(ii) Standardized Materials

Standardized materials are a special type of reconstruction material. To meet the needs of reconstruction at different sites, these materials are pre-designed into various components that replicate major structures of the chest wall. During Surgery, they can be assembled on-site as needed to fulfill different reconstruction purposes. Strictly speaking, MatrixRIB is a type of standardized material. It can be trimmed, assembled, and shaped during Surgery to meet specific Surgical needs. There are also other standardized materials in clinical use. These include various components that replicate parts of the sternum and ribs, which can be temporarily assembled according to Surgical requirements. The purpose of designing standardized materials is to offer greater flexibility in meeting reconstruction demands, aiming to come as close as possible to personalized solutions. If the components are well-designed, this type of material can be very practical.

(iii) Custom-designed materials

Custom-designed materials refer to what we have recently termed “digital materials." This is an entirely new concept and does not refer to a single specific material, but rather a category of specially designed materials. The term "digital" highlights the digitally-driven processing involved in their creation [14,15]. The digital aspect underscores the high precision and customization of the design.

Digital materials are custom-made reconstruction materials developed through a series of digital processes based on the specific characteristics of the lesion. Digitalization and personalization are the most distinctive features of this class of materials.

The production of digital materials requires a series of specific processes [15]. The first step is obtaining the patient's original data, usually through CT scans, which provide data primarily in DICOM format. The second step involves constructing a complete 3D image of the chest wall based on this original data. This 3D image not only includes a three- dimensional view of the lesion but also shows the entire chest wall and other thoracic structures. The third step is to simulate the Surgical resection range on the 3D image and design the shape of the reconstruction material accordingly. The fourth step is to fabricate the reconstruction material based on the design plan.

Throughout the process, every step and component are centered around the patient's lesion data, ensuring a fully digital workflow. Thus, these are referred to as digital materials. There are various manufacturing techniques available for producing the final material CNC machining can be used, or it can be directly fabricated with a 3D printer, a method that has gained significant attention in recent years. Materials produced through

The latter are referred to as 3D-printed materials, though they still fall under the broader category of digital materials [16,17].

Digital materials are characterized by a distinct level of personalization, which manifests on three levels: ① Targeted to a specific patient; ② Tailored to a specific lesion; ③ Designed for a specific Surgical procedure. Due to this high degree of personalization, digital materials are believed to best meet Surgical requirements and are therefore considered the theoretically most ideal reconstruction materials.

However, digital materials also come with a number of practical issues. First, the personalized nature of these materials is an idealistic goal envisioned by the designers. If this goal can be fully realized, then such materials would indeed be the best option. However, the fabrication process requires close cooperation and communication between the Surgeon and the material engineers. If there is a lack of adequate interaction and mutual understanding between the two, the resulting material may deviate from the intended personalization, making it far from ideal. In clinical practice, such situations are not uncommon; in fact, they occur quite frequently, thereby significantly undermining the advantages of personalization. Second, the design and manufacturing process demands the full involvement of the Surgeon, which can consume a considerable amount of their time and energy, ultimately affecting clinical duties. Third, the production process is lengthy and complex, requiring the patient to wait a long time before the Surgery can be performed. Fourth, over- personalization may actually complicate the Surgery. Instead of facilitating the procedure, it can restrict the Surgeon's operational flexibility. For example, in the case of sternum and first rib defects, if the design insists on reconstructing the first rib along with the sternum solely for the sake of personalization, the digital material design could pose major Surgical challenges and risks, potentially even leading to Surgical failure. Therefore, although digital materials offer many advantages, they are not perfect. Their application must be guided by a balanced and comprehensive evaluation of various practical factors to ensure optimal use.

Considering the complexity of reconstructing the sternum and surrounding structures, digital materials can be given priority for reconstruction in this area. However, for reconstruction Surgeries involving only the lateral chest wall, which primarily focus on the ribs, digital materials offer no particular advantage. In contrast, MatrixRIB is a more rational choice [11]. Given the various superior qualities of MatrixRIB, if no better reconstruction materials are available, this material is virtually universal and could be considered the most ideal option. Even for sternal reconstruction, it can produce excellent results.

In conclusion, there are various materials available for chest wall reconstruction, each with its own characteristics. These features can meet the requirements of reconstructive Surgery from different angles and levels. In actual Surgical practice, it is essential to select appropriate materials based on the specific characteristics of the Surgery. Only in this way can the success of the operation be ensured; otherwise, it may seriously affect the Surgical outcome.

REFERENCES

[1] Foroulis, C. N., A. D. Kleontas, G. Tagarakis, et al. 2016. "Massive Chest Wall Resection and Reconstruction for Malignant Disease." *OncoTargets and Therapy* 9: 2349–2358.

[2] Raz, D. J., S. L. Clancy, et al. 2017. "Surgical Management of the Radiated Chest Wall and Its Complications." *Thoracic Surgery Clinics* 27 (2): 171–179.

[3] Sanna, S., J. Brandolini, A. Pardolesi, et al. 2017. "Materials and Techniques in Chest Wall Reconstruction: A Review." *Journal of Visualized Surgery* 3: 95.

[4] Seder, C. W., and G. Rocco. 2016. "Chest Wall Reconstruction After Extended Resection." *Journal of Thoracic Disease* 8 (Suppl 11): S863–S871.

[5] Sandler, G., and A. Hayes-Jordan. 2018. "Chest Wall Reconstruction After Tumor Resection." *Seminars in Pediatric Surgery* 27 (3): 200–206.

[6] Ferraro, P., S. Cugno, M. Liberman, et al. 2010. "Principles of Chest Wall Resection and Reconstruction." *Thoracic Surgery Clinics* 20 (4): 465–473.

[7] Rocco, G. 2011. "Chest Wall Resection and Reconstruction According to the

Principles of Biomimesis." *Seminars in Thoracic and Cardiovascular Surgery* 23 (4): 307–313.
[8] Salo, J. T. K., and E. J. Tukiainen. 2018. "Oncologic Resection and Reconstruction of the Chest Wall: A 19-Year Single-Center Experience." *Plastic and Reconstructive Surgery* 142 (2): 536–547.
[9] Harati, K., J. Kolbenschlag, B. Behr, et al. 2015. "Thoracic Wall Reconstruction After Tumor Resection." *Frontiers in Oncology* 5: 247.
[10] Mao, N., C. Zuo, Y. Zhou, et al. 2005. "Surgical Treatment of Chest Wall Tumors." *Chinese Journal of Clinical Thoracic and Cardiovascular Surgery* 12 (4): 299–300.
[11] Wang, W. 2018. "Application of MatrixRIB Repair Material in Complex Chest Wall Surgeries." *Thoracic Deformity Surgery Expert*, April 17, 2018.
[12] Aghajanzadeh, M., A. Alavi, G. Aghajanzadeh, et al. 2015. "Chest Wall Reconstruction Using a Two-Layer Prolene Mesh and Bone Cement Sandwich Technique." *Indian Journal of Surgery* 77 (Suppl 1): 39–43.
[13] Du, R., N. Yu, X. Long, et al. 2018. "Advances in the Application of Chest Wall Reconstruction Materials." *Journal of the Chinese Academy of Medical Sciences* 40 (2): 289–293.
[14] Wang, W. 2019. "Broad and Narrow Definitions of Digital Materials." *Thoracic Deformity Surgery Expert*, November 23, 2019.
[15] Wang, W. 2019. "Personalized Characteristics of Digital Materials." *Thoracic Deformity Surgery Expert*, November 24, 2019.
[16] Smelt, J., A. Pontiki, M. Jahangiri, et al. 2020. "Three-Dimensional Printing for Chest Wall Reconstruction in Thoracic Surgery." *Thoracic and Cardiovascular Surgeon* 68 (4): 352–356.
[17] Aragon, J., and I. P. Mendez. 2016. "Dynamic 3D-Printed Titanium Prosthesis: A Novel Design for Large Chest Wall Resection and Reconstruction." *Journal of Thoracic Disease* 8 (6): E385–E389.

Sternal tumors are relatively rare, with a low incidence accounting for only about 15% of chest wall tumors and less than 1% of all bone tumors [1]. These tumors can affect any part of the sternum. They may be primary tumors originating in the sternum or metastatic tumors that have spread from other locations. Once a sternal tumor develops, it can adversely affect not only the sternum itself but also the entire chest wall and thoracic cavity, and therefore must be appropriately treated.

The sternum has a rich blood supply, making it a common site for metastatic tumors [2,3]. Additionally, myelomas and cartilage-derived tumors are also prone to develop in the sternum. Views on the incidence and nature of sternal tumors vary; some authors believe malignant tumors, especially metastases and multiple myeloma, are more common, while others suggest benign tumors predominate. Common benign tumors include chondromas, osteochondromas, desmoid tumors, and fibrous dysplasia, whereas malignant tumors include rhabdomyosarcoma, lymphoma, osteosarcoma, and chondrosarcoma, the latter being the most frequently observed malignant type [1,4].

The sternum is an important structure of the human body with five main functions: First, it serves as the primary load-bearing structure of the chest. Located at the front of the torso, it is the only bony structure in the front center of the body, working together with the thoracic vertebrae to support the weight of the torso, including not only the chest but also the abdominal structures. When the body is upright, the torso's weight is borne by both the sternum and the spine. Second, the sternum plays a crucial role in maintaining body balance. While the body's main supporting structures are located on the back, the front abdominal wall lacks bony support; the sternum, positioned centrally on the chest wall, complements the spine to help maintain balance. Third, it provides stability to the thoracic cage. Most structures of the thorax attach directly or indirectly to the sternum, which supports and stabilizes the ribs and costal cartilages, creating a unified and stable thoracic structure. Fourth, the sternum protects the internal organs of the thoracic cavity. As the strongest bony structure of the anterior chest wall, its large surface area and dense bone provide direct protection for the organs within the chest. Fifth, it maintains the normal appearance of the chest wall. A proper chest appearance depends on all bony structures being aligned on the same plane and positioned correctly. The sternum offers suitable attachment points for these structures, ensuring their proper arrangement and thus the normal external contour of the chest wall, making the sternum essential for maintaining its appearance.

The sternum is a vital component of the thoracic cage and plays an extremely important physiological role. When a sternal tumor occurs, the structure of the sternum is damaged, impairing its physiological functions, which can affect multiple aspects of the human body and pose serious health risks. The dangers of sternal tumors can be summarized in two categories: physiological and psychological. The physiological dangers include three aspects: first, damage or loss of the sternum's own function; second, its impact on the function of the thoracic cage; and third, its systemic effects on the body. A sternal tumor directly destroys the sternum's structure, inevitably impairing its physiological functions, affecting all five basic functions previously mentioned. Since the sternum is an essential part of the thoracic cage, any lesion in the sternum will affect the thoracic cage and consequently its functions. From a systemic perspective, sternal tumors, as a type of tumor in the human body, inevitably impact overall health. Thus, the physiological dangers of sternal tumors should not be underestimated. In addition to physical harm, such tumors also pose psychological threats to patients. These arise not only from changes in the appearance of the chest wall but more significantly from the fear associated with having a tumor. While psychological harm may not directly manifest as physical dysfunction, it can potentially be even more dangerous.

The harm caused by sternal tumors can lead to various clinical symptoms in patients, with pain being the most common symptom. The pain is usually localized, clearly defined, and generally situated near the lesion. It is often a dull ache, with stabbing pain being rare. If the tumor invades surrounding structures, the pain may become more widespread and its nature may change. When the tumor is confined to the sternum, respiratory symptoms typically do not occur. However, if the tumor grows large enough to extend into the thoracic cavity, related symptoms may appear, such as breathing difficulties and coughing. If the heart or major blood vessels are compressed, circulatory symptoms may develop, including chest tightness, palpitations, and shortness of breath. When the sternal tumor has distant metastases or is itself a metastatic lesion from another site, symptoms may arise in other parts of the body, along with pronounced systemic symptoms.

The sternum is located superficially, so when a tumor occurs, it is easily detected. The most obvious sign is a local mass, which can appear in any part of the sternum, most commonly in the body and manubrium, with occasional reports of tumors involving the xiphoid process. The tumor can infiltrate laterally, affecting the costal cartilages and even the ribs. It can also spread superficially or deeply; superficially, it may invade the skin, causing related skin signs, while deeply, it can invade the mediastinum and affect its various structures. In severe cases, the tumor may invade the thoracic cavity, involving the lungs, pericardium, or diaphragm, and the patient will show corresponding signs.

In most cases, a physical examination can detect a sternal tumor, but imaging studies are necessary to provide clinical evidence. X-rays can offer the simplest information, while detailed tumor data requires CT scans. CT imaging can precisely determine the tumor's location, size, internal structure, extent of invasion, and relationship with surrounding tissues[5]. The ideal examination is a three-dimensional reconstruction, which provides all necessary information about the tumor in relation to the thoracic cage and chest.

The diagnosis of sternal tumors is relatively straightforward and can be confirmed based on clinical manifestations and examination results. Differential diagnosis requires distinguishing sternal tumors from other space-occupying lesions occurring in the sternum. Considering that the treatment principles for all space-occupying lesions are basically the same, if the differential diagnosis is difficult to achieve, decisive Surgical intervention is necessary.

Once a sternal tumor is confirmed, Surgery is often required. Contraindications mainly include: ① sternal tumors with widespread systemic metastases; ② sternal metastases combined with metastatic lesions in other parts of the body; and ③ sternal tumors in patients whose overall condition does not permit Surgery. Surgery for sternal tumors primarily involves two aspects: tumor resection and chest wall reconstruction.

1. Resection of Sternal Tumors

Due to the sternum's unique anatomical location with mediastinal structures lying posteriorly, internal thoracic arteries on both sides, and special structures above it requires considerable Surgical skill to safely perform tumor resection, as improper handling can pose serious risks [6,7]. One of the key Surgical considerations is the extent of resection. There are varying opinions in the literature regarding this: some suggest extending 2 cm beyond the tumor, while others recommend 3 cm. These views differ in credibility and are often inconsistent. Theoretically, a wider resection margin is more ideal; however, the sternum's limited length and proximity to critical structures mean that excessively removing healthy tissue may lead to unnecessary damage. Furthermore, when discussing fixed resection margins, many overlook critical factors such as the patient's body size, the tumor's actual size, and its malignancy level. Ignoring these variables and relying on a fixed resection margin lacks scientific validity and practical value. The correct approach is to base Surgical decisions on the specific intraoperative situation and, when conditions permit, remove as much of the tumor and surrounding tissue as possible. This represents the most rational and individualized method.

(1) Resection of Lower Sternal Tumors

When resecting tumors located in the lower sternum, it is necessary to cut the costal arch, the costal cartilages or ribs on both sides, and then transect the sternum horizontally. A midline incision is generally used, extending laterally while preserving as much soft tissue as possible. The xiphoid process is exposed first, followed by exposure of the coastal arches on both sides. After cutting the costal arches, the costal cartilages and ribs are successively severed upward. The sternum is then transected above the upper margin of the tumor, and the tumor is removed along with any necessary adjacent structures on both sides.

(2) Resection of Middle Sternal Tumors

For tumors located in the middle portion of the sternum, a mid-sternal resection can be performed. The incision remains a midline one, and the pleural cavity is first accessed through an intercostal space on one side. A finger is used to explore the deep extent of the tumor. The corresponding costal cartilages and ribs on both sides of the chest wall are then severed, and the sternum is transected horizontally slightly above and below the tumor margins. Given the limited length of the sternum, achieving complete resection of tumors in this region often leaves minimal residual sternal structure. In such cases, resection should not be limited just to preserve part of the sternum. If the remaining portions are very short, it is advisable to remove all the residual sternal structures.

(3) Resection of Upper Sternal Tumors

Tumors located in the upper sternum pose more complex Surgical challenges due to the presence of major blood vessels behind this area and the sternoclavicular joints on both sides above. A midline incision is still used. The pleural cavities are first entered through the intercostal spaces on both sides, followed by upward and downward cutting of the costal cartilages or ribs. The sternum is then transected horizontally at an appropriate point below the tumor. The upper portion of the sternum, along with the tumor, is lifted, and adhesions between the posterior aspect of the tumor and mediastinal structures are carefully freed. The sternoclavicular joints are incised, and the entire tumor mass, together with the upper sternum and any connected structures, is resected Upper sternal tumors often require removal of the manubrium. Some Surgeons are overly conservative due to concerns about damaging the sternoclavicular joints, sometimes to the extent that even the minimum resection needed is not achieved. This conservative approach clearly contradicts the fundamental principles of tumor removal. Although the sternoclavicular joint is a semi-mobile joint that contributes somewhat to clavicle movement and by extension, to upper limb mobility, its functional importance is limited. Even if this joint is compromised, upper limb movement is generally not significantly affected. Considering the serious threat posed by malignant tumors, compromising some upper limb mobility is fully justified if it ensures complete tumor resection. Therefore, if necessary, during Surgery, the sternoclavicular joint should be sacrificed without hesitation; this is the most rational and effective approach.Tumors in the upper sternum may also involve two additional critical structures: the clavicle and the first rib. If the tumor invades the sternoclavicular joint or directly infiltrates the clavicle, the medial portion of the affected clavicle must be resected; this is a basic requirement for effective tumor removal. However, clavicle resection is a relatively risky procedure because numerous blood vessels and nerves pass between the clavicle and the first rib. To perform this operation safely, the medial clavicle can be fully elevated and then dissected from its posterior side under direct visualization, which allows for a safer Surgical approach. The 1 rib and clavicle are not parallel; they intersect spatially, with the subclavian vessels and nerves running between them. If direct resection of the first rib is necessary, the procedure also carries significant risk. In cases where the Surgeon lacks sufficient confidence in performing this step safely, it is often better to refrain from resecting the first rib.

(4) Total Sternotomy

When the sternal tumor is extensive, involving the entire length of the sternum, or when only a small portion of the sternum remains after tumor resection, a total sternotomy may be considered [8]. The specific Surgical procedure involves making a midline incision to fully expose the tumor and the entire sternum. Depending on the extent of resection required, the incision may extend to expose the lateral chest wall. Once exposure is complete, the procedure begins with the area that is easiest to operate on, and the corresponding structures are sequentially resected until the entire sternum and tumor are removed.

2. Chest Wall Reconstruction

After resection of a sternal tumor, the sternum is no longer intact. The respected structures often include portions of the coastal cartilage on both sides and even parts of the ribs. At this point, reconstruction of these structures is necessary [9,10]. In the past, various reconstruction methods were used, often treating the defect as a whole without considering the specific shapes of the sternum, costal cartilage, and other individual structures. Such methods are relatively simple and can ensure partial restoration of the function of the sternum and thoracic cage. If the procedural details are carefully designed, satisfactory results can be achieved

In recent years, some procedures have reconstructed the sternum and ribs separately, and such approaches undoubtedly have clear advantages. However, this method requires specialized materials. MatrixRIB is a relatively ideal material that can be conveniently used for anterior chest wall reconstruction (Figures 3-5-1 and 3-5-2). A material that has gained more attention in recent years is custom-designed material, also known as digital material [7,11]. This type of material is designed based on the personalized contour of the chest wall defect after resection, taking into account not only the reconstruction of the defect but also the detailed structures of the sternum, costal cartilage, and ribs.

If well-designed, such materials can essentially restore the normal structure of the chest wall, making them a relatively satisfactory option (Figure 3-5-3).

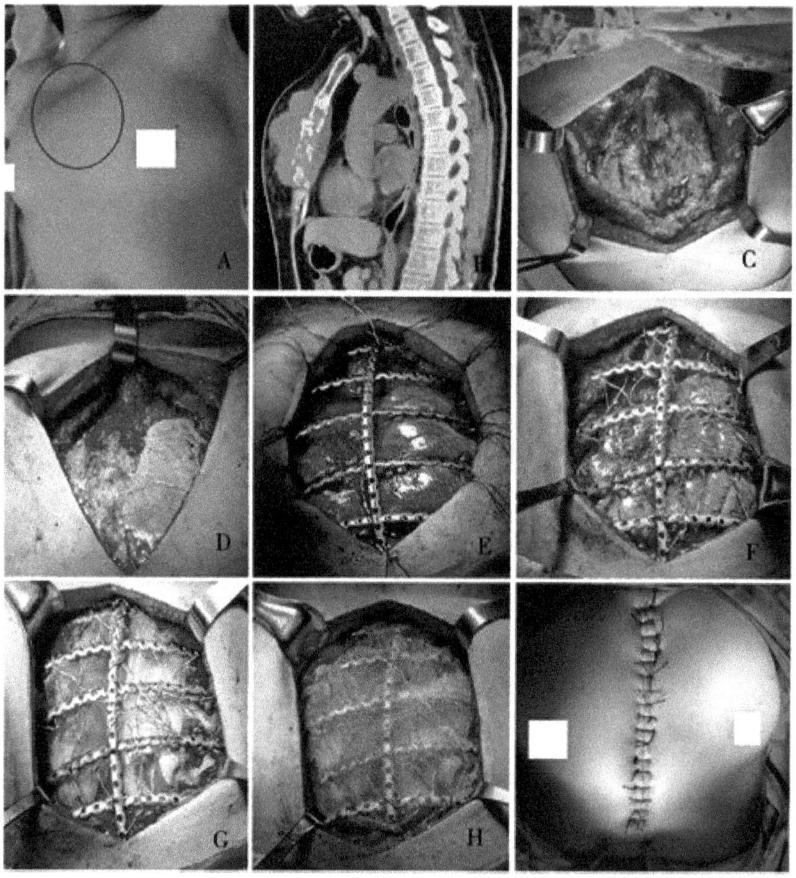

Figure 3-5-1 Chest wall reconstruction with MatrixRIB after sternum tumor resection (A. Location of the sternal tumor on the body surface; B. CT scan showing the position of the sternal tumor; C. Midline incision on the anterior chest wall to expose the sternal tumor; D. Resection of the tumor along with adequate surrounding bony structures; E. reconstruction of bony structures including costal cartilage, ribs, and sternum using MatrixRIB; F. Wire mesh woven between gaps to reduce the empty space; G, H. Fibrous membranes placed on both inner and outer sides of MatrixRIB; I. Postoperative appearance of the chest wall)

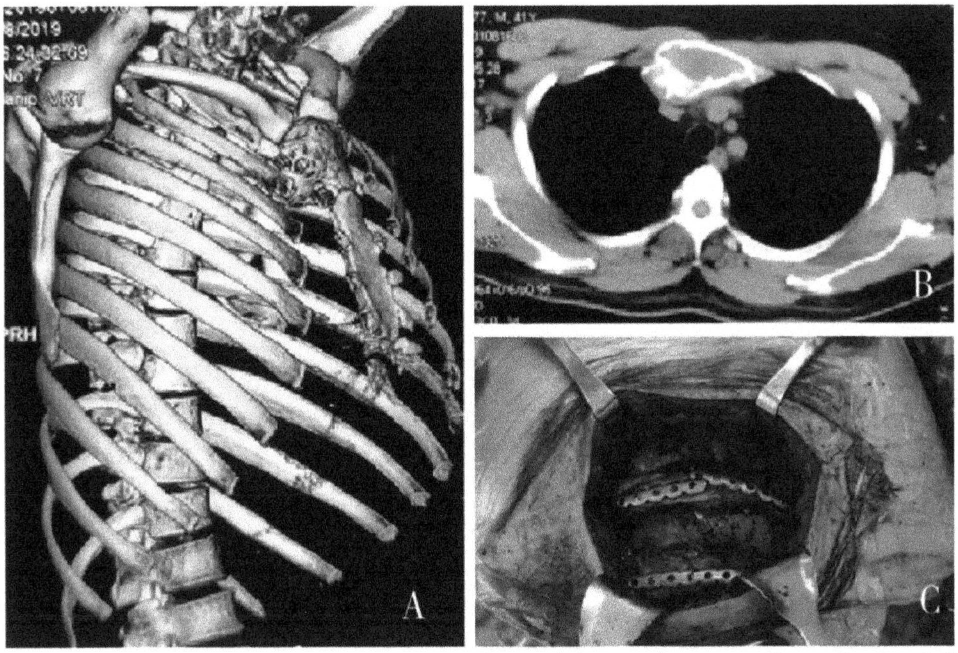

Figure 3-5-2 Chest wall reconstruction with autologous rib and MatrixRIB after sternal tumor resection (A. 3D reconstruction image showing the tumor located at the manubrium of the sternum; B. CT cross-sectional image showing the tumor location; C. After tumor resection, a rib was harvested from the right chest wall, divided into two segments, placed horizontally in the center of the defect, and then fixed using MatrixRIB to complete the reconstruction of the bony chest wall structure.)

During the reconstruction process, the following issues need attention:① Management of the sternoclavicular joint. After resection of the sternoclavicular joint, the artificial material needs to be fixed onto the clavicle. To accommodate the movement of the clavicle, some materials are designed with a movable joint to replace the function of the sternoclavicular joint. Such a design has certain advantages, but it is not necessarily essential. If a movable joint is not included in the design, it can still be managed appropriately depending on the specific case. The material can be directly fixed on the clavicle, which generally does not significantly affect the movement of the upper limbs. ② Treatment of the clavicle. When the sternoclavicular joint is removed or the clavicle is partially removed, it is considered a more reasonable approach to directly fix the artificial material to the clavicle. However, the operation of fixing the clavicle is sometimes very difficult, especially considering the blood vessels and nerves below the middle of the clavicle. Fixing the clavicle is not only difficult but also risky. At this time, you can consider leaving the free end of the clavicle alone without any treatment. This approach seems unreasonable on the surface, but in fact, it is a very reasonable approach. ③ Treatment of the first rib. The 1 rib is located in a concealed position, and after its costal cartilage is removed, the remaining portion of the rib lies directly beneath the clavicle, close to the subclavian vessels and nerves. Attempting to reconstruct the resected portion of the first rib is not only technically difficult but also carries significant risk. Therefore, it is reasonable to leave the residual end of the first rib unreconstructed and free, without any further intervention.④ Fixation of the material. Fixation methods are usually well considered during the design of reconstruction materials. Most materials are designed to be fixed using screws or nails. However, such designs are often overly idealistic, as in many real-world Surgical cases, the bony structures are not suitable for this type of fixation. In such situations, alternative measures must be taken. The ideal solution is to use steel wire fixation, which often yields very good results.⑤

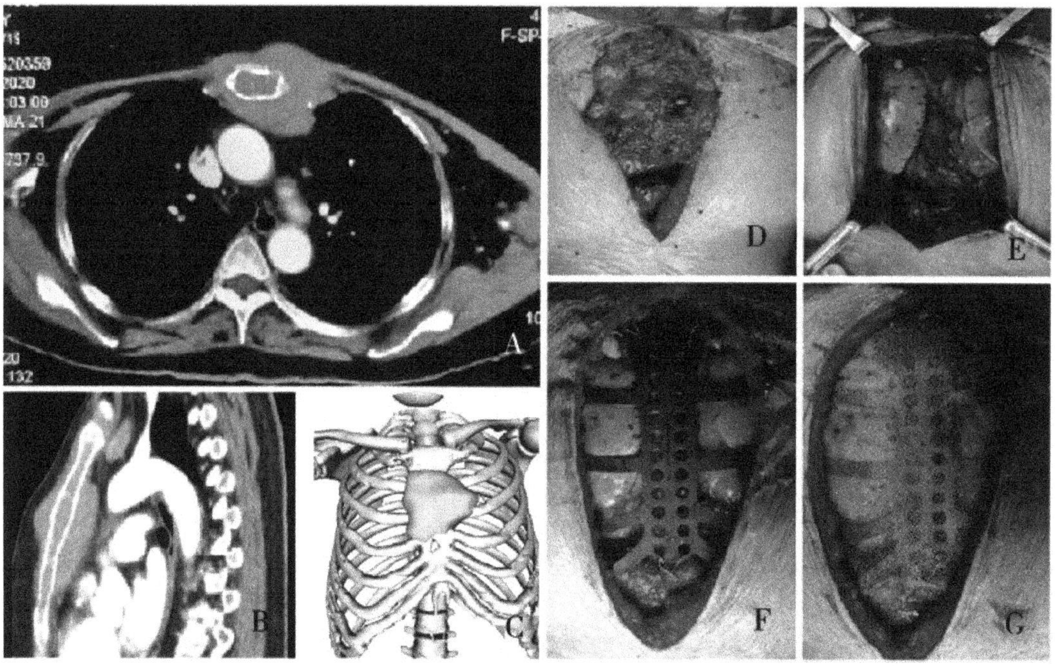

Figure 3-5-3 Chest wall reconstruction with digital material after sternal tumor resection(A. CT cross-sectional image of the sternal tumor; B. CT sagittal image showing the tumor location on the sternum; C. 3D reconstruction image of the thorax showing the tumor's location and its relation to surrounding structures; D. Midline incision made on the anterior chest wall to expose the tumor; E. Resection of the sternal tumor along with adequate surrounding bony structures; F. Chest wall bony structure reconstructed using digital materials; G. Digital material covered with fibrous membrane, incision closed, and Surgery completed.)

Management of intercostal gaps. Some artificial materials are designed only with the sternum, costal cartilage, and rib structures in mind, without considering the intercostal structures. The intercostal structures consist primarily of the intercostal muscles, which are generally not taken into account during bony structure reconstruction. Even when soft tissue reconstruction is performed, the issue of reconstructing intercostal muscles is usually overlooked. In some cases, the intercostal gaps between reconstruction materials are quite wide, and since there are no other structures in between, this essentially still constitutes a defect in the chest wall. If these gaps are not addressed, corresponding postoperative complications may arise. To prevent such issues, these overly wide gaps can be reconstructed during Surgery by weaving steel wire across them, thereby narrowing the gaps, which aligns better with physiological needs. ⑥ Padding issue. After fixing the artificial material, the inner surface of the material. Some artificial materials are designed only with the sternum, costal cartilage, and rib structures in mind, without considering the intercostal structures. The intercostal structures consist primarily of the intercostal muscles, which are generally not taken into account during bony structure reconstruction. Even when soft tissue reconstruction is performed, the issue of reconstructing intercostal muscles is usually overlooked.in some cases, the intercostal gaps between reconstruction materials are quite wide, and since there are no other structures in between, this essentially still constitutes a defect in the chest wall. If these gaps are not addressed, corresponding postoperative complications may arise. To prevent such issues, these overly wide gaps can be reconstructed during Surgery by weaving steel wire across them, thereby narrowing the gaps, which aligns better with physiological needs.

The above reconstruction procedures are entirely focused on bony structure reconstruction. The next step should be the reconstruction of soft tissue. In sternal tumor resection Surgeries, the pectoralis major muscle is the best source of soft tissue, so it must be preserved during tumor removal whenever possible. However, in some cases, the sternal tumor may invade the pectoralis major, making it necessary to respect the affected portion of the muscle during the tumor excision. This makes soft tissue reconstruction even more critical and relevant. In typical procedures, the pectoralis major should be mobilized as much as possible and used to cover the reconstructed materials. If, after mobilization, the pectoralis major is still insufficient to meet Surgical needs, other soft tissue materials must be considered for coverage.

Another important aspect of chest wall reconstruction is the reconstruction of the skin. If a sternal tumor extensively invades the skin, skin reconstruction becomes necessary. This is typically done using various types of flaps. As long as the flap is well-designed, it generally meets the Surgical requirements. Throughout the entire reconstruction process, aesthetic considerations are involved in every step. If each procedure is carefully and thoughtfully planned, the final outcome can achieve both functional success and a satisfactory appearance.

If the outcome not only meets the requirements for disease treatment but also fulfills aesthetic expectations, it represents the highest level of Surgical excellence. However, in actual Surgical practice, it is often difficult to fully balance both goals. Since the lesion is of a tumorous nature, curing the disease must always be the top priority. On this basis, if a satisfactory aesthetic result can also be achieved, it would be the best possible outcome. However, if aesthetic considerations compromise the thorough removal of the tumor, it can lead to very adverse consequences, and the patient may pay a heavy price for it.

REFERENCES

[1] Tang, L., W. He, N. Chen, et al. 2021. "Advances in the Clinical Diagnosis and Treatment of Primary Sternal Tumors." *Chinese Journal of Surgical Oncology* 13 (2): 200–205.

[2] Sponholz, S., N. Baldes, M. Schirren, et al. 2018. "Sternal Resection for Breast Cancer Metastases." *Thoracic and Cardiovascular Surgeon* 66 (2): 164–169.

[3] Haraguchi, S., Y. Yamashita, K. Yamashita, et al. 2004. "Sternal Resection for Metastasis from Thyroid Carcinoma and Reconstruction with Marlex and Stainless-Steel Mesh." *Japanese Journal of Thoracic and Cardiovascular Surgery* 52 (4): 209–212.

[4] Chapelier, A. 2010. "Resection and Reconstruction for Primary Sternal Tumors." *Thoracic Surgery Clinics* 20 (4): 529–534.

[5] Chen, Y., T. Lu, and L. Cai. 2005. "CT Diagnosis of Sternal Tumors." *Radiologic Practice* 20 (6): 511–513.

[6] Zhang, Y., J. Li, Y. Hao, et al. 2014. "Titanium Mesh Reconstruction After Sternal Tumor Resection: A Preliminary Study." *Chinese Journal of Orthopaedics* 34 (11): 1145–1150.

[7] Dzian, A., J. Zivcak, R. Penciak, et al. 2018. "Implantation of a 3D-Printed Titanium Sternum in a Patient with a Sternal Tumor." *World Journal of Surgical Oncology* 16 (1): 7.

[8] Wang, W. 2021. "Total Sternum Resection with MatrixRIB Chest Wall Reconstruction." *Thoracic Deformity Surgery Expert*, October 9, 2021.

[9] Drinnon, K. D., S. Sherali, C. T. Cox, et al. 2020. "Sternal Tumor Resection and Reconstruction Using Iliac Crest Autograft." *Plastic and Reconstructive Surgery Global Open* 8 (8): e3002.

[10] Sandri, A., G. Donati, C. D. Blanc, et al. 2020. "Anterior Chest Wall Resection and Sternal Body Wedge for Primary Tumors: Reconstruction with Biological Mesh and Titanium Plates." *Journal of Thoracic Disease* 12 (1): 17–21.

[11] Wang, W. 2019. "Personalized Characteristics of Digital Materials." *Thoracic Deformity Surgery Expert*, November 24, 2019.

Rib tumors are one of the primary research focuses among chest wall tumors and refer to tumors originating in the ribs; in a broader sense, they also include tumors arising from the costal cartilage. In the early stages, the tumor occurs in a single rib, but as it continues to grow, it may involve multiple ribs and adjacent structures. Benign rib tumors are more common, while malignant tumors are most frequently metastatic tumors and multiple myeloma [1]. The biological characteristics of these tumors vary, and so do their potential harms to humans; these characteristics determine the diagnosis, treatment, and prognosis of the tumors.

1. Basic concepts:

Rib tumors can be either benign or malignant. Benign tumors are generally well-localized, often encapsulated, and have clear boundaries from surrounding structures. In contrast, malignant tumors grow invasively and have poorly defined margins. Rib tumors can occur in any of the ribs as well as in the costal cartilage. In the early stages, the tumor is usually confined to a localized area of a single rib [2]. As it grows, the tumor can expand in all directions. It may first grow longitudinally along the rib, then laterally to adjacent ribs, and also in a three-dimensional manner, extending both deeper into the body and outward toward the surface. structures that may be invaded by the tumor include the sternum, spine, scapula, clavicle, lungs, and mediastinum. Tumors in the lower ribs can also invade the diaphragm, and may extend into the abdominal wall or even the abdominal cavity.

The harm caused by rib tumors primarily falls into two categories: local and systemic. Local harm arises mainly from the tumor's pressure and invasive growth in the surrounding area, while systemic harm is associated with certain broader effects the tumor may have on the body. Most rib tumors are relatively localized and do not cause systemic issues. However, if the tumor becomes severe, affects vital organs such as the heart and lungs, or secretes specific substances, it can lead to serious systemic consequences. The main clinical manifestation of rib tumors is pain, typically localized. If the tumor invades thoracic organs, symptoms related to the respiratory or circulatory systems may occur. A common physical sign is a localized mass, often found on the anterior or lateral chest wall, fixed to one or more ribs. This mass usually has limited mobility and may be accompanied by changes in the overlying skin

The examination of rib tumors can be conducted through basic physical examination and imaging studies. Physical examination helps to gather general information about the tumor, but detailed information must be obtained through imaging techniques. X-ray examination is the most basic form of assessment, while CT scanning is considered the fundamental diagnostic tool. CT scans can clearly define the tumor's location, size, internal structure, and its relationship with surrounding structures [3]. Three-dimensional reconstruction imaging provides even more detailed information about the tumor itself, the chest wall, and the thoracic cavity. This information plays a crucial role in the diagnosis and treatment of rib tumors.

The diagnosis of rib tumors is relatively simple. The diseases that need to be differentiated are mainly sternal tumors and metastases from intrathoracic tumors. Metastatic tumors: Sternal tumors originate primarily from the sternum and may subsequently grow toward the costal cartilage and ribs. In contrast, tumors that metastasize to the ribs from within the thoracic cavity originate inside the chest. A rough distinction can usually be made based on the patient's medical history. However, if distinguishing between them is difficult, it is acceptable not to differentiate, as the origin does not affect the Surgical procedure.

The nature of a rib tumor can only be definitively determined through cytological examination. Although it is relatively easy to obtain this information before Surgery, it is not strictly necessary. Overemphasizing cytological testing may increase the patient's discomfort, add to their financial burden, and potentially delay Surgery. Therefore, it should not be made a mandatory requirement

Rib tumors are mostly located near the body surface and are relatively easy to detect due to their obvious symptoms and signs. Once the diagnosis is confirmed, Surgery should be performed as early as possible.

2. Surgery for Rib Tumors

Surgery for rib tumors also has two fundamental aspects: first is disease treatment, and second is reconstruction. Disease treatment requires complete removal of the tumor along with the surrounding invaded structures, while reconstruction involves repairing the chest wall defect left after tumor removal.

(1) Resection Surgery

The Surgical removal of rib tumors directly reflects the curative aspect of treatment. The extent of resection can be determined based on the actual condition. Most literature suggests that the resection margin should exceed the lesion by 3 cm; however, this recommendation lacks reliable evidence and should not be rigidly applied. The surrounding structures to be removed include the ribs, costal cartilage, and soft tissues around the lesion [4,5]. If the sternum or intrathoracic organs are involved, If involved, corresponding resection of the sternum or intrathoracic organs is also necessary. The fundamental principle of resection is clear: to be as thorough as possible. However, because the chest wall is surrounded by many vital structures, when these structures are invaded, complete resection may not be feasible. In such cases, the goal should be to perform the widest possible resection. This type of resection is not considered curative but rather a palliative Surgery. Although palliative Surgery is not thorough, it is equally important. First, it can alleviate the condition and buy time for thorough treatment; secondly, it can partially eliminate the lesions and play a partial therapeutic role.

During Surgery, the appropriate incision should first be selected based on the tumor's location. Generally, a standard thoracic incision specifically, the posterolateral thoracotomy is used, which meets the needs for most rib tumor resections. If the tumor is located on the anterior chest wall, especially the upper part, an anterior chest wall incision may be considered, placed directly over the tumor surface. For smaller tumors that slightly protrude on the body surface without skin damage, an incision can be made directly over the tumor. However, if the tumor is large, significantly protruding, or if the skin is obviously invaded or ulcerated, a spindle-shaped (elliptical) incision is required. This must balance thorough removal of the lesion while preserving as much skin as possible to avoid compromising wound closure.

After the skin incision is completed, the tumor needs to be carefully freed. If the tumor has an intact capsule, resection can be performed along the capsule. However, if the boundaries with surrounding tissues are unclear, all suspicious tissues should be removed as thoroughly as possible. An important part of freeing the tumor is to expose the surface of the bony structures, which prepares for entering the thoracic cavity to complete the subsequent resection. Once the outer part of the tumor is fully freed, the surgeon enters the chest through a normal intercostal space, using their finger to explore the tumor's location on the thoracic cavity side, and then sequentially frees the healthy ribs around the tumor. The ribs are cut using rib shears, removing the tumor together with the affected ribs and surrounding structures. After the tumor resection, a corresponding defect appears in the chest wall, which requires reconstruction, also known as chest wall repair according to the needs.

(2) Reconstructive Surgery

Regarding the indications for chest wall reconstruction, there are various opinions in the literature. Some believe reconstruction is only necessary when three or more ribs are removed. Others set criteria based on the defect size, suggesting reconstruction is appropriate when the defect exceeds 6 cm × 6 cm. Some base the decision on the location of the rib resection, as different rib areas have different Surgical requirements. In reality, no matter how many ribs are removed, it always damages the ribs themselves and affects the integrity of the thoracic cage. Therefore, whenever conditions allow and suitable materials are available, reconstruction should be performed regardless of how many ribs are resected. Of course, if conditions do not permit or basic reconstruction materials are unavailable, the situation might be different. However, an undeniable fact is that when there is a rib defect, the chest wall locally becomes noticeably softened. Even if there is no physiological functional impairment, the patient often feels very uncomfortable. Therefore, reconstruction should be done as much as possible whenever there is a defect. Like defects in other parts of the chest wall, reconstruction after rib tumor resection also involves three main components: reconstruction of the bony structure, soft tissue reconstruction, and skin reconstruction.

Like chest wall defects in other parts, reconstruction after rib tumor resection still includes three aspects, namely, bone structure reconstruction, soft tissue reconstruction and skin reconstruction. The key to bone structure reconstruction is the selection of materials. In the past, there were many materials used in clinical practice, including plate-like structures, strip-like structures, membrane-like structures, and some people directly used steel wire for mesh reconstruction. Different materials will result in different reconstruction effects. The ideal reconstruction effect needs to meet two requirements: one is the restoration of structure, and the other is the restoration of spatial relationship. For ribs, both requirements are important because only when both requirements are met at the same time can the reconstructed chest wall have good function. At present, the most ideal material in clinical practice is MatrixRIB [6]. The shape of this material is the shape of a normal rib, with sufficient strength and good elasticity. There are products of different specifications to choose from. Not only can it be used as needed, but it can also be cut and shaped according to the needs of the operation (Figure 3-6-1). These advantages make MatrixRIB the preferred material for rib reconstruction. In recent years, some have attempted to use so-called 3D-printed materials [7], with their biggest selling point being customized design. This feature seems to offer a certain superiority over conventional materials. However, when compared with MatrixRIB, 3D-printed materials have no real advantages. MatrixRIB already possesses the natural rib shape and can easily meet all Surgical requirements, advantages that 3D-printed materials lack. Moreover, considering the complexities of processing involved with 3D printing, these materials become even less favorable in practical clinical applications.

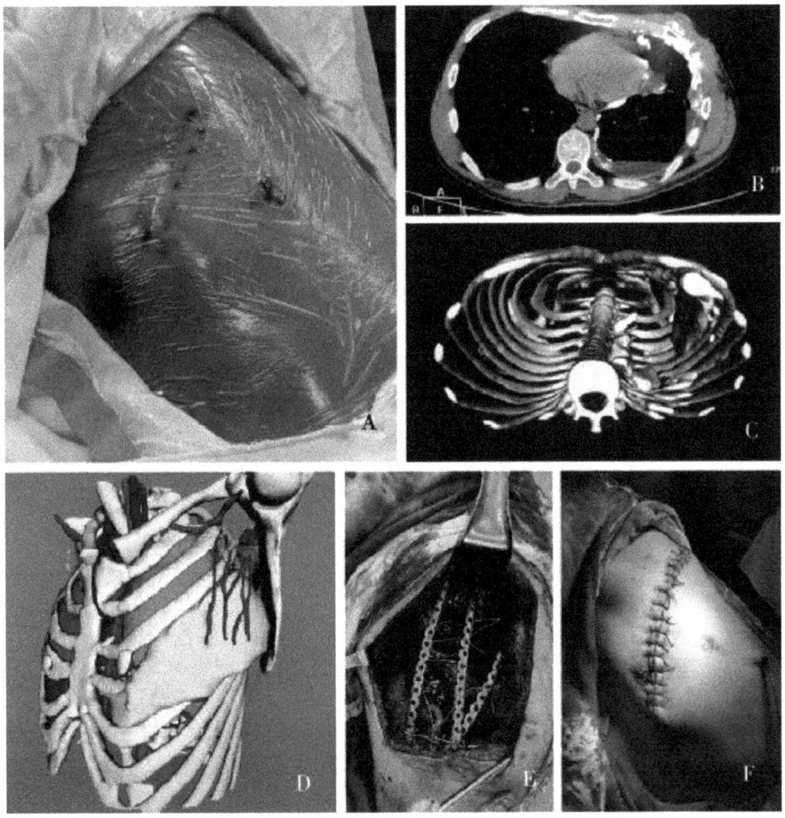

Figure 3-6-1 Rib tumor resection and reconstruction (A Appearance of the chest wall of a patient with rib tumor; B. CT cross-sectional image showing the location of the rib tumor; C, D, and three-dimensional reconstruction images showing the location of the rib tumor; E. reconstruction of the chest wall bony structure using MatrixRIB; F. Appearance of the chest wall after Surgery)

When using MatrixRIB, first determine the length of MatrixRIB according to the size of the defect. After the length is determined, shape the MatrixRIB according to the curvature of the target rib, and then fix it in sequence. There are two ways to fix it. You can use the original screws or directly use steel wire to tie the MatrixRIB to the rib. When doing fixation, some special skills should be remembered: ① Do not stick to the inherent direction of the rib. The most ideal reconstruction is to replace each rib with MatrixRIB and reconstruct it completely according to the original rib running direction and position characteristics. However, in actual operation, due to
If ideal reconstruction cannot be performed due to the extent of the lesion's impact on the rib or due to the outcomes of rib resection, then a reasonable compromise must be made. In such cases, one end of the MatrixRIB can be fixed to the remaining rib stump, while the other end can be secured to the sternum, another rib, or any other relatively firm structure. These adaptations are perfectly valid Surgical options. They do not violate any fundamental principles and can ensure the successful completion of the operation even under

challenging conditions.If the length of a single Matrix RIB is insufficient, then it can be extended or connected appropriately using Surgical techniques to ensure proper anatomical and functional reconstruction.②Use two plates connected together. MatrixRIB comes in different lengths and specifications, generally able to meet the reconstruction needs of defects of various sizes. However, when the defect area is large, the length of MatrixRIB may not meet the Surgical requirements. At this time, two MatrixRIB plates can be joined end to end; only the two holes in the middle need to be tied and fixed to achieve a good docking effect. After such treatment, it can meet the reconstruction needs of defects of almost all sizes. ③ MatrixRIB can be flexibly assembled as needed. During tumor removal, the removal of bony structures can only be done according to the needs of the condition, and the remaining ribs after removal may not necessarily have two residual ends available. At this time, the reconstruction cannot be too rigid; the fixed position of MatrixRIB Flexible options is available. If necessary, both ends of the MatrixRIB can even be fixed onto another MatrixRIB.④ Wiring mesh between MatrixRIBs: Following MatrixRIB reconstruction, wide gaps often remain between the plates. These gaps should be addressed by weaving a mesh using steel wire between the MatrixRIBs. This mesh serves two main purposes: Directly to narrow or eliminate excessive gaps between plates. Indirectly: to further stabilize the MatrixRIBs by integrating them into a unified structural framework, firmly connected to the surrounding chest wall. This technique significantly enhances the stability and integrity of the reconstruction. Additionally, the wiring mesh helps mimic the function of intercostal structures, complementing the fibrous membrane often placed beneath MatrixRIBs for added protection and structural support.

MatrixRIB reconstruction falls under the category of bony structure reconstruction. Once this step is completed, the next crucial phase is soft tissue reconstruction. One of the key procedures in this stage is the placement of a fibrous membrane lining on the thoracic side of the MatrixRIB. As mentioned earlier, although the fibrous membrane is not a true soft tissue, it functions as a substitute for the intercostal muscles, and is thus considered part of soft tissue reconstruction.

The fibrous membrane can be placed before MatrixRIB fixation, but doing so may hinder the exposure of the rib ends that need to be fixed. Since gaps typically remain between MatrixRIB plates after bony reconstruction, the fibrous membrane can also be inserted through these gaps onto the thoracic side and then sutured into place. This technique is simple and effective; its primary goal is to separate the MatrixRIB from lung tissue, thereby preventing postoperative complications.

True soft tissue reconstruction involves covering the rigid implants with biological tissue, which promotes wound healing and contributes to a more aesthetically pleasing outcome. The most common soft tissue sources are muscle flaps. In cases where subcutaneous fat is sufficiently abundant, it may be used for coverage. In female patients, breast tissue may also be considered for coverage, provided that the breast structure is not compromised.

For small defects, soft tissues from the surrounding chest wall are usually adequate. However, for large defects, tissue from more distant sites is needed. The most commonly used options include the pectoralis major muscle flap or the latissimus dorsi muscle flap. If these are still insufficient, reconstruction must rely on free flaps harvested from even more distant donor sites.

In most cases, soft tissue loss corresponds closely to skin loss. If there is no extensive skin damage, the soft tissue coverage is generally sufficient. However, in extreme cases where subcutaneous soft tissue is minimal, using it to cover reconstruction materials may not affect wound healing but can lead to a poor aesthetic result postoperatively. Appearance and the patient's subjective experience may also be affected, so at this point, soft tissue reconstruction must not be casually omitted.

The primary goal of skin reconstruction is to ensure that the incision can be satisfactorily sutured. If the defect is too large, flap reconstruction is required. The first choice should be nearby skin flaps, selected together with muscle flaps. This not only ensures adequate blood supply but also results in a better appearance, and of course, fulfills the requirements for soft tissue reconstruction. The preferred flaps are still local myocutaneous flaps, such as the pectoralis major or latissimus dorsi myocutaneous flaps. If such flaps cannot meet the Surgical needs, then flaps must be taken from more distant areas.

3 Rib tumor Surgery in special areas

The ribs make up the majority of the chest wall, and every segment of the ribs can develop tumors. A tumor arising in the mid-portion of a rib may be surrounded by other healthy ribs. In such cases, tumor removal and reconstruction are straightforward. However, tumors located at the edges of the ribs involve adjacent structures. When these surrounding structures are invaded, the Surgery becomes more complicated. At that point, considerations extend beyond just the tumor and the ribs; many other practical issues must also be addressed.

(1) 1- Rib Tumor Surgery

A 1-rib tumor is a tumor in a special location, and because it involves numerous issues, it is discussed separately. The 1 rib lies immediately beneath the clavicle; the clavicle crosses the mid-portion of the first rib, and at that crossing the subclavian vessels and nerves pass through. Broadly speaking, if a tumor in this region is relatively localized, it is classified as a definite first-rib tumor [8–10]. If the mass is large and infiltrates deeply into the pulmonary apex, its clinical presentation mirrors that of a superior sulcus (Pancoast) carcinoma [11]. Surgery in this area has always been the most challenging procedure in traditional thoracic Surgery (Fig. 3-6-2). The fundamental reasons for its difficulty are twofold: first, the abundance of critical surrounding structures makes the Surgical risk extremely high; second, local exposure is difficult, rendering the operation very demanding.

Considering the Surgical risks and difficulty, the procedure must be carried out with caution, and the most important issue is protecting the sub clavicular structures (Fig. 3-6-3). If the mass is too large and its relationship to surrounding structures is unclear, Surgery may be abandoned in favor of primary chemoradiotherapy. Alternatively, chemoradiotherapy can be administered first, with Surgery performed after the tumor has shrunk. During Surgery, the tumor should still be resected as completely as possible, including any suspicious surrounding tissues. However, if the tumor lies too close to or has already invaded the vessels and nerves, forced resection should not be attempted. In specific cases, local measures can be taken as needed. If the clavicle is involved, partial claviculectomy may be performed.

After resection of the 1st rib, reconstruction of this rib is very difficult due to its deep location. Considering that it is covered anteriorly by the clavicle, even without reconstruction there is no obvious functional deficit; therefore, reconstruction of the 1st rib may be omitted. In other procedures such as resection of a tumor in the upper half of the sternum if the 1st rib cartilage or part of the 1st rib is removed, reconstruction of that rib likewise is not required. If the tumor is extensive and the resection range is wide, bony reconstruction can begin from the 2nd rib. Anterior to the 1st rib runs the pectoralis major muscle, and the 1st rib itself serves as an attachment point for the pectoralis major. If the lesion has not invaded the pectoralis major, there is generally no deficiency in soft-tissue coverage at this location. If the tumor can be removed smoothly, simply closing the incision will usually suffice to complete the Surgery. If the soft tissue and skin are invaded, intraoperative management should be tailored to the actual situation.

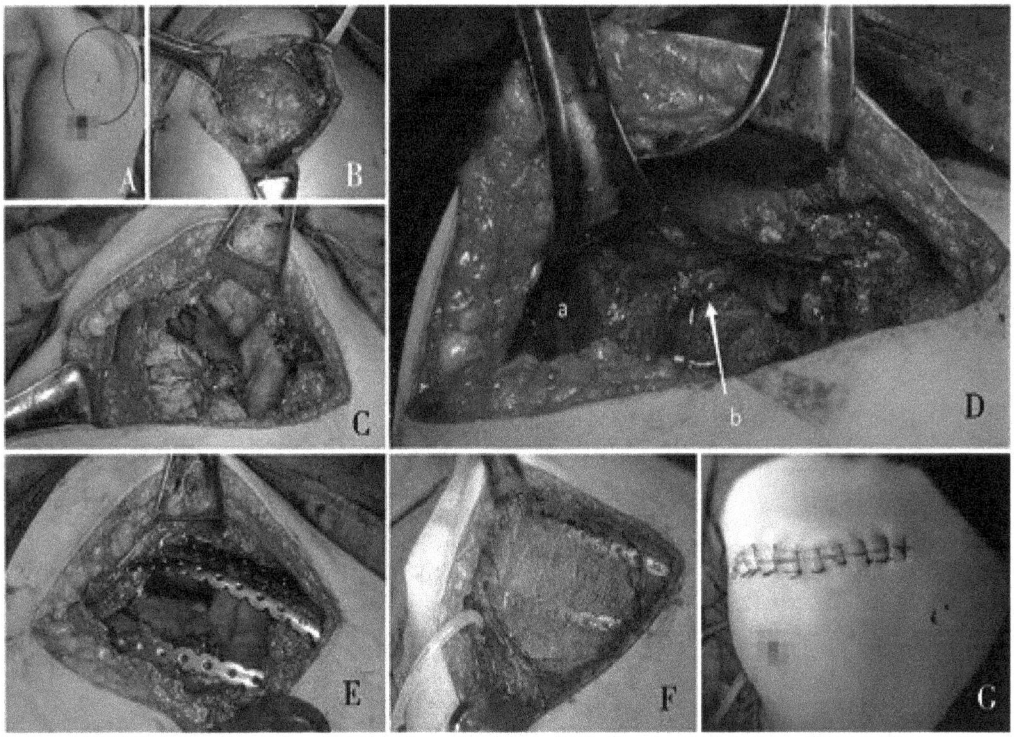

Figure 3-6-2 Chest Wall Tumor Resection and reconstruction Involving the 1st Rib The patient's right 1st, 2nd, and 3rd costal cartilages and ribs were involved, with the tumor growing into the thoracic cavity and invading the right upper lobe. After tumor resection, reconstruction was performed using MatrixRIB. A) Tumor location ; B) Exposure of the tumor; C) Surgical field after tumor resection D) Relationship between the residual 1st rib and the subclavian vein (a = subclavian vein; b = residual 1st rib end) (E) reconstruction of three ribs with MatrixRIB ; D) Relationship between the residual 1st rib and the subclavian vein (a = subclavian vein; b = residual 1st rib end) ;E) reconstruction of three ribs with MatrixRIB ; F) Fibermembrane covering the MatrixRIB G) Postoperative appearance of the chest wall)

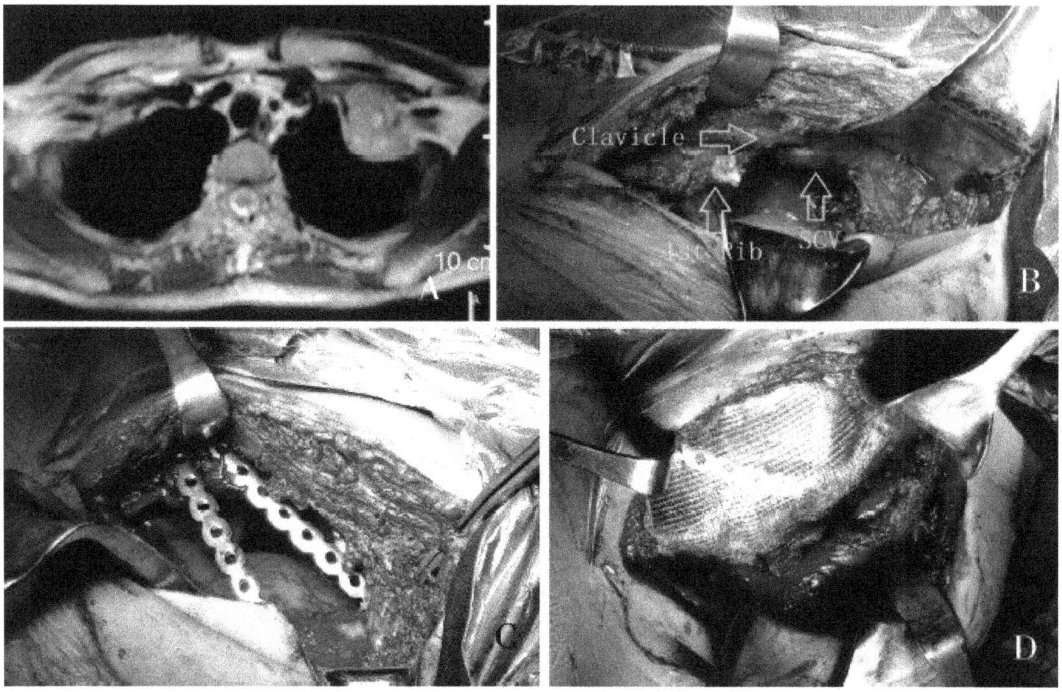

Figure 3-6-3, a left first-rib tumor is first identified on a CT cross-section A). Once the tumor and involved rib segment are resected, the Surgical field B) clearly exposes the subclavian vein alongside the residual first-rib stump. To restore chest-wall integrity, a MatrixRIB implant is contoured and secured in place C), after which a fiber membrane is draped over the reconstruction to fill residual gaps and reinforce fixation D) before final closure of the incision

(2) Rib tumors involving the sternum

Some tumors can simultaneously involve the ribs and the sternum, and such cases are actually not uncommon. The tumor may originate from the ribs or from the sternum. For such tumors, both the rib and sternum lesions need to be removed together. During reconstruction, both structures must be reconstructed simultaneously. Since the sternum is an important load-bearing structure of the anterior chest wall, its reconstruction is particularly important. reconstruction involving the sternum can use digital materials or other materials such as MatrixRIB. As long as the design is reasonable, satisfactory results can be achieved (Figure3-6-4).

(3) Rib tumors near the thoracic spine

If a rib tumor occurs near the thoracic vertebrae, it may directly invade the vertebrae (Figure 3-6-5) [12]. When removing the tumor, the affected part of the thoracic vertebra must also be excised. However, resection of the vertebra should be done with caution; it must not compromise the stability of the spine or damage the spinal cord. During reconstruction, if there is a suitable part of the vertebra available for fixation, it will facilitate the reconstruction procedure (Figure 3-6-6). If no suitable fixation point is available on the vertebra, the reconstruction material can be fixed vertically, that is, anchored to the healthy ribs above and below. This method can also achieve satisfactory results.

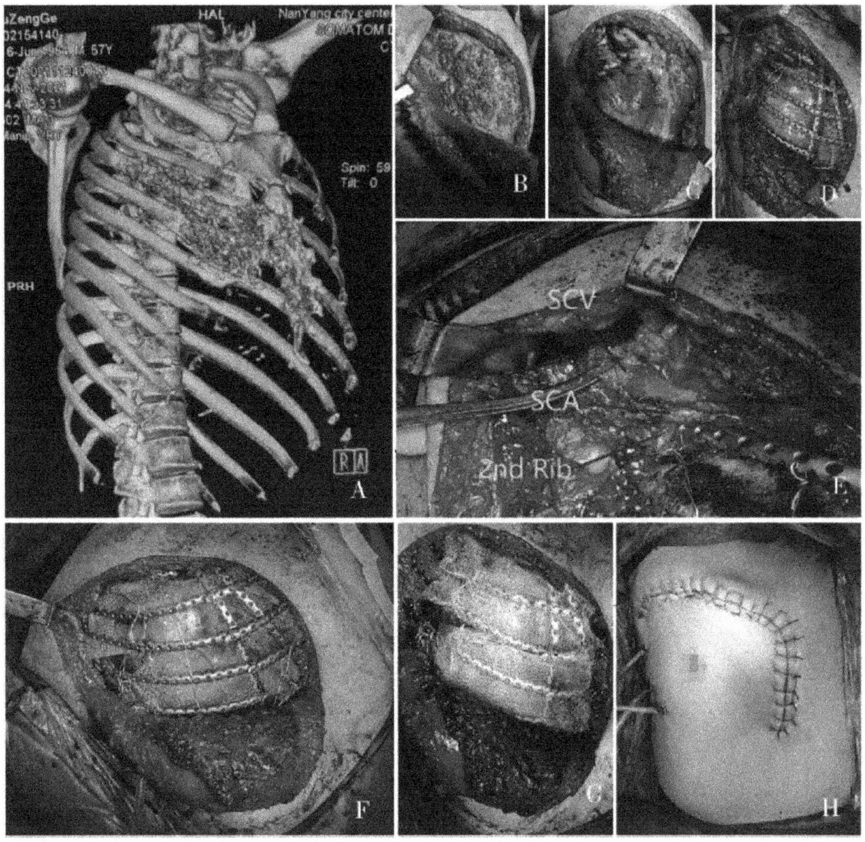

Figure 3-6-4 Resection of Rib and Sternal Tumor with Chest Wall reconstruction Surgery. The patient had involvement of the right 2, 3, 4, 5 ribs along with most of the sternum. After tumor resection, chest wall reconstruction was performed using MatrixRIB. (A. 3D reconstruction image of the chest wall; B. Exposure of the tumor site on the chest wall; C. Complete resection of the tumor; D. reconstruction of ribs and sternum using MatrixRIB; E. Relationship of the 2nd rib with the subclavian vein (SCV) and subclavian artery (SCA); F, G. Fibrous membrane used as a liner on both the inner and outer sides of the MatrixRIB; H. Postoperative appearance of the chest wall after incision closure.)

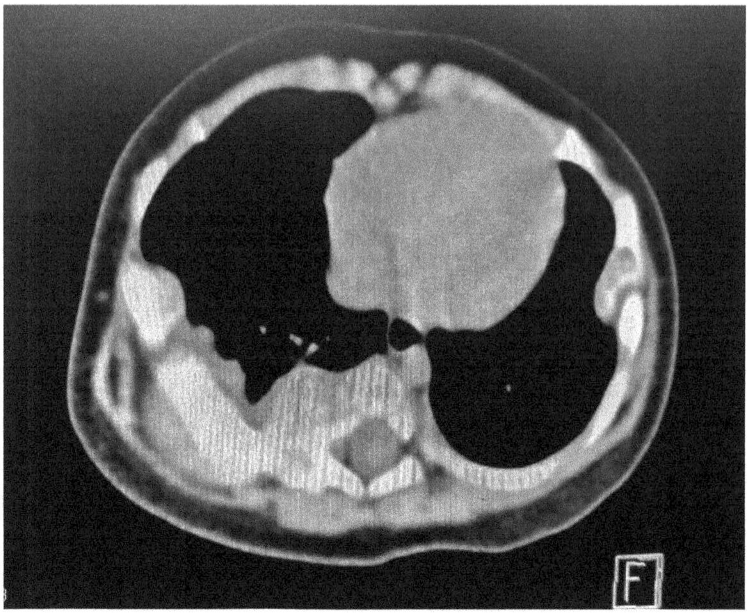

Figure 3-6-5 Rib Tumor invades spine

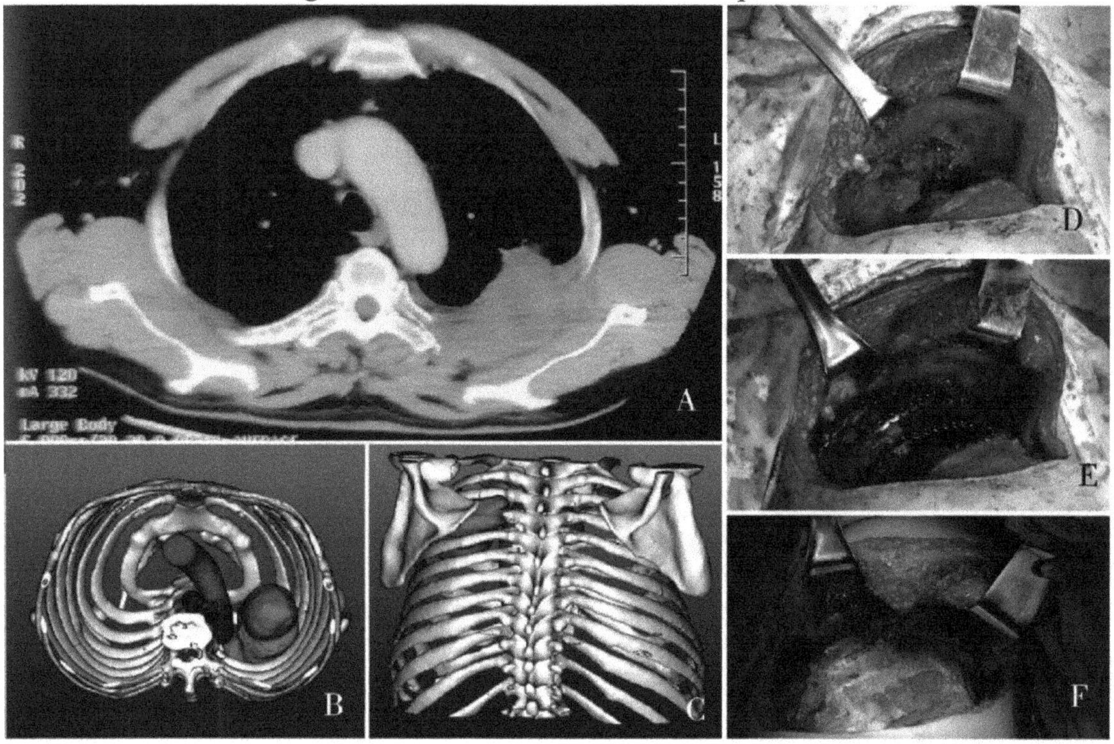

Figure 3-6-6 Surgery for rib tumor adjacent to spine (A. CT cross-sectional image showing the location of rib tumor; B, C. 3D reconstruction images showing the location of rib tumor; D. Resection of rib tumor; E. Chest wall reconstruction with MatrixRIB; F. Covering MatrixRIB with fibrous membrane and closing the incision)

(4) Rib tumor deep to the scapula

The scapula is a fixed-position bone, so when a rib tumor occurs on its deep surface, Surgical **exposure is often quite difficult** [1,13]. In such situations, the main challenge lies in achieving adequate exposure of the tumor. There are two main approaches to obtaining satisfactory exposure: first, making a sufficiently large incision, and second, applying effective and well-planned retraction. An arc-shaped incision that curves around the inferior angle of the scapula can increase the mobility of the scapula. A key point in retraction is to pull the scapula backward (toward the dorsal side), which often results in better exposure of the operative field (Figures 3-6-7 and 3-6-8).

Some severe rib tumors may invade the scapula. In such cases, exposure becomes even more challenging, but it can still be achieved using the two approaches mentioned earlier: making a sufficiently large incision and applying proper retraction. Once adequate exposure is achieved, the rib tumor can be resected first, followed by the removal of the tumor- invaded portion on the deep surface of the scapula. This removal should be as thorough as possible. If necessary, even the periosteum or cortical bone may need to be removed.

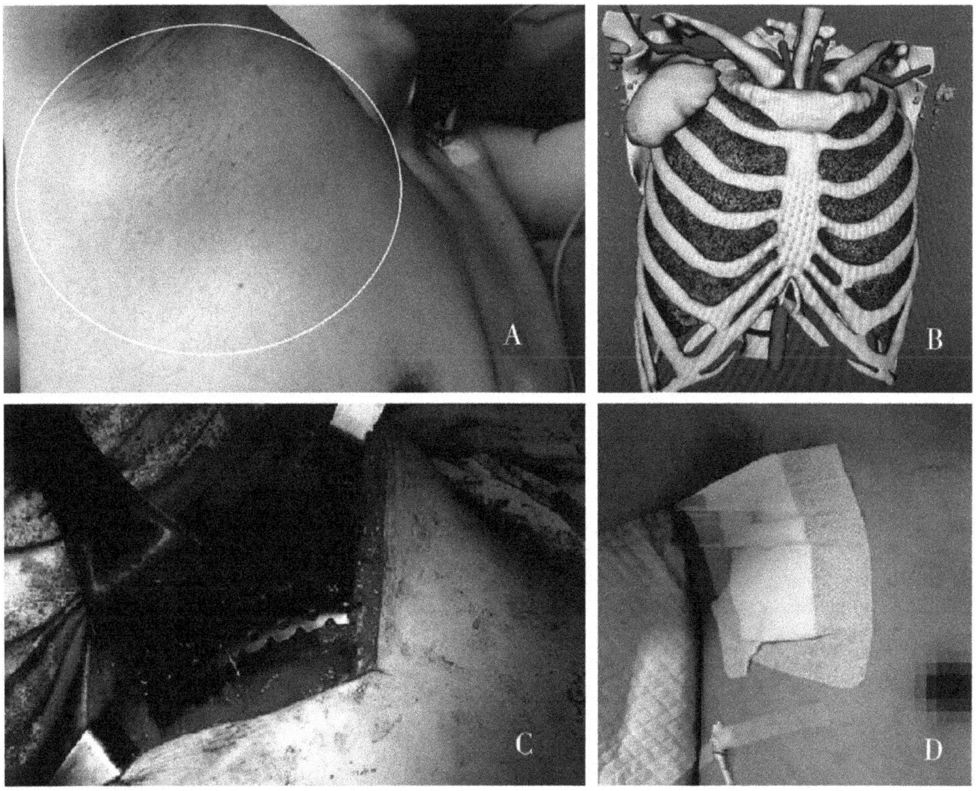

Figure 3-6-7 Rib Tumor on the Deep Surface of the Scapula. (A. The tumor is located beneath the scapula and can be palpated through the armpit; B. 3D

reconstruction image showing the tumor location; C. Chest wall reconstruction using MatrixRIB after tumor resection; D. Postoperative appearance of the chest wall.)

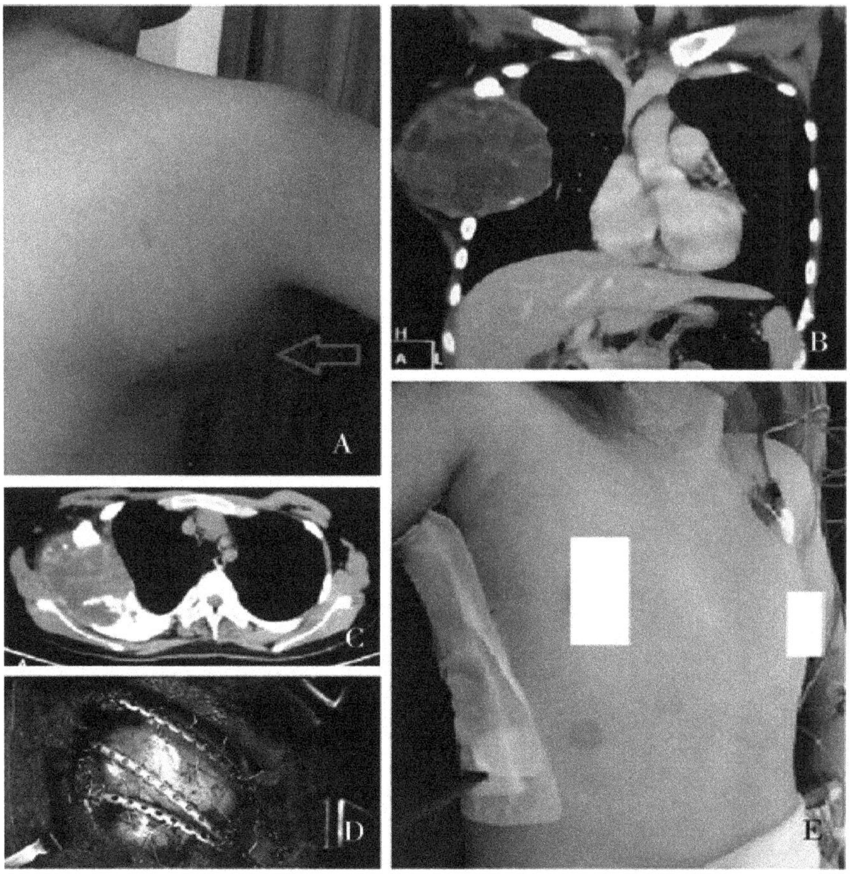

Figure 3-6-8 Rib Tumor on the Deep Surface of the Scapula. (A. Surface location of the chest wall tumor;B, C. CT images showing the location of the chest wall tumor; D. Resection of the chest wall tumor followed by reconstruction with MatrixRIB; E. Postoperative appearance of the chest wall.)

(5) Rib tumor located deep in the breast

For female patients, if there is a breast in front of the rib tumor on the anterior chest wall, it will be difficult to remove the tumor because it is impossible to make an incision directly on the tumor surface. In this case, a larger incision is often required on the lateral chest wall or below the breast to complete the exposure and operation of the tumor (Figure 3-6-9).

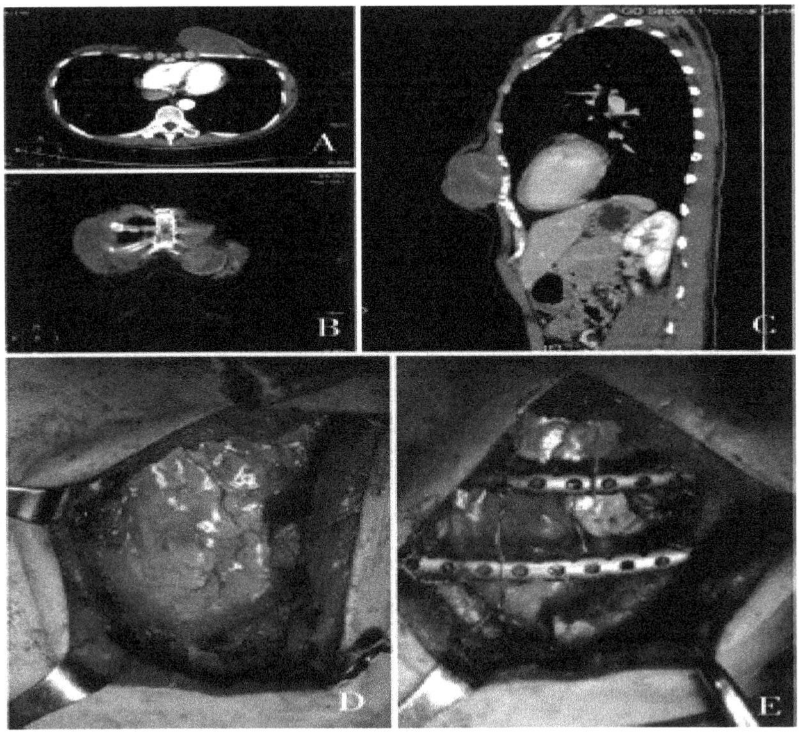

Figure 3-6-9 Resection of Rib Tumor Beneath the Breast and Chest Wall reconstruction. (A, B, C. CT images show the chest wall tumor located beneath the left breast; D. An incision is made around the breast tissue to expose the tumor, and the tumor along with sufficient surrounding bony structures is resected; E. The chest wall is reconstructed using MatrixRIB.)

3. Surgical Outcomes

The effect of rib tumor Surgery is determined by the nature of the Surgery. In other words, the effect of Surgery depends on two aspects: the effect of curing the disease and the effect of plastic Surgery. Since there is no unified standard to measure the two, a comprehensive judgment is needed. For benign tumors, the effect of plastic Surgery is something that needs to be emphasized. But for malignant tumors, For malignant tumors, the therapeutic outcome becomes virtually the sole criterion for evaluating the success of the Surgery. Regardless of the type of rib tumor, as long as the resection is thorough, good therapeutic results can generally be expected. However, even with complete removal, malignant tumors do not always guarantee favorable outcomes. These cases often require additional postoperative treatments, such as chemotherapy or radiotherapy. Only when the tumor is fully eradicated can the Surgery be considered truly successful in terms of its therapeutic effect.

REFERENCES

[1] Yu, H., X. Chen, and Y. Guo. 2014. "A Discussion on Minimally Invasive Resection of High-Position Rib Tumors on the Deep Surface of the Scapula." *Practical Oncology Journal* 28 (2): 154–156.

[2] Manjunatha, H. K., A. S. Ramaswamy, and B. S. Kumar. 2012. "Aggressive Giant Cell Tumor of the Anterior Arc of the Rib." *Journal of Cytology* 29 (1): 51–53.

[3] Fan, G., M. Qian, J. Gong, et al. 2005. "CT Analysis of Rib Tumors." *Journal of Clinical Radiology* 24 (3): 246–248.

[4] Shah, A., H. Ma, X. Sun, et al. 2012. "Primary Parosteal Osteosarcoma of the Rib." *Interactive Cardiovascular and Thoracic Surgery* 15 (1): 169–170.

[5] Krishnamurthy, A., and A. Arulmolichelvan. 2017. "Management Challenges in an Unusual Case of Primary Osteosarcoma of the Rib in an Adult Patient." *Indian Journal of Surgery* 79 (4): 363–366.

[6] Wang, W. 2021. "Matrix-Rib Reconstruction Surgery (14-Year-Old Girl): Chest Wall Tumor Resection and Reconstruction." *Thoracic Deformity Surgery Expert*, February 8, 2021.

[7] Hoang, D., D. Perrault, M. Stevanovic, et al. 2016. "Surgical Applications of Three-Dimensional Printing: A Review of the Current Literature and How to Get Started." *Annals of Translational Medicine* 4 (23): 456.

[8] Huang, Z., Y. Li, and P. Yao. 2006. "Diagnosis and Treatment Experience of Axillary Approach for First Rib Tumor Resection." *Anhui Medical Journal* 27 (4): 320–321.

[9] Zhang, D., J. Jiang, and J. Zhang. 2016. "Surgical Approach for Giant Aneurysmal Bone Cyst of the First Rib." *Modern Oncology* 24 (23): 3823–3825.

[10] Matsunobu, T., A. Maekawa, A. Nabeshima, et al. 2021. "Giant Cell Tumor of the First Rib Treated with Preoperative Denosumab and Surgery via a Transmanubrial Approach." *American Journal of Case Reports* 22: e931796.

[11] Palumbo, V. D., S. Fazzotta, F. Fatica, et al. 2019. "Pancoast Tumour: Current Therapeutic Options." *Clinical Therapeutics* 170 (4): E291–E294.

[12] Xu, N., R. Xu, W. Ma, et al. 2011. "Langerhans Cell Histiocytosis Causing Pathologic Fractures of T3 and T4 with Incomplete Paralysis." *Zhongguo Gushang (Chinese Journal of Orthopaedic Trauma)* 24 (10): 848–850.

[13] Wang, W. 2021. "Resection of a Giant Chest Wall Tumor on the Deep Surface of the Scapula with MatrixRIB Reconstruction." *Thoracic Deformity Surgery Expert*, September 6, 2021.

The chest wall is composed of three basic structures: bony structures, soft tissue, and skin. The previous sections focused on tumors of the bony structures. This section will introduce tumors of the soft tissue and skin. These two types are among the most common chest wall tumors. In the early stages, they do not invade deeper structures and are relatively independent tumors. However, if they invade deeper structures especially when the bony structures are affected management becomes more complex. When that happens, it brings us back to the discussion in the earlier text. This illustrates a fundamental principle: the chest wall is an organic whole. Pathological changes in any one structure cannot exist independently; over time, they will spread to other structures, eventually leading to the same outcome pathological changes involving the entire chest wall. From this perspective, it may seem unnecessary to study a particular structure in isolation. However, it must be clearly understood that the progression of disease is a gradual process, and not every patient seeks medical attention only at the final stage. In the early stages of the disease, the pathological changes still bear the imprint of their tissue of origin. At this point, diagnosis and treatment will certainly differ significantly, which gives special importance to research based on the tissue origin of the lesions. This section's independent study of soft tissue and skin tumors precisely reflects the significance of such research

1. Soft Tissue Tumors

The soft tissues of the chest wall are distributed throughout every part of the chest wall, filling every corner. When soft tissue tumors occur, they can arise in any location on the chest wall. In terms of origin, soft tissue tumors can develop from any type of tissue that makes up the chest wall, including muscle, fat, nerves, blood vessels, and pleura. Each type of tissue is composed of different cells, and these cells can serve as more specific origins of tumors [1–3]. Tumors of different origins exhibit significantly different fundamental characteristics. For example, tumors originating from muscle or nerve tissue will display features of their tissue origin on multiple levels. These characteristics are of great importance for understanding and treating tumors

Soft tissue tumors can be either benign or malignant. Among all chest wall tumors, malignant tumors account for 50% - 80%, of which approximately 45% are malignant soft tissue tumors. In certain populations, the incidence rate of chest wall soft tissue tumors is 2.2/100,000 [4].

Benign tumors exhibit the typical characteristics of non-cancerous growths:

they grow in a localized manner, are encapsulated, grow slowly, do not metastasize to distant sites, do not infiltrate surrounding tissues, and do not invade bony structures or the skin. In contrast, malignant tumors tend to grow invasively, have poorly defined boundaries, grow rapidly, may invade bones and skin, and often spread to distant parts of the body

Soft tissue tumors can be primary tumors or metastases from other parts of the body. Metastatic tumors are generally malignant tumors.

Benign soft tissue tumors may have no obvious symptoms. Occasionally, there may be pain, but it is usually mild, such as a dull ache or soreness, with stabbing pain being rare. The most significant clinical sign is a localized mass. In the early stages the mass may not be prominent and is often discovered incidentally. malignant soft tissue tumors, on the other hand, may cause noticeable pain. The local sign is also a mass, which may enlarge within a short period. When the tumor invades the skin, local skin abnormalities may appear, and in severe cases, ulceration or rupture may occur. If the tumor compresses nearby veins and obstructs local venous return, for the examination of soft tissue tumors, physical examination should be performed first, which usually provides the most basic information. Soft tissue tumors may be located deep within the chest wall or beneath special anatomical structures, making them difficult to detect, and physical examination alone may not yield effective findings. To gain more understanding of the tumor, imaging studies are necessary, such as X-rays.

Examination is the most basic form of imaging and can roughly identify the tumor's location and its relationship with surrounding structures. However, since soft tissues have poor contrast on X-ray images, the amount of information obtained is limited. The most valuable examination is CT, as it can clearly show the tumor's location, size, and internal structure, and it can also clarify the relationship between the tumor and surrounding structures, which is why CT is an essential examination for soft tissue tumors. In addition, MRI and ultrasound can also be performed. MRI functions similarly to CT and may provide better results for certain types of tumors. Ultrasound is considered a particularly useful test; it can determine the tumor's location, size, neighboring relationships, and also assess blood supply, even allowing for a preliminary assessment of the nature of the tumor. In addition to the imaging tests mentioned above, cytological examination can also be performed before Surgery to determine the tumor's nature. Since most tumors are located superficially, cytological sampling is relatively easy to perform. This can involve a simple needle aspiration or a partial excisional biopsy

Soft tissue tumors of the chest wall that are located superficially are relatively easy to diagnose. However, tumors located in certain special areas may be difficult to detect due to the obstruction of superficial structures. For example, soft tissue tumors located on the back, especially those beneath the scapula, are not easily discovered and are typically only identified when symptoms become obvious or when the tumor grows large. Similarly, tumors on the anterior chest wall, if located deep beneath the breast tissue in women, are also difficult to detect. Diagnosing tumors in these areas can be challenging. However, with the aid of imaging examinations, diagnosis becomes much easier.

The differential diagnosis of soft tissue tumors of the chest wall primarily involves distinguishing them from benign chest wall conditions, particularly chronic infectious lesions. Chronic infections may present as localized abscesses or osteomyelitis, and in severe cases, skin ulceration may occur. This needs to be differentiated from malignant soft tissue tumors that invade the skin. Infections typically have a history of local infection and present with prominent local symptoms. In contrast, malignant tumors usually present first as a mass, followed later by skin changes. Tuberculous abscesses, a form of chronic infection, may lack obvious local symptoms but often have a history of tuberculosis and are accompanied by systemic symptoms. In comparison, soft tissue tumors of the chest wall tend to show more prominent local symptoms but generally do not cause systemic symptoms.

Soft tissue tumors located in the deep layer of the anterior chest wall beneath the breast must be differentiated from breast tumors. Breast tumors are typically more superficial and exhibit greater mobility. However, if a breast tumor is deeply situated and invades deeper structures, it becomes difficult to distinguish from a soft tissue tumor of the chest wall. In such cases, imaging studies such as CT, MRI, or ultrasound can assist in making an accurate differential diagnosis.

Once a soft tissue tumor is confirmed, Surgery should generally be performed as early as possible provided there are no significant contraindications. The main contraindications include:①Distant metastasis: If the soft tissue tumor has spread to distant organs, Surgery is typically not considered. However, if the metastasis is isolated, both the primary tumor and the metastatic site may be Surgically removed, depending on the clinical situation.② Multiple tumors in various parts of the body: Some tumors, such as neurofibromas, may occur in multiple locations throughout the body. In such cases, a chest wall tumor is only part of a systemic disease, and Surgery might not be beneficial unless the lesion causes specific symptoms or complications. In such cases, the chest wall lesion is only part of a systemic disease, so resection offers little benefit and Surgery is generally not recommended. However, in special circumstances if the chest wall tumor causes severe local effects, surgery may still be justified (Figure 3-7-1).③Concurrent metastases in other body regions. If the soft tissue tumor originates from a primary lesion elsewhere in the body that has already metastasized to multiple sites, a chest wall metastasis is not a suitable target for Surgery. ④Tumor invasion too extensive for reconstruction. Here the limitation to Surgery is not the tumor itself but technical feasibility if resection would leave a defect too large to reconstruct (for example, massive skin loss or extensive bony destruction), the operation cannot be undertaken lightly. ⑤Poor overall patient condition. If the patient's general health status precludes

Surgery, then operative treatment is not possible.
The specific Surgical technique for chest wall soft tissue tumors depends on the tumor's characteristics. For well-circumscribed tumors particularly, those preoperatively diagnosed as benign simple excision of the lesion may suffice. However, for malignant tumors, a wide excision is required. In addition to removing the tumor itself, a margin of surrounding suspicious tissue must also be respected. This excision encompasses two dimensions: horizontally, tissues within a specified distance beyond the tumor's edge are removed; and vertically, resection extends both superficially toward the skin and deeply toward the underlying structures. If the tumor's infiltration is extensive, even deep bony structures must be included in the resection.

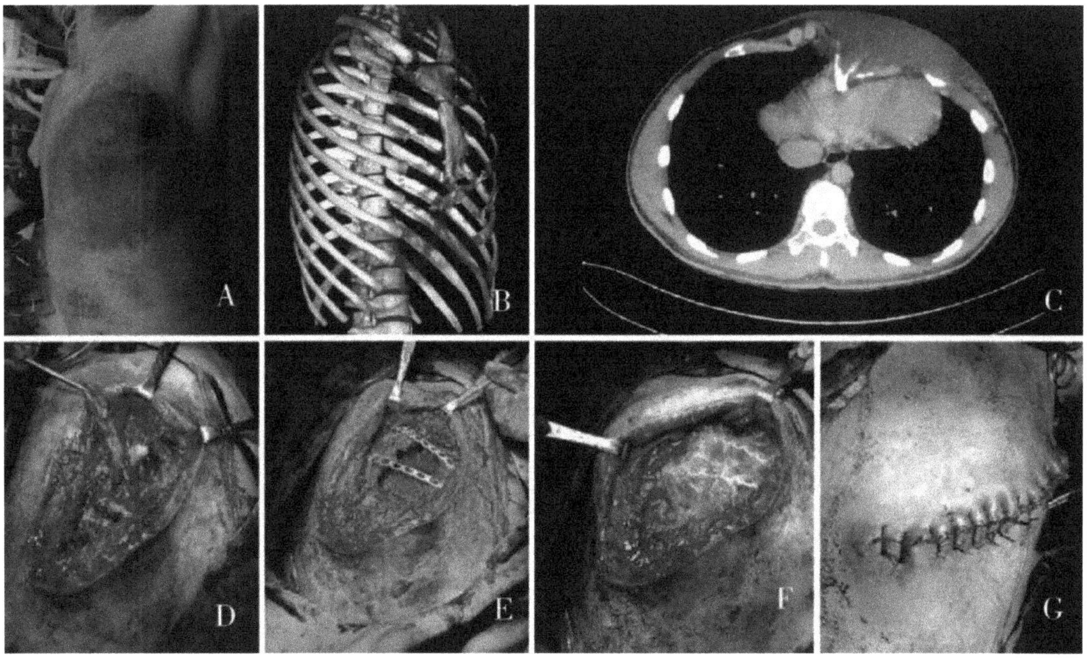

Figure 3-7-1 Resection of Chest Wall Neurofibroma and Chest Wall reconstruction. (A. The tumor extensively invades the chest wall, mainly located on the left anterior chest wall; B. 3D reconstruction shows involvement of the bony structures on the left chest wall, with loss of normal anatomy; C. The chest wall in the precordial area is sunken, with bony destruction and protrusion of structures toward the heart, significantly affecting cardiac function and causing symptoms;D. Tumor is resected; E. Repair materials are used to reconstruct the bony structure; F. A fiber membrane is used as a liner; G. The incision is closed.)

The overlying skin is also excised. After resection of an isolated or well-circumscribed tumor, there is generally no significant defect, so the wound and skin can be directly sutured without the need for soft tissue or skin reconstruction. However, for patients requiring wide excision, reconstruction must be performed in the same manner as for bony-structure tumor resections. reconstruction again involves three components: bony structure, soft tissue, and skin. Essentially, at this stage the nature of the Surgery is almost identical, and the specific techniques used are exactly the same as those for bony-structure reconstruction.

Because they are superficially located, malignant soft-tissue tumors may invade more extensively than malignant tumors of bony structures and are more prone to cause skin destruction; the soft-tissue damage itself may also be more severe. Therefore, Surgery must include not only skin reconstruction but also soft-tissue reconstruction [5-7]. The ideal approach is to use a musculocutaneous flap preferentially from adjacent tissues, which usually suffice. If the defect is too large, a pedicled musculocutaneous flap harvested from a more distant site can be employed.

The prognosis of soft tissue tumors is related to many factors [8-10]: ① The nature of the tumor. If a benign tumor is completely removed, a radical cure can be achieved. The prognosis of a malignant tumor is related to the degree of malignancy. Low-grade malignant tumors have a satisfactory prognosis, while low-grade malignant tumors are prone to recurrence and metastasis. ② The size of the tumor. The larger the tumor, the worse the prognosis. ③ The extent of resection. When the extent of tumor resection is larger, the prognosis is often more satisfactory. ④ Auxiliary treatment. In addition to Surgery, malignant tumors also require postoperative adjuvant treatment. Auxiliary treatment can often consolidate the therapeutic effect and achieve better results. ⑤ The patient's condition. If the patient's general condition is poor, the prognosis is often poor.

2. Skin Tumors

Skin tumors can develop on any part of the body, with exposed sites showing the highest incidence. Although the chest wall is not directly exposed, its large surface area and wide extent make it a relatively common location for skin tumors. In clinical practice, however, chest-wall skin tumors appear to be rare, a perception that stems from patient referral patterns. Patients with skin lesions typically present first to dermatology or plastic-reconstructive clinics, and traditional thoracic-Surgery outpatient departments seldom see these cases, creating the false impression that chest-wall skin tumors are uncommon.

Chest wall skin tumors can occur in the skin of any part of the chest wall. Tumors can be benign or malignant, with benign tumors being more common in women than in men. Based on the tissue source, skin tumors can be divided into [11]: ① melanocytic tumors; ② epithelial cell tumors; ③ skin connective tissue tumors; ④ hematopoietic tissue tumors; ⑤ skin appendage tumors; ⑥ cysts; ⑦ skin metastatic cancer. Among them, melanocytic tumors and epithelial cell tumors account for the majority.

Skin malignancies can be divided into malignant melanoma and non-melanoma skin tumors. Malignant melanoma is the least common, but it is extremely malignant. The most common non-melanoma skin tumors are basal cell carcinoma and squamous cell carcinoma [12-14].

Benign skin tumors are not very harmful, grow slowly, and are relatively localized. Malignant tumors are very harmful, highly destructive, grow rapidly, and can grow in an invasive manner. In severe cases, local skin breaks may occur, and necrotic tissue or fluid may flow out.

Benign skin tumors are not very harmful, grow slowly, and are relatively localized. Malignant tumors are very harmful, highly destructive, grow rapidly, and can grow in an invasive manner. In severe cases, local skin breaks may occur, and necrotic tissue or fluid may flow out. There are also virus infection foci. Some symptomatic neoplasms are not tumors, but may become malignant.

Once a skin tumor is diagnosed, it should be treated. Early benign tumors can be treated with conservative treatment to remove the lesions. The chest wall Surgeon can do it alone or in cooperation with the dermatology and cosmetology departments. If the lesion is large, Surgical removal is required.

Malignant skin tumors require direct Surgical removal. Early malignant tumors only need to remove the lesion. If the tumor is extensive and invades deeper structures, the deep structures and even the bone structures need to be removed together, and the removal range also needs to include other suspicious structures around it.

After the removal of a skin tumor, a skin defect is inevitably present, and soft tissue defects are also unavoidable. If the excision is more extensive, there may also be defects in bony structures. Small areas of skin and soft tissue defects do not require special reconstruction; simply closing the Surgical field and skin incision is sufficient. However, if the defect is large, reconstruction of the affected structures is necessary.

The prognosis of skin tumors also depends on numerous factors, including tumor-related factors, systemic factors,

and treatment-related factors. Overall, benign and low-grade malignant tumors have a good prognosis, while the higher the malignancy, the poorer the prognosis

The prognosis of skin tumors is also influenced by numerous factors, including tumor-specific factors, systemic factors, and treatment-related factors. Generally speaking, benign and low-grade malignant tumors have a favorable prognosis, while the higher the malignancy, the poorer the prognosis. The better the patient's overall health and immunity, the more favorable the outcome. Additionally, the more complete the tumor resection, the better the prognosis. If the tumor is large and cannot be completely removed, the prognosis is poor.

REFERENCES

[1] Batihan, G., O. Usluer, S. O. Kaya, et al. 2018. "Atypical Deep Somatic Soft-Tissue Leiomyoma of the Extrathoracic Chest Wall: First Case in the Literature." *BMJ Case Reports* 11 (1): e226668.

[2] Sirivella, S., and I. Gielchinsky. 2013. "Treatment Outcomes in 23 Thoracic Primitive Neuroectodermal Tumours: A Retrospective Study." *Interactive Cardiovascular and Thoracic Surgery* 17 (2): 273–279.

[3] Davis, C. H., H. Yammine, P. G. Khaitan, et al. 2016. "A Multidisciplinary Approach to Giant Soft Tissue Sarcoma of the Chest Wall: A Case Report." *International Journal of Surgery Case Reports* 28: 211–213.

[4] Yoon, S. H., J. C. Jung, I. K. Park, et al. 2019. "Clinical Outcomes of Surgical Treatment for Primary Chest Wall Soft Tissue Sarcoma." *Korean Journal of Thoracic and Cardiovascular Surgery* 52 (3): 148–154.

[5] Sakamoto, A., T. Noguchi, and S. Matsuda. 2021. "Thoracoabdominal Flap Reconstruction After Resection of Superficial Soft-Tissue Sarcomas in the Chest Wall." *Journal of Surgical Case Reports* 2021 (1): rjaa571.

[6] Morgan, R. F., M. T. Edgerton, H. J. Wanebo, et al. 1988. "Reconstruction of Full-Thickness Chest Wall Defects." *Annals of Surgery* 207 (6): 707–716.

[7] Sanna, S., J. Brandolini, A. Pardolesi, et al. 2017. "Materials and Techniques in Chest Wall Reconstruction: A Review." *Journal of Visualized Surgery* 3: 95.

[8] Soerensen, T. R., M. Raedkjaer, P. H. Jorgensen, et al. 2019. "Soft Tissue Sarcomas of the Thoracic Wall: Higher Mortality and Local Recurrence—A Single-Institution Long-Term Follow-Up Study." *International Journal of Surgical Oncology* 2019: 2350157.

[9] Van Geel, A. N., M. W. J. M. Wouters, T. E. Lans, et al. 2011. "Chest Wall Resection for Adult Soft Tissue Sarcomas and Chondrosarcomas: Analysis of Prognostic Factors." *World Journal of Surgery* 35 (1): 63–69.

[10] Harati, K., J. Kolbenschlag, J. Böhm, et al. 2018. "Long-Term Outcomes of Patients with Soft Tissue Sarcoma of the Chest Wall: Prognostic Significance of Microscopic Margins." *Oncology Letters* 15 (2): 2179–2187.

[11] Men, Y., Q. Zhang, B. Zhang, et al. 2016. "Retrospective Analysis of 4,695 Cases of Solitary Skin Tumors." *Peking University Medical Journal* 48 (2): 377–379.

[12] Liu, Z., Q. Zhang, W. Wu, et al. 2018. "Retrospective Analysis of 518 Cases of Malignant Skin Tumors and Precancerous Lesions." *Journal of Capital Medical University* 39 (4): 602–606.

[13] Santos, P. J. F., C. Prendergast, and A. Leis. 2016. "Giant Anterior Chest Wall Basal Cell Carcinoma: An Approach to Palliative Reconstruction." *Case Reports in Oncology Medicine* 2016: 5067817.

[14] Berking, C., A. Hauschild, O. Köbl, et al. 2014. "Basal Cell Carcinoma: Treatments for the Commonest Skin Cancer." *Deutsches Ärzteblatt International* 111 (22): 389–395.

The thoracic inlet is an important anatomical region due to the presence of numerous critical structures passing through it. When a tumor develops in this area, it can affect many of these structures and lead to severe functional impairments, often with serious consequences. In the past, Surgeries in this region were primarily performed by specialists from different medical fields. Each specialty has its own principles and methods for handling such cases, with unique strengths as well as limitations. Thoracic wall Surgery focuses on the chest wall, and most procedures involving the thoracic inlet fall within the scope of thoracic wall Surgery. Utilizing thoracic wall Surgical techniques to treat tumors in this area allows for the integration of expertise from multiple specialties, which is beneficial for effective tumor treatment.

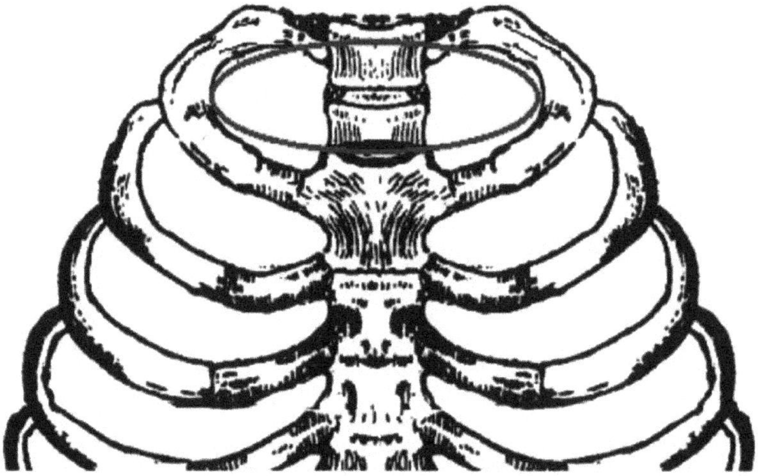

Figure 3-8-1 The location and the structure of the upper opening of the thorax

1. Anatomical structure of the upper opening of the thorax

The thoracic inlet is an important anatomical passage bounded by the upper border of the sternum, the 1 rib, and the body of the 1 thoracic vertebra (Figure 3-8-1). When studying tumors that occur in the thoracic inlet, it is necessary to consider the interactions among the various structures. Therefore, the scope of the thoracic inlet is slightly expanded to include several important surrounding structures, such as the clavicle, adjacent vertebrae, and nearby ribs. Together, these form the broader concept of the thoracic inlet. This book discusses the thoracic inlet in this expanded sense.

The contents of the upper opening refer to the upper opening of the thorax in a broad sense.

The structures inside and near the upper opening of the thorax are closely integrated, and there are orderly and complex connections between them. In order to better reveal these connections, we study them as a whole. In general, the upper opening of the thorax and its surrounding structures can be divided into three categories: ① Structures that directly participate in the formation of the upper opening of the thorax. There are four types of such structures, namely the manubrium of the sternum, the clavicle, the 1 rib and the thoracic vertebrae. These structures together surround the upper opening of the thorax from different directions. ② Structures passing through the upper opening of the thorax. The main structures of the neck and chest communication pass through the upper opening of the thorax. These structures can be divided into two parts: one is the contents of the upper mediastinum, and the other is the apex of the lung. The main contents of the upper mediastinum include blood vessels, nerves, trachea and esophagus, and the apex of the lung is a part of the upper lobe of the lung, located on the upper part of the plane above the first rib. ③ Nearby structures. All structures located near the upper opening of the thorax are in this category, including nearby bones, muscles, nerves, blood vessels and other structures. It is important to emphasize that the neurovascular sheath leading to the upper limb is a particularly critical structure near the thoracic inlet. Although it is not located within the thoracic inlet itself, it lies at the upper outer side of the inlet. Because this structure is susceptible to invasion by various types of tumors, it warrants special attention. The thoracic inlet region contains a wide variety of structures that involve multiple medical specialties. Although there is some overlap between these
specialties, clinical practice tends to be compartmentalized, which can hinder effective management. By bringing these structures together under the scope of thoracic wall Surgery, a more integrated approach is established, which undoubtedly facilitates the treatment of tumors in this region.

2. Types of Tumors in the Thoracic Inlet

Tumors may occur in the upper thoracic opening itself and all nearby structures, and all of these tumors fall within the scope of this section. These tumors can be divided into the following categories based on their location: ① Clavicle tumors; ② 1 rib tumors; ③ Stem-manubrium tumors; ④ Vertebral tumors; ⑤ Lung apex tumors; ⑥ Other tumors. These tumors can be benign or malignant, have different histological origins, and can be primary tumors or metastatic tumors.

3. Differentiation of Some Special Concepts

(1) Thoracic Outlet

In clinical practice, the term "thoracic outlet" is often encountered. Many people mistakenly equate the thoracic inlet with the thoracic outlet, but these are actually two entirely different concepts. The thoracic outlet refers to the passageway between the lateral aspect of the clavicle and the 1 rib. This channel directly connects the supraclavicular fossa to the axilla [1-3]. Despite its name, the so-called "thoracic outlet" is not actually related to the thoracic cavity; rather, it is a passage adjacent to the thoracic inlet (Figure 3-8-2). Clearly, the term itself is logically flawed and somewhat misleading. The concept of the thoracic outlet comes from orthopaedics or hand Surgery, not from thoracic Surgery. However, some thoracic Surgeons may be misled by the literal meaning of the term and incorrectly assume that the thoracic outlet is the same as the thoracic inlet; this is a misconception that needs to be corrected.

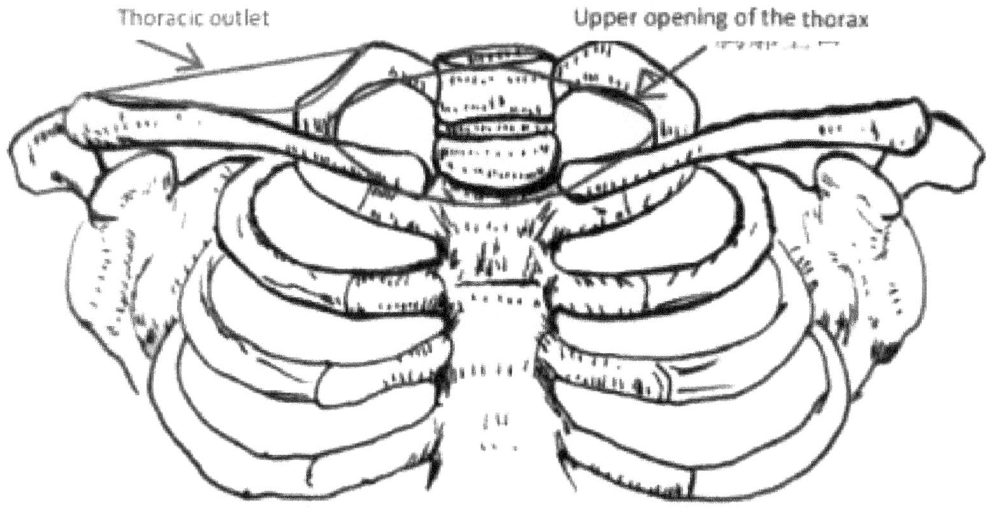

Figure 3-8-2 Thoracic outlet and upper thoracic opening

The most important structures within the thoracic outlet are the brachial plexus nerves and the subclavian vessels that supply the upper limb. These structures originate from the upper inner region of the thoracic inlet, pass obliquely across the top of the thoracic inlet, and then travel downward and outward, closely following the upper edge of the first rib to enter the axilla. Because these structures pass over the top and outer side of the thoracic inlet not through its interior, they are considered adjacent to the thoracic inlet, rather than being part of the thoracic inlet itself (Figure 3-8-3).

Figure 3-8-3 Structures passing through the thoracic outlet

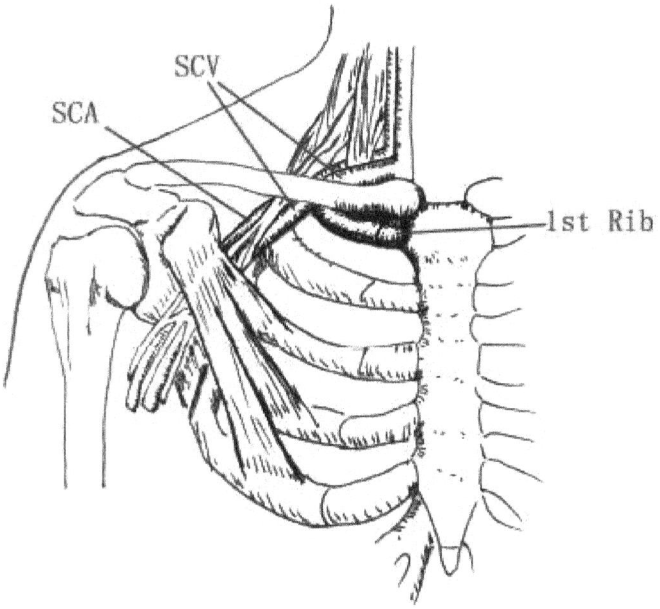

(2) Thoracic Outlet Syndrome

Thoracic outlet syndrome refers to a condition in which various lesions near the thoracic outlet compress the brachial plexus nerves and subclavian artery and vein, resulting in a range of neurological and vascular symptoms affecting the upper limb. These symptoms may include pain, numbness, weakness in the shoulder, arm, and hand, as well as muscle atrophy, coldness in the hand, cyanosis, and weakened radial pulse. The causes of this syndrome are diverse. While tumors can be a cause, it is more commonly due to benign conditions, such as cervical rib anomalies, abnormal positioning of the first rib, or trauma. Although this condition is named after the "thoracic outlet," it is primarily managed by orthopaedic Surgeons or hand Surgeons, with minimal involvement from thoracic surgeons[2,3].

(3) Pancoast Tumor

The lung apex is an anatomical region referring to the portion of the lung that extends above the clavicle and the upper edge of the 1 rib. The top of the lung apex is rounded and blunt, located approximately 2-3 cm above the inner and middle 1/3 of the clavicle and 2-4 cm above the 1 rib. Normally, the apex of the lung fills the very top of the thoracic cavity and sits centrally within the thoracic outlet. A Pancoast tumor refers to a malignant tumor located in this area. Once cancer develops in the lung apex, it can easily invade the chest wall and affect the critical structures around the thoracic outlet, leading to serious complications.

(4) Superior Pulcus Tumor

The superior pulmonary sulcus is an anatomical term referring to the impression left on the upper lobe of the lung by the subclavian artery. This impression is very limited in scope and only involves a small area at the lung apex. A cancer that occurs in this specific region is referred to as a superior sulcus tumor.By anatomical definition, the superior sulcus tumor is just a subtype of apical lung cancer (Pancoast tumor). However, aside from carcinoma in situ, malignant tumors tend to progress quickly, and tumors originating in the superior sulcus can infiltrate or spread to the entire lung apex within a short time. Thus, in clinical practice, it's rare to find tumors strictly confined to the superior sulcus; most are categorized as apical lung cancers[4].

(5) Pancoast Tumor

Named after the American radiologist Pancoast, this term does not refer to a specific tumor type, but rather to any tumor occurring near the thoracic inlet. This region includes the lung apex and surrounding structures. Such tumors may be primary, metastatic, or even non-malignant.

(6) Pancoast syndrome

This syndrome refers to a series of clinical manifestations caused by Pancoast tumors. There are three main manifestations: ① Shoulder pain; ② Clinical manifestations caused by involvement of the C8-T1 nerve roots, mainly abnormalities in the distribution area of the ulnar nerve of the upper limb; ③ Clinical manifestations caused by involvement of the sympathetic ganglia, which is the so-called Horner syndrome. This syndrome is relatively typical. Once it occurs, Pancoast tumors are often considered. The manifestations of this syndrome are similar to thoracic outlet syndrome, but they are not exactly the same. Pane coast syndrome is caused by tumors at the upper thoracic opening, and thoracic outlet syndrome is caused by lesions at the thoracic outlet. Since the upper thoracic opening is adjacent to the thoracic outlet, local tumors may overlap, so the two may have some of the same symptoms, but they are not the same disease.

(7) Thoracic Outlet Tumor Resection

As the name implies, this tumor is a tumor that occurs at the thoracic outlet. The tumor here is not the same as the thoracic outlet tumor and should not be mistaken for the thoracic outlet tumor.

(8) Tumors at the cervicothoracic junction

Although there is no clear anatomical definition of the cervicothoracic junction, it is roughly the area near the upper opening of the thorax. Tumors at this location are basically similar to tumors at the upper opening of the thorax and Pancoast tumors, and are a general term for a large category of tumors.

4. Clinical Manifestations

The early clinical manifestations of thoracic superior opening tumors are not typical. If the tumor is confined to a small area, it may not affect other surrounding structures and thus may not produce obvious symptoms. However, if the tumor continues to grow and starts to involve nearby structures, certain distinctive symptoms may appear. A typical manifestation is Pancoast syndrome [6], which is a common symptom that occurs when tumors at the thoracic inlet progress to a certain stage. In addition to these general symptoms, each type of tumor may also present with its own unique signs. For example, A tumor of the manubrium (upper part of the sternum) may compress the superior vena cava, resulting in venous return obstruction in the upper limbs and neck. A clavicle tumor can lead to more local symptoms and also affect the upper limbs.

Tumors of the clavicle and the 1 rib may compress the subclavian vessels and nerves, and such tumors can also be considered thoracic outlet tumors. When the compression caused by the tumor is severe, it can lead to thoracic outlet syndrome. Pancoast tumors (tumors at the apex of the lung) fall under the category of peripheral lung cancers. These tumors typically do not cause noticeable respiratory symptoms in the early stages. Symptoms only appear when the tumor invades the hilum of the lung (the central area where bronchi, blood vessels, and nerves enter and leave the lung).

5. Examinations

The local structure of the upper opening of the thorax is complex. Once a tumor occurs, it often affects multiple structures, so there are high requirements for examination. Physical examination can detect early superficial tumors, such as first rib tumors, clavicle tumors, sternal manubrium tumors, etc., but it is difficult to detect deep tumors. Further examination requires imaging examination. X-ray examination can roughly show the location of the tumor. The most commonly used and most effective examination is CT examination, which can display tumor information from all angles (Figure 3-8-4). If conditions permit, three-dimensional reconstruction examination can be performed, which can not only more intuitively reveal local information, but also help to clarify the relationship between important structures.

The above examinations are structural examinations. In addition to these examinations, some functional examinations should also be considered, with the focus on functional examinations of the brachial plexus. Based on these examinations, the extent of nerve involvement can be roughly determined.

6.Diagnosis and differential diagnosis

The clinical manifestations of early thoracic superior opening tumors are atypical, and diagnosis is difficult without relevant examinations. After obvious local masses or Pancoast syndrome occur, diagnosis is easier and can be confirmed through relevant examinations.

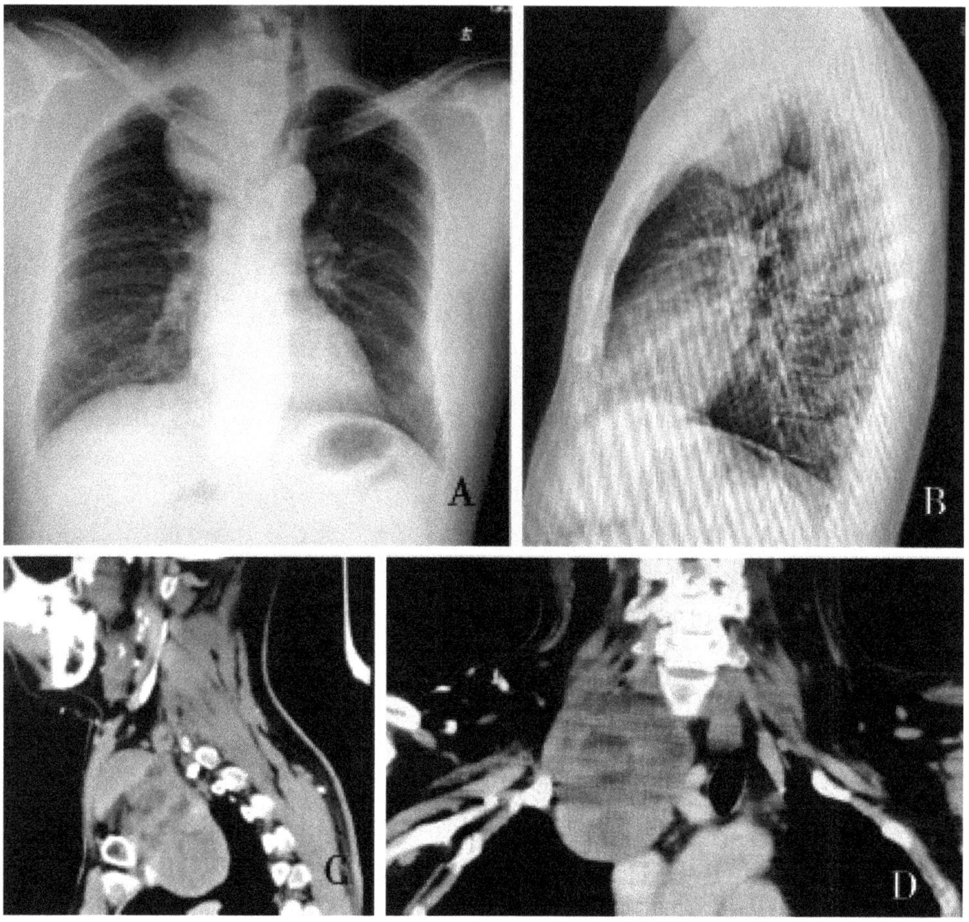

Figure 3-8-4: X-ray and CT Imaging of Thoracic Inlet Tumors. (A. Frontal X-ray view shows the approximate location of the tumor. B. Lateral X-ray view reveals that the tumor is located at the apex of the thoracic cavity. C, D. CT scans clearly display the precise position of the tumor)

Thoracic cavity tumors include all tumors occurring in the thoracic cavity and surrounding structures. Due to the complexity of the local structure, in order to facilitate treatment, the following contents need to be clarified when making a diagnosis: ① The primary structure of the tumor; ② The structure invaded by the tumor; ③ The function of blood vessels and nerves.

Differential diagnosis should first be made from some benign lesions, including cervical and thoracic deformities, rib deformities, tuberculosis, injuries, and lesions caused by other special reasons. Although these lesions do not have the harm of tumors, they may have symptoms similar to Pancoast syndrome and are easily confused with thoracic upper opening tumors, so imaging examinations are needed for differentiation.

Differential diagnosis also needs to be made from the lesions that cause thoracic outlet syndrome. The lesions that cause the latter may be located near the upper thoracic opening or not in this area. In addition, the lesions may be benign and not necessarily tumors.

7.Surgical Treatment

(1) Indications for Surgery

Once a thoracic inlet tumor is diagnosed, Surgical treatment is generally required unless there are specific contraindications. These contraindications are mostly technical in nature. Some tumors present high Surgical difficulty and risk, which may initially be deemed inoperable. However, such contraindications are often relative, not absolute. As Surgical techniques and technologies continue to improve, many conditions that were once considered Surgical contraindications may no longer be so.

(2) Preoperative preparation

Since the tumor may invade important structures, some people suggest using appropriate radiotherapy and chemotherapy for preoperative preparation in order to achieve better Surgical results. This approach is reasonable, but not necessary. Most tumors can be directly removed.

(3) Incision selection

The greatest difficulty of the upper thoracic opening tumor is exposure. In order to obtain a good exposure effect, a suitable incision must be used. The choice of incision needs to be determined based on the location of the tumor and the invasion. If the tumor occurs in a relatively superficial structure, such as the clavicle, the first rib or the sternal manubrium, the incision can be directly selected on the surface of these structures. If the tumor of these structures invades the deep structure, resulting in the deep structure of the upper thoracic opening being affected, the incision needs to be designed differently.
Some thoracic Surgeons choose to expand the chest incision, which generally makes it difficult to reveal the area around the upper opening of the thorax. In order to obtain a good exposure effect, some special incisions are used in clinical practice.

1. Posterior chest incision [4]. An incision is made from the 7th cervical spinous process downward, through the posterior midline of the scapula, around the inferior angle of the scapula and upward to the anterior axillary line. The size of the incision can be determined according to the need for lesion exposure. First, the rib structure is exposed, and the intercostal space to enter the chest is selected according to the operation needs. After the specific ribs are removed, the incision is opened with a spreader to complete the lesion exposure. This incision has a good exposure effect on lung lesions and a satisfactory exposure effect on subclavian structures. It

can meet the needs of various tumor resections.

2. Cervical-thoracic combined incision [4,9]. An incision is made from the outside of the neck downward, to the vicinity of the sternoclavicular joint, around the subclavian, and then a horizontal incision is made outward. The sternoclavicular joint is cut open, and part of the clavicle or the first rib is removed as needed, and then the lesion is exposed. Considering the role of the sternoclavicular joint, some people use the method of splitting the sternum to protect this joint. Such an incision has a certain rationality. However, if the tumor is extensive and a partial clavicle resection is required, such an operation is not very meaningful.
3. Other incisions [10-12]. The occurrence of tumors in the upper thoracic opening is complex, and a single incision is sometimes difficult to achieve satisfactory results. During the specific operation, other incisions can be designed according to Surgical needs. There is no fixed pattern for this type of incision. As long as the tumor resection operation can be completed without damaging important structures, it is a reasonable incision.

(4) Tumor resection

Early tumor resection is relatively simple. If it invades other surrounding structures, the tumor itself and all the invaded structures need to be removed together. The basic principles of tumor resection are: ① Remove all of it as much as possible; ② Protect important structures as much as possible; ③ If there is a risk of complete tumor resection, it can be partially removed.

The operation of tumor resection is the core content of the operation, and certain skills are required for specific operations: ① There must be a reasonable order. Generally, it should start from the most easily exposed part. As the resection operation proceeds, the difficult-to-expose parts will gradually be exposed. ② There must be a reasonable method. Direct resection is the simplest operation method, but because it involves important structures such as blood vessels, direct resection may lead to uncontrollable complications. Therefore, important structures should be treated first, and then resection should be performed to ensure the safety of the operation. ③ There must be an appropriate degree. Tumors at the upper opening of the thorax are closely related to surrounding structures, and surrounding structures are often invaded. Do not be too radical when resecting the tumor, otherwise it may lead to extremely serious complications.

(5) Chest wall reconstruction

During the process of exposing and removing the tumor, the ribs or sternum may be partially removed, and the chest wall will have obvious defects after the removal. Since the defect will affect the integrity of the chest after Surgery, reconstruction is required. reconstruction is not required after the 1 rib is removed. If the ribs below the 2 ribs are removed, reconstruction is generally required after Surgery. The sternum is an important structure of the chest. After the upper half of the sternum is removed, reconstruction must be performed after Surgery. The reconstruction method needs to be determined according to the structure removed, and the focus is on the choice of materials. You can choose digital materials or MatrixRIB. The specific choice needs to be determined according to the actual situation (Figure 3-8-5).

(6) Management of Special Situations

1. Vascular Involvement: When a tumor invades major blood vessels and cannot be effectively separated from them, vascular grafting is necessary. In some cases, certain veins may be ligated without reconstruction, but this is not the preferred approach. If feasible, vascular grafting should always be performed to maintain proper blood flow and reduce complications.
2. Sternoclavicular Joint Involvement: The sternoclavicular joint plays a role in upper limb movement. However, when this joint is invaded by a tumor, preserving it serves no functional purpose and it must be respected. After resection, upper limb function is generally not significantly impaired, so there is no need to intentionally preserve this joint during Surgery.

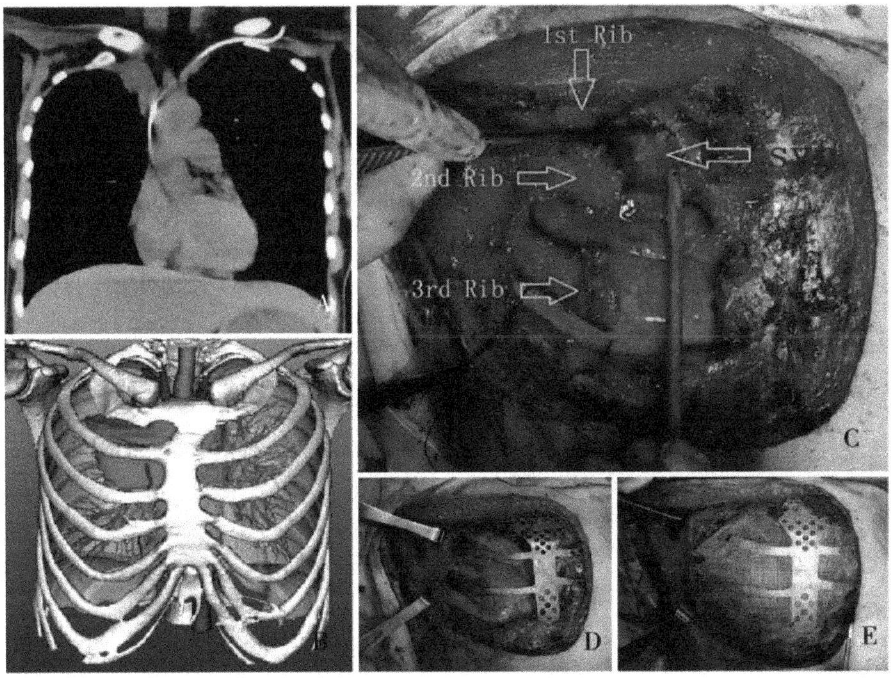

Figure 3-8-5 Surgical resection and chest wall reconstruction of thoracic outlet tumor (A. CT examination shows that the tumor is located near the thoracic outlet; B. Three-dimensional reconstruction shows that the tumor is located on the right anterior chest wall, involving the sternum, the 1, 2, 3 ribs and costal cartilages on the right side; C. The upper half of the sternum, the 1, 2, 3, costal

cartilages on the right side and part of the ribs are removed, and the tumor is completely removed. The figure shows that the tumor is adhered to the superior vena cava; D. The chest wall is reconstructed with digital materials; E. The digital materials are covered with fiber membranes)

3. Clavicle Involvement: The clavicle serves multiple functions, mainly facilitating movement of the shoulder and upper limb. If the clavicle itself is affected by a tumor or requires removal for better Surgical exposure, partial resection is acceptable. Reconstruction of the clavicle after resection is not necessary, and the free end can be left without special treatment.
4. Management of Thoracic Vertebral Lesions: If the thoracic spine is affected, it is necessary to remove the lesion. However, the extent of resection must be approached with caution; over-resection can lead to serious complications.

(7) Surgical Risks and Difficulties

Tumors of the Thoracic Inlet are a very special category of tumors, primarily due to the Surgical risks and complexity involved.The risk of Surgery is mainly related to potential damage to blood vessels and nerves, with vascular injury being particularly serious. The blood vessels involved fall into two main categories: those supplying the head and neck, and those supplying the upper limbs. Injury to these vessels can lead to massive bleeding, posing a direct threat to life, and represents the greatest Surgical risk. ① Difficulty of Exposure: Exposing the lesion requires specific Surgical approaches. Conventional thoracic incisions are typically located lower on the chest, making it difficult to adequately expose lesions in this region. Even with specially designed incisions, exposure remains challenging. ② Difficulty of Resection: The thoracic inlet contains many important structures. Lesions are often located among these structures or may directly invade them, making direct resection of the tumor highly difficult. ③ Difficulty of reconstruction: The thoracic inlet is surrounded by numerous anatomical structures with complex spatial relationships. reconstructingtive Surgery in this area is influenced by many factors, which adds significant difficulty to the procedure.

The traditional focus of thoracic Surgery is within the thoracic cavity, but Surgeries for tumors of the thoracic inlet often extend beyond the thoracic cavity. Therefore, thoracic Surgeons frequently encounter significant difficulties when treating tumors in this area. If such Surgeries are performed by chest wall Surgeons, there are many advantages:① Tumor Location is Closer to the Chest Wall: Although these lesions are located at the thoracic inlet, the tumors themselves are closer to the chest wall. Many of the structures involved belong to the chest wall, which is precisely the area of expertise for chest wall Surgery. ② Extensive Involvement of Chest Wall Structures: Due to the limited scope of the thoracic inlet tumors, they often grow toward superficial areas, leading to invasion of chest wall structures. Since invasion of chest wall structures falls under chest wall Surgery, this makes chest wall Surgeons better suited to treat these lesions.③ Most Surgeries Require Resection of Chest Wall Structures: During exposure and resection of the lesions, multiple chest wall structures need to be removed, making the Surgery more similar to chest wall Surgery. ④Postoperative reconstruction is Essentially Chest Wall reconstruction: Because the resected structures involve many chest wall components, reconstruction primarily focuses on the chest wall, which is the domain of chest wall Surgery. ⑤ The Surgical Philosophy of Chest Wall Surgery is More Suitable for Completing the Operation: Chest wall Surgery not only aims at disease treatment but also incorporates reconstructive principles. For these tumors, curing the disease is naturally the primary goal. However, without reconstructive awareness, many structural and functional problems will occur postoperatively. Therefore, the chest wall Surgical approach is better suited to these operations. ⑥ Management of Certain Special Structures Also Falls Within the Scope of Chest Wall Surgery: Surgeries at the thoracic inlet involve various special structures such as the clavicle and thoracic vertebrae, which are typically outside the purview of thoracic Surgery. However, these structures are familiar territory in chest wall Surgery and are frequently addressed in chest wall procedures. Thus, these structures can be considered part of the chest wall Surgery domain.

8. Prognosis

Although the structure of the thoracic inlet is complex, early-stage tumors are often confined to certain specific structures and do not necessarily affect the surrounding tissues. If Surgery can be performed in a timely manner, good outcomes can be achieved. However, in clinical practice, most diagnosed tumors are not in the early stages. Due to the involvement of multiple structures, Surgery becomes not only complex but also difficult to achieve complete resection, which will significantly affect the prognosis. In other words, the prognosis of some Surgeries is not ideal. Nevertheless, this does not negate the value of Surgery. For most patients, if the diagnosis is clear and there are no obvious contraindications, Surgery should be performed as thoroughly as possible. of course, Surgery does not necessarily have to be forced. If the Surgery is too difficult, it can be combined with radiotherapy and chemotherapy, which often yields good results.

REFERENCES

[1] Connolly, M. R., and H. G. Auchincloss. 2021. "Anatomy and Embryology of the Thoracic Outlet." *Thoracic Surgery Clinics* 31 (1): 1–10.

[2] Li, N., G. Dierks, H. E. Verveke, et al. 2021. "Thoracic Outlet Syndrome: A Narrative Review." *Journal of Clinical Medicine* 10 (5): 962.

[3] Jones, M. R., A. Prabhakar, O. Viswanath, et al. 2019. "Thoracic Outlet Syndrome: A Comprehensive Review of Pathophysiology, Diagnosis, and Treatment." *Pain and Therapy* 8 (1): 5–18.

[4] Marulli, G., L. Battistella, M. Mammana, et al. 2016. "Superior Sulcus Tumors (Pancoast Tumors)." *Annals of Translational Medicine* 4 (12): 239.

[5] Panagopoulos, N., V. Leivaditis, E. Koletsis, et al. 2014. "Pancoast Tumors: Characteristics and Preoperative Assessment." *Journal of Thoracic Disease* 6 (Suppl 1): S108–S115.

[6] Das, A., S. Choudhury, S. Basuthakur, et al. 2014. "Pancoast's Syndrome Due to Fungal Abscess in the Apex of the Lung in an Immunocompetent Individual: A Case Report and Review of the Literature." *Case Reports in Pulmonology* 2014: 581876.

[7] Gehman, K. E., I. Currie, D. Ahmad, et al. 1998. "Desmoid Tumor of the Thoracic Outlet: An Unusual Cause of Thoracic Outlet Syndrome." *Canadian Journal of Surgery* 41 (5): 404–406.

[8] Pan, X., C. Gu, R. Wang, et al. 2017. "Transmanubrial Osteomuscular Sparing Approach for Resection of Cervicothoracic Lesions." *Journal of Thoracic Disease* 9 (9): 3062–3068.

[9] Parissis, H., and V. Young. 2010. "Treatment of Pancoast Tumors from the Surgeon's Perspective: Reappraisal of the Anterior-Manubrial Sternal Approach." *Journal of Cardiothoracic Surgery* 5: 102.

[10] Christison-Lagay, E. R., D. G. Darcy, E. J. Stanelle, et al. 2014. "'Trap-Door' and 'Clamshell' Surgical Approaches for the Management of Pediatric Tumors of the Cervicothoracic Junction and Mediastinum." *Journal of Pediatric Surgery* 49 (1): 172–177.

[11] Kawai, N., T. Kawaguchi, M. Yasukawa, et al. 2017. "Less Invasive Approach to Pancoast Tumor in a Partitioned Incision." *Annals of Thoracic and Cardiovascular Surgery* 23 (3): 161–163.

[12] Oka, S., K. Kobayashi, H. Matsumiya, et al. 2017. "An Effective and Safe Surgical Approach for a Superior Sulcus Tumor: A Case Report." *International Journal of Surgery Case Reports* 37: 87–89.

The chest wall, as part of the trunk, is an organic whole but not a closed structure. It is closely connected with various surrounding structures. The surrounding structures related to the chest wall can be roughly divided into five categories:

① Internal structures: These mainly refer to various structures inside the thoracic cavity, including the lungs, heart, major blood vessels, trachea, esophagus, and so on. ② Anterior structures: The chest wall itself is located on the outer surface of the trunk, so logically, there should be no other structures in front of it. However, due to traditional specialty divisions, the breast is classified under general Surgery or as a separate specialty. Therefore, the anterior structures of the chest wall specifically refer to the female breast. ③ Posterior structures: The spine is located behind the chest wall and should technically be considered part of it. However, it is customarily assigned to other specialties. The scapula is also located posteriorly and, like the spine, belongs to other specialties. ④ Superior structures: These mainly refer to the neck and other structures above it, with the clavicle being the most closely related. Although the clavicle is tightly adjacent to the chest wall, it is never considered part of the chest wall. ⑤ Inferior structures: These primarily include the diaphragm and structures of the abdominal cavity, of course including the abdominal wall. The chest wall is closely connected with these surrounding structures, and diseases can affect each other.

Chest wall lesions may invade adjacent structures, and lesions of surrounding structures may also invade the chest wall. Chest wall tumors are common lesions occurring in the chest wall. These lesions can infiltrate surrounding structures, leading to serious consequences. Conversely, tumors originating in surrounding structures can also invade the chest wall [1]. From the perspective of traditional specialty divisions, tumors originating from surrounding structures belong to other specialties and are not part of conventional thoracic Surgery. If these tumors are confined to their primary sites without invading the chest wall, each specialty usually has complete treatment methods for them. However, once the chest wall is invaded, intervention by chest wall Surgeons is required. In the past, thoracic Surgeons have done some work addressing these situations. Although somewhat effective, these efforts were not specialized. With the emergence of the concept of chest wall Surgery, the perspective on these diseases has broadened and deepened compared to traditional thoracic Surgery.

Consequently, some diseases that originally did not belong to thoracic Surgery may now be included within the scope of chest wall Surgery. This represents the biggest difference between chest wall Surgery and traditional thoracic Surgery. Because of this difference, new concepts and approaches have arisen for treating certain diseases. Regarding tumors of surrounding structures, if the chest wall is not invaded, chest wall Surgeons may not be concerned with the disease. But once the chest wall is invaded, the entire disease falls within the scope of chest wall Surgery and becomes a chest wall Surgical disease.

1. Intrathoracic Tumors Invading the Chest Wall

Intrathoracic tumors and chest wall tumors have always belonged to the same discipline, which has been beneficial for tumor diagnosis and treatment. After the emergence of chest wall Surgery as a specialty, intrathoracic tumors no longer fall under the scope of chest wall Surgery. This division is more conducive to precise tumor treatment. However, for intrathoracic tumors that invade the chest wall, excessive subdivision is actually detrimental to tumor treatment. At this point, chest wall Surgery should adopt an inclusive approach toward such tumors and consider them as part of this specialty for management. This attitude will be more beneficial for the treatment of the tumor. When the tumor is confined within the thoracic cavity, it has no relation to chest wall surgery and does not require the attention of chest wall Surgeons. However, once the tumor invades the chest wall and requires treatment of the chest wall lesion, chest wall Surgeons should decisively undertake the treatment of these tumors. The treatment of such tumors includes two main parts: first, management of the intrathoracic lesion; second, management of the chest wall lesion. Treatment of the intrathoracic lesion primarily involves direct resection. When special structures or organ functions are involved, corresponding measures can be taken as needed. Resection of the chest wall lesion must follow the general principles of chest wall tumor management prioritizing disease control first and reconstruction second. The intrathoracic lesion is addressed first, followed by treatment of the chest wall lesion, ultimately achieving an ideal outcome.

In the past, when managing such tumors, the focus was primarily on treating the intrathoracic lesions. The treatment of the invaded chest wall was often unprofessional, mostly limited to resection with little reconstruction of the resected structures. Ideally, thoracic Surgeons should have a clear understanding of the importance of reconstruction. However, during the era when thoracic Surgeons generally paid little attention to chest wall diseases, this shortcoming was not criticized and was at most regarded as a necessary cost of tumor treatment. Thoracic Surgeons originally had great advantages in managing these tumors, but outdated concepts hindered satisfactory tumor treatment. This situation creates an opportunity for chest wall Surgeons to develop this area of work. The specialty of chest wall Surgery emphasizes the characteristics of chest wall orthopaedics and chest wall reconstruction, which is clearly beyond the scope of general thoracic Surgery. By applying orthopaedic and reconstructive concepts to chest wall Surgery, Surgical outcomes are inevitably more distinctive and superior.

Intrathoracic tumors invading the chest wall most commonly originate from the lung [1-4], with peripheral lung cancer being the most frequent. Such tumors can infiltrate the chest wall even at an early stage. Some central lung cancers may also invade the chest wall in advanced stages, but this usually occurs later. The invasion of the chest wall begins from the parietal pleura and can gradually extend into the deeper structures of the chest wall. Both soft tissue and bony structures may be involved. In the most severe cases, the invasion can extend through the entire thickness of the chest wall up to the skin. Malignant tumors from the mediastinum can also infiltrate the chest wall. Tumors in the anterior mediastinum often directly invade the sternum, and when the invasion is extensive, they may also affect the costal cartilages and even the ribs. Tumors in the posterior mediastinum may invade the posterior chest wall and may simultaneously involve the spine. The broader the invasion, the more complicated the management becomes.

When intrathoracic tumors invade the chest wall, it is important to differentiate this from metastatic tumors within the thoracic cavity. Invasion involves a continuous lesion with no separation between the primary tumor and the invaded area. In contrast, metastatic tumors are distinct from the primary lesion with no direct anatomical connection between them. Metastatic tumors are often solitary lesions and may even exhibit some features of benign tumors, but in essence, they are malignant.

In recent years, with the development of thoracoscopic techniques, the resection of tumors confined to the thoracic cavity is generally performed under thoracoscopy. However, when a tumor invades the chest wall, the invaded chest wall structures must be respected, and such resections are typically performed through an open incision. This provides convenience for exposing the intrathoracic tumor. These Surgeries do not require thoracoscopy; all procedures can be completed through an open approach (Figure 3-9-1). Such Surgeries offer good exposure, intuitive operation, and are relatively straightforward to perform. For some more localized tumors, thoracoscopic Surgery has been attempted, where the lung tumor is first resected, followed by resection of the chest wall tumor from inside the thoracic cavity.

Although this approach is minimally invasive, it is not recommended because it is difficult to ensure complete resection and impossible to perform chest wall reconstruction, limiting its clinical value [4].In most cases, intrathoracic tumors with chest wall invasion can be easily exposed, but tumors in certain special locations such as deep within the breast or on the deep surface of the scapula require careful incision design, since a direct incision on the tumor surface is not feasible, to ensure smooth completion of the Surgery.

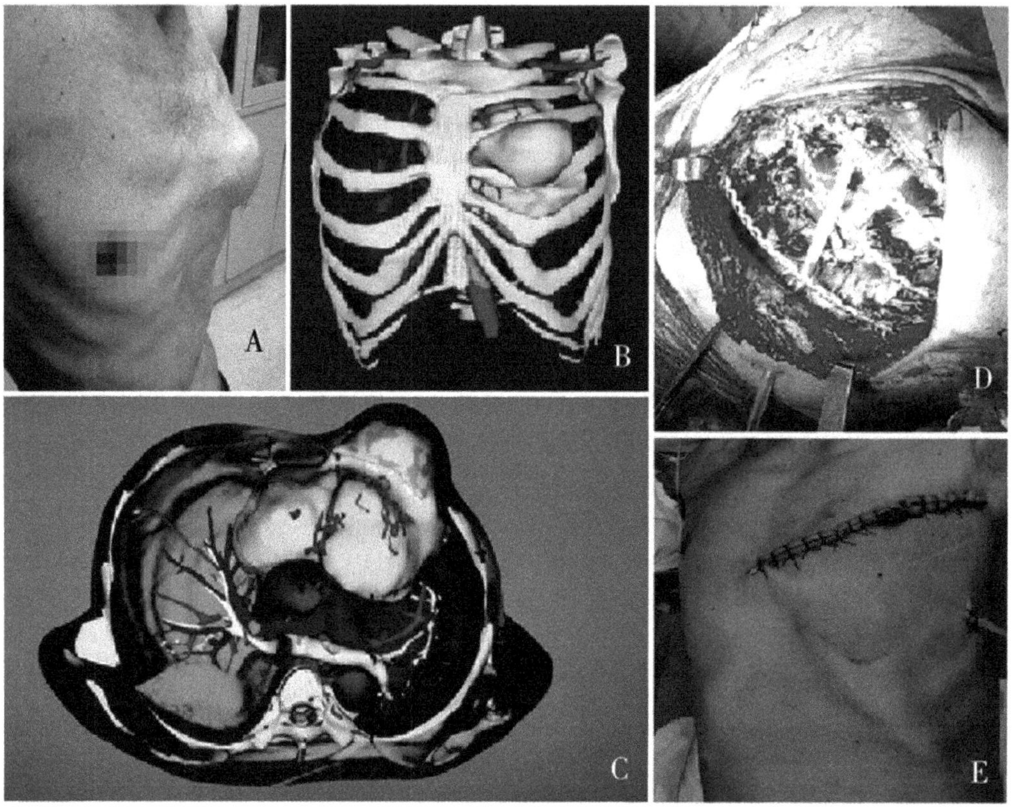

Figure 3-9-1 Intrathoracic Tumor Invading the Chest Wall (A. The chest wall surface shows a visible chest wall tumor; B, C. Three-dimensional reconstructed images indicate the tumor originates from the thoracic cavity, with the primary lesion located in the mediastinum; D. The chest wall tumor along with the primary lesion is resected together, and the chest wall is reconstructed using MatrixRIB; E. Postoperative appearance of the chest wall.

2. Breast Tumors Invading the Deep Structures of the Chest Wall

The breasts are located on the anterior lateral sides of the chest wall and, based purely on their position, are truly part of the chest wall structures. However, since breast Surgery has long been established as an independent and well-developed specialty, including breast diseases under chest wall Surgery would not only cause conflicts but is also unnecessary. That said, there is considerable overlap between breast diseases and chest wall Surgery, especially in cases of advanced breast tumors invading the deep structures of the chest wall. Such cases are more appropriately managed by chest wall Surgeons.

According to the standard treatment methods for breast cancer, when the deep structures of the chest wall are invaded, radical or extended radical mastectomy not only involves removing the breast tissue but also resecting chest wall muscles and sometimes multiple ribs [5]. However, when breast Surgeons manage breast cancer invading deep structures, two possible outcomes may arise: first, insufficient resection leading to tumor recurrence (Figure 3-9-2);

second, excessive resection resulting in chest wall defects. The first approach is overly conservative, while the second is overly aggressive. Both outcomes are related to a lack of specialized knowledge.

During radical or extended radical mastectomy for breast cancer, varying degrees of chest wall defects may occur. Typically, breast Surgeons do not address these defects. This approach is unacceptable from the perspective of chest wall Surgeons. The harm caused by chest wall defects is obvious; they pose a clear risk, not only affecting the stability and integrity of the chest wall but also potentially impairing wound healing, leading to a series of complications. Therefore, the breast Surgeons' approach to managing these tumors is not perfect. However, if this work is carried out by chest wall Surgeons, the results are entirely different. The main difference lies in the management of chest wall defects. When breast Surgeons treat this particular disease, their primary concern is disease control, eliminating the harm caused by breast cancer with little attention to the postoperative appearance, shape, or function of the chest wall. Even when some cosmetic considerations of the breast are taken into account during resection, this is incomplete reconstruction or cannot be called reconstruction at all. In fact, breast Surgery shares many similarities with traditional thoracic Surgery, with almost all procedures aimed solely at curing the disease. There is nothing wrong with curing the disease, but it may not fully meet the patients' needs. As living standards continue to improve, people increasingly desire not only treatment but also aesthetic outcomes. Continuing to perform Surgery based solely on disease treatment standards will seem outdated. Since its inception, chest wall Surgery has embraced reconstruction as one of its missions. This is not only a characteristic of chest wall Surgery but also its strength, giving it greater vitality.

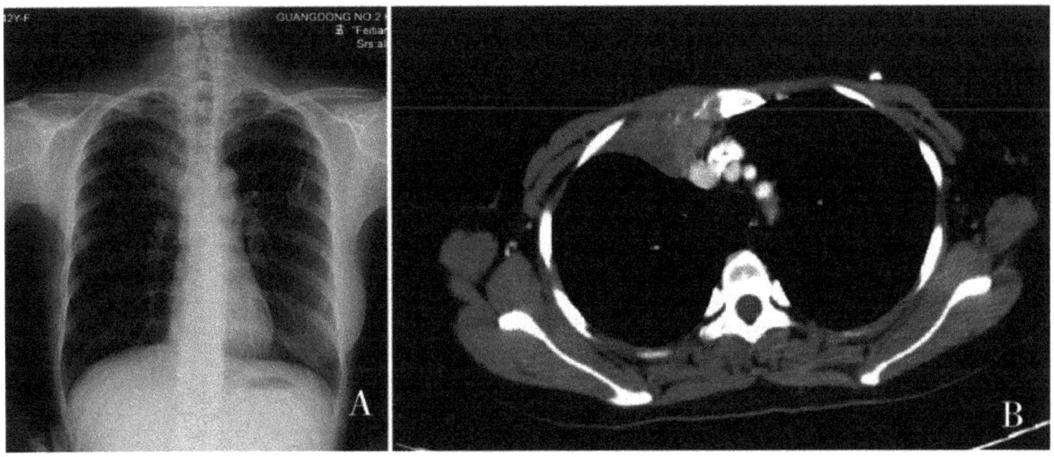

Figure 3-9-2 Tumor Recurrence Caused by Insufficient Resection Range in Breast Cancer Surgery. The tumor invades the deep structures of the chest wall, extending into the thoracic cavity. (A. No obvious lesion seen on the X-ray frontal view; B. CT cross-sectional image shows the tumor crossing the entire

thickness of the chest wall and invading intrathoracic structures.)

Reconstruction in Surgeries for breast cancer invading the chest wall involves two main aspects: first, the reconstruction of the deep structures of the chest wall, and second, the aesthetic appearance of the chest wall. As mentioned above, reconstruction of the deep structures primarily involves rebuilding the bony framework, which poses no difficulty for chest wall Surgeons [5]. However, addressing cosmetic concerns can sometimes exceed the capabilities of chest wall Surgery alone. In such cases, further management should be based on the patient's individual needs. If the patient has no aesthetic concerns, no additional procedures are necessary; if they do, multidisciplinary collaboration with other specialties is recommended. It is important to consider objective limitations regarding appearance. For example, if the entire breast is removed and there is a large area of local skin defect, restoring a normal chest wall appearance may be unrealistic. Additionally, given the likelihood of postoperative treatments such as radiotherapy, placing excessive emphasis on cosmetic appearance may not be necessary. In these cases, careful and thorough reconstruction of the deep structures is sufficient.

3. Clavicle Tumors Invading the Chest Wall

The clavicle is traditionally a focus of orthopaedic Surgery, but due to its special location, it often involves chest wall Surgery. Tumors of the clavicle and sternum can invade each other, making the disease particularly complex [6]. Tumors in the upper segment of the sternum may invade the sternoclavicular joint or the clavicle itself. Managing such cases is not difficult for chest wall Surgeons and is part of their routine work. Conversely, when tumors originate in the clavicle, they can also affect chest wall structures. The area of involvement may extend beyond the sternum to the 1 and 2 ribs, and even invade the thoracic cavity (Figure 3-9-3). Such cases are challenging for orthopaedic Surgeons to manage, but the results are certainly different when handled by chest wall Surgeons. For this reason, it may be more reasonable to consider clavicle tumors as part of chest wall tumor pathology.

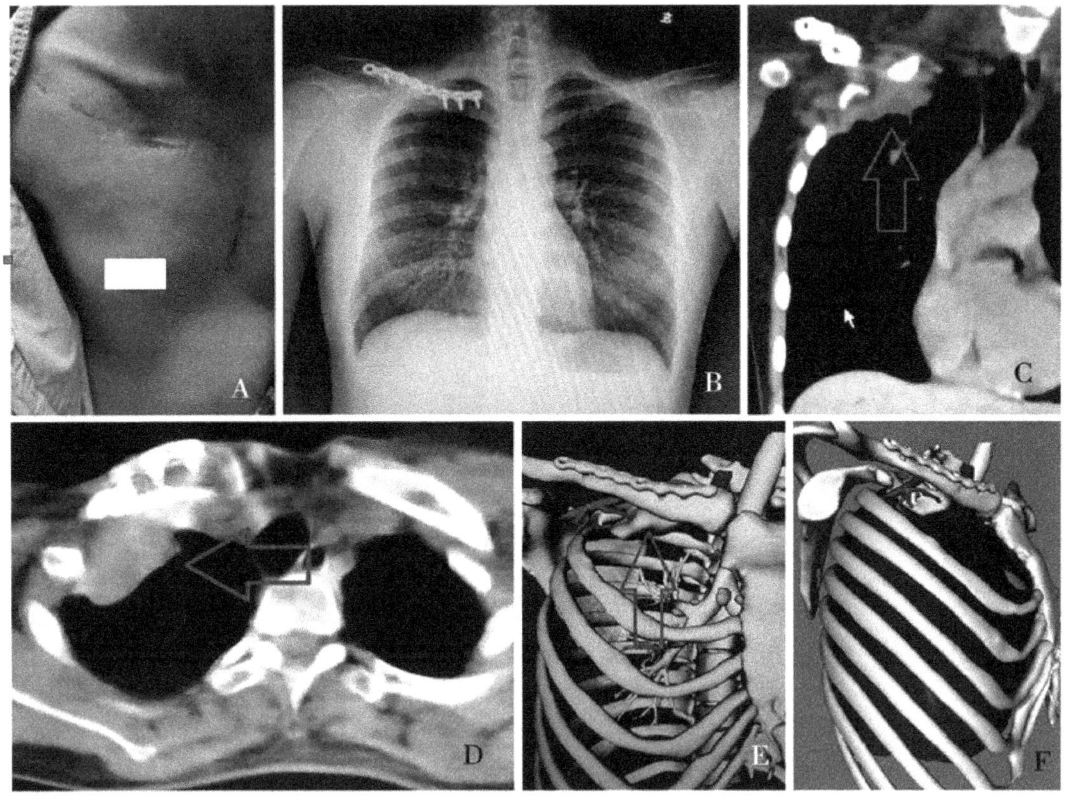

Figure 3-9-3 Clavicle Tumor Recurrence Invading the Chest Wall The patient is an adult female who underwent tumor resection for a clavicle tumor 5 years ago, during which a custom steel plate was used to fix the clavicle. 2 years ago, the tumor recurred, located at the top of the thoracic cage, and underwent tumor resection again. The tumor recurred once more afterward. (A. The chest wall shows an old Surgical scar. B. The X-ray frontal view shows the clavicle fixation plate, with no obvious tumor lesions visible. C, D. CT scans reveal tumor recurrence located at the top of the thoracic cage E, F Three-dimensional reconstruction images display the location of the recurrent tumor)

The treatment for clavicle tumors is direct resection. Since the clavicle has certain functions, some believe that reconstruction of the clavicle is necessary, while others do not support this approach. Those who oppose reconstruction argue that although the clavicle has a function, it is not essential, and its removal has very limited impact on upper limb function. Therefore, direct resection without reconstruction is acceptable. Regardless of whether clavicle reconstruction is performed, from the perspective of chest wall Surgery, there is no technical difficulty. The key point is that if the clavicle tumor invades the chest wall, it must be treated by chest wall Surgeons to ensure a more professional approach and achieve better outcomes.

In the specific procedure, the incision should first be designed according to the tumor's location, taking into account both the clavicle lesion and the chest wall lesion. After fully exposing the tumor structures, depending on the actual situation, the clavicle tumor can be resected first, or the chest wall lesion can be removed first. During resection, handling of the subclavian vessels and nerves may be required. If the tumor invades these structures, forced resection is not possible. Once the lesion is completely removed, reconstruction of the chest wall should be considered. Simple resection of the 1 rib may not require reconstruction. However, if the 2 ribs or the upper segment of the sternum is involved, chest wall reconstruction is necessary. This is the fundamental principle of the Surgery.

Clavicular tumors invading the chest wall are part of thoracic inlet tumors. Due to the complexity of the structures involved, Surgery often presents significant challenges [7]. However, as long as the technical requirements are strictly followed during the operation, generally satisfactory Surgical outcomes can be achieved.

4.Scapular Tumors Invading the Chest Wall

The scapula is also a structure traditionally managed by orthopaedics. Scapular tumors are discussed here for the same reason as clavicle tumors because they may invade chest wall structures [8]. A purely scapular tumor may have no relation to the chest wall structures. However, if it is a malignant tumor infiltrating the anterior chest wall structures, involvement of chest wall Surgeons is required for treatment.

Scapular tumors themselves involve many complex orthopaedic issues and are considered challenging tumors within orthopaedics. If chest wall Surgeons do not have the capability to independently complete such Surgeries, they can collaborate with orthopaedic Surgeons to carry out the related procedures. However, the management of lesions involving chest wall invasion must be undertaken by chest wall Surgeons.

The areas affected by scapular tumors invading the chest wall are mainly located on the dorsal (back) chest wall. Due to the obstruction caused by the scapula itself, exposure is very difficult. However, if the scapula needs to be removed because of the tumor, exposure will no longer be difficult, and the operation at that point is relatively simpler.

When resecting chest wall lesions that involve removal of bony structures, reconstruction is necessary postoperatively. Previously, some believed that local defects of certain ribs on the back could be left unreconstructed; however, this view is questionable. If part of the scapula is removed, the defect in the dorsal chest wall will be largely exposed and therefore requires reconstruction. reconstruction Surgery is not complicated and can be easily performed using materials specifically designed for rib reconstruction.

5.Tumors of the Thoracic Spine Invading the Chest Wall

The thoracic vertebrae are also components that form part of the chest wall;

however, this part of the structure was initially classified under orthopaedics and later reassigned to the department of spine Surgery. The thoracic vertebra is also a component of the chest wall, but this part of the structure originally belongs to orthopaedics and later was classified under spine Surgery. When tumors occur in the thoracic vertebra, their management requires very specialized knowledge and skills; otherwise, it can be not only dangerous but also negatively impact Surgical outcomes. However, since these tumors exist on the chest wall, they have close connections with chest wall Surgery. If the tumor is large and invades the chest wall, even if the chest wall Surgeon cannot complete the operation alone, their participation is necessary. Only through such collaboration can the best Surgical outcomes be achieved [9].

6. Tumors of the Upper Abdomen Invading the Chest Wall

The upper abdomen is adjacent to the chest, and if a tumor infiltrates surrounding tissues, it may invade the chest wall [10]. The principle of treatment in such cases remains the resection of the lesion combined with chest wall reconstruction. Since the structures in the upper abdomen are complex, the treatment of tumors in this region requires more specialized knowledge. Therefore, chest wall Surgeons should closely cooperate with specialists from relevant disciplines to jointly complete the tumor treatment.

The above provides a general overview of tumors from other possible sites that may invade the chest wall. Although these tumors differ in location and origin, once they invade the chest wall, the fundamental Surgical principles remain the same, that is, thorough resection of the lesion combined with reconstruction must be performed. It is important to recognize that if a tumor invades the chest wall, it indicates that the tumor is already quite advanced. This situation demands higher requirements for treatment. At this point, consideration should not be limited to Surgery alone but also include the possibility of comprehensive treatment.

The chest wall exists as part of the human trunk and is an important component of the body. Although chest wall Surgery has been established as an independent specialty, it still needs to interact with other disciplines. As an emerging field, maintaining a humble attitude and learning from well-established specialties is a mindset that must always be upheld. However, innovation is the very essence and vitality of this new specialty.

If one rigidly sticks to old conventions, it will not only hinder the development of the discipline but may also carry some outdated practices into the new specialty's work.

The types of tumors mentioned above traditionally belong to other specialties, and chest wall Surgeons may not need to pay attention to them. However, if the involvement of chest wall Surgeons significantly improves the level of tumor treatment and leads to greater patient satisfaction, this precisely highlights the advantages of the chest wall Surgery specialty.

The chest wall Surgery specialty's separation from thoracic Surgery is not simply to inherit certain clinical work related to chest wall diseases. During the development of the specialty, it is the responsibility and obligation to include diseases that are more conducive to its own development and treatment within its scope. There has never been a unified standard for disease classification. Cross-disciplinary development is for the progress of the specialty, and always embracing challenges with an open and inclusive mindset will enable chest wall Surgery to advance to a higher level.

REFERENCES

[1] Filosso, P. L., A. Sandri, F. Guerrera, et al. 2016. "Primary Lung Tumors Invading the Chest Wall." *Journal of Thoracic Disease* 8 (Suppl 11): S855–S862.

[2] Lanuti, M. 2017. "Surgical Management of Lung Cancer Involving the Chest Wall." *Thoracic Surgery Clinics* 27 (2): 195–199.

[3] Santhos, H. T. A., A. J. Lopes, C. Higa, et al. 2014. "Lung Cancer with Chest Wall Invasion: Retrospective Analysis Comparing En Bloc Resection and 'Resection in Bird Cage.'" *Journal of Cardiothoracic Surgery* 9: 57.

[4] D'Agnol, G., R. Oliveira, and P. A. Ugalde. 2018. "Video-Assisted Thoracoscopic Surgery Lobectomy with Chest Wall Resection." *Journal of Thoracic Disease* 10 (Suppl 22): S2656–S2663.

[5] Chaudhry, I. U., A. Asban, T. Mahboub, et al. 2013. "Recurrent Phyllodes Sarcoma of Breast with Complete Chest Wall Invasion: A Multidisciplinary Approach for Radical Resection." *BMJ Case Reports* 2013: bcr2012008110.

[6] Zhu, Dongdong, Zhanquan Yang, Bing Guan, et al. 2006. "Surgical Treatment of Tumors Involving Both Clavicle and Sternum: Analysis of 12 Cases." *Chinese Journal of Otorhinolaryngology Head and Neck Surgery* 41 (11): 848–850.

[7] Parissis, H., and V. Young. 2010. "Treatment of Pancoast Tumors from the Surgeon's Perspective: Reappraisal of the Anterior-Manubrial Sternal Approach." *Journal of Cardiothoracic Surgery* 5: 102.

[8] Chun, D., J. Cho, I. H. Choi, et al. 2018. "Osteochondroma of the Ventral Scapula Associated with Chest Pain Due to Rib Cage Compression: A Case Report." *Medicine (Baltimore)* 97 (17): e0510.

[9] Yu, H., R. Shi, Z. G. Peng, et al. 2018. "Primary Malignancy in Giant Cell Tumor of Thoracic Vertebrae: A Case Report." *Medicine (Baltimore)* 97 (28): e11484.

[10] Cai, Xiaoyan, Qilong Chen, and Yiping Mou. 2013. "Extended Resection and Reconstruction of Abdominal Wall Tumors at the Thoracoabdominal Junction." *Chinese Journal of Hernia and Abdominal Wall Surgery (Electronic Edition)* 7 (3): 208–209.

CHAPTER 4

CHEST WALL DEFECTS

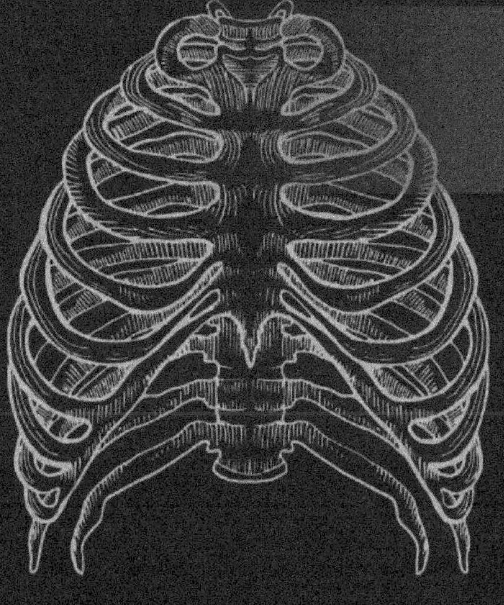

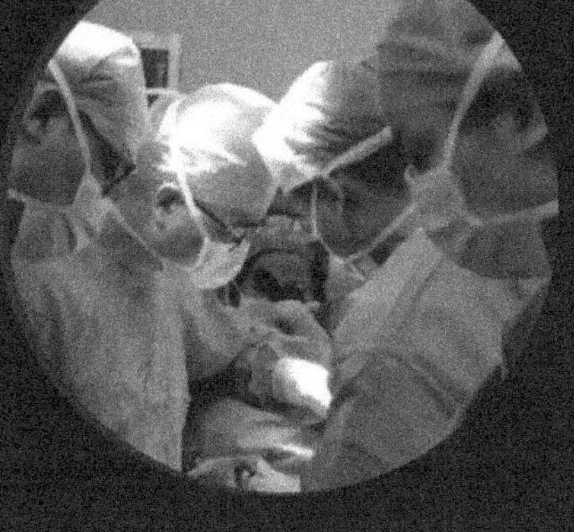

Section 1

BASIC CONCEPTS OF CHEST WALL DEFECTS

The chest wall is an integrated whole, and an intact chest wall requires the combined integrity of skin, soft tissue, and bony structure. When any one of these three components is partially missing, the chest wall becomes incomplete, resulting in a defect [1,2]. Chest wall defects are one of the most fundamental conditions in chest wall Surgery. Due to the loss of chest wall integrity, various corresponding functions are affected. Patients not only present with abnormal chest wall appearance but may also develop various symptoms, and in most cases, Surgical treatment is required.

1. Classification

Chest wall defect refers to the loss of chest wall structure. Due to the complex composition of the chest wall, defects can present in many different forms. To better study chest wall defects, classification is necessary. Different classification criteria can lead to different classification outcomes.

(1) Classification Based on Tissue Origin:

The chest wall has a complex tissue structure, which can generally be divided into three categories: skin, soft tissue, and bony structure [1]. Each type of tissue may develop defects. Therefore, based on tissue origin, chest wall defects can be classified into skin defects, soft tissue defects, and bony structure defects. Skin defects mainly involve localized loss of skin and can occur in any part of the chest wall. When skin integrity is compromised, the subcutaneous tissue becomes exposed to the surface, leading to a series of complications that often cause the patient considerable discomfort. Soft tissue defects occur in the deeper layers of the chest wall and may exist independently or in combination with defects of other structures. Independent soft tissue defects may involve loss of muscle or other soft tissues. Due to coverage by the skin, such defects are not easily detected. In clinical practice, soft tissue defects are often accompanied by skin defects, which represent a more severe form of chest wall defect. Even more serious cases involve the bony structure as well, resulting in full-thickness chest wall defects. Soft tissue defects can affect both appearance and function. Bony structure defects are most commonly seen in the ribs and costal cartilage, while sternal defects are relatively rare and usually localized. Small bony defects may not affect appearance or thoracic function, but larger defects can have significant impacts and are among the more frequently encountered types in clinical practice.

(2) Classification Based on the Involved Layers:
Chest wall defects can be relatively superficial or may involve deeper structures. According to the extent of tissue involvement, they can be classified as incomplete defects and complete defects. Incomplete defects refer to defects that do not penetrate the entire thickness of the chest wall, such as isolated skin defects or bony structure defects. These defects involve only certain layers of the chest wall and do not affect the full thickness. Complete defects refer to the loss of the entire thickness of the chest wall, with the defect extending from inside the thoracic cavity to the outside, exposing the thoracic organs within the defect [3,4]. Because the pressure inside the thoracic cavity may be affected by the defect, respiratory and circulatory functions can be impacted. This is the most severe type of defect. In most cases, defects do not involve the full thickness, but severe trauma or infections can lead to complete defects. Patients with such conditions are often critically ill and may even face life-threatening situations.

(3) Classification Based on the Cause of Onset
Many causes can lead to chest wall defects, but some defects have unknown causes. Based on the cause of onset, chest wall defects can be divided into primary defects and secondary defects. Primary defects have no obvious cause and may be congenital, present in the chest wall from birth. Secondary defects have clear causes such as trauma, infection, Surgery or other factors. There is a clear causal relationship between
these factors and the defects.
Among the five basic diseases in chest wall Surgery, defects are described as an independent disease entity. However, in many cases, defects can occur as part of other chest wall Surgical conditions, such as chest wall infections. When infections cause sinus tracts or localized necrosis, chest wall defects may develop [5]. Additionally, during the treatment of other chest wall diseases, defects may be intentionally created, such as during the resection of chest wall tumors. Since tumors often involve various chest wall structures, removing these structures results in intraoperative chest wall defects. Therefore, one important aspect of chest wall tumor Surgery is defect reconstruction [6]. Such defects can be considered temporary Surgical occurrences and are not classified as independent defects. In some chest wall tumor Surgeries, due to insufficient Surgeon awareness or lack of reconstructive techniques, tumor resection may be performed without reconstruction, resulting in secondary chest wall defects. This is a secondary condition caused by Surgery.
In general, secondary chest wall defects can be divided into several specific types: ① Secondary to trauma: These defects can involve all layers of the chest wall, varying in depth and extent, with irregular shapes. They mainly occur in severe chest wall injuries [7].② Secondary to various Surgeries: After the removal of chest wall lesions, if reconstruction is not performed, secondary

defects may remain. This is the most common type of chest wall defect.③ Secondary to infection: Some chest wall infections progress to a severe stage, causing local necrosis and ulceration, ultimately resulting in obvious defects. ④ Secondary to other treatments: The most common example is chest wall defects caused by radiotherapy following breast cancer Surgery [8,9]. The lesion initially undergoes necrosis, followed by ulceration, leading to large-area defects. This is a frequently encountered serious secondary defect in clinical practice.

Primary defects have unknown causes and commonly include the following two types: ①Isolated primary defects: These defects represent congenital absence of chest wall structures and are not associated with other congenital diseases; they have no specific names. Primary defects can involve different structures. Primary skin defects are almost never reported. Although skin defects can appear in other congenital malformations, they are not considered independent diseases. Soft tissue lies in the deeper layers beneath the surface, and its defects are generally difficult to detect, making it hard to classify as an isolated defect. The most commonly seen primary defects in clinical practice are bony structure defects, which may involve the sternum, ribs, or costal cartilage. ② Defects associated with other congenital diseases: These defects are primary but not isolated; they occur as part of other malformations. For example, in Poland syndrome, there is absence of ribs and chest wall deformities

Defects associated with other congenital diseases include rib absence in Poland syndrome and thoracic dysplasia syndrome, localized defects in sternal clefts, and full-thickness chest wall defects where the heart is ectopic or internal organs are exposed on the body surface. These are all considered primary chest wall defects. In patients with Poland syndrome, unilateral absence of ribs and costal cartilage can cause localized defects and chest wall depressions, which may be accompanied by deformities in other structures [10]. Thoracic dysplasia syndrome primarily involves scoliosis and may be combined with unilateral rib absence, resulting in large localized defects [11]. In patients with sternal clefts, varying degrees of sternal fissures occur, with a lack of bony structures in the fissure area, representing another type of defect [12]. In foetuses with thoracic and thoracoabdominal ectopia cordis, the heart protrudes on the body surface due to full-thickness chest wall absence, which is among the most severe chest wall defects [3]. An extremely rare full-thickness chest wall defect is thoracostomies, where internal organs are exposed through a defect in the chest wall [4]. The chest wall defects in all these diseases are well-defined, but since the defects do not exist independently, they require discussion within the context of the associated conditions and will not be repeated in this section.

2. Hazards

Like other chest wall Surgical diseases, the hazards of chest wall defects primarily come from two aspects: Physiological Impact and Psychological

Impact [13]. Physiological impact: The main issue is the disruption of thoracic integrity. The most significant consequence is paradoxical respiration, which directly impairs respiratory function. In severe cases, circulatory function may also be affected. Psychological impact: This mainly stems from the effect on physical appearance, with skin defects having the most pronounced influence. Large bony structure defects can result in severe thoracic deformities, significantly affecting the overall appearance of the chest.

3.Clinical Manifestations

After a defect occurs, patients may exhibit a variety of symptoms, which are mainly related to the location and extent of the defect. In cases of isolated skin defects, there is usually a visible opening with exposure of deeper structures, accompanied by localized pain. If there is no associated deep soft tissue defect especially if the pleura remains intact there are generally no significant respiratory symptoms. Bony structure defects are the most commonly seen in clinical practice. These present with localized chest wall softening, visible paradoxical respiration, and palpable defect boundaries. If the defect is large, respiratory symptoms may be present. When a full-thickness chest wall defect occurs, it is classified as a complete defect. In such cases, the thoracic cavity is exposed to the external environment, leading to severe impairment of respiratory function and symptoms of significant hypoxia.

4.Examinations

Once a defect is identified, appropriate examinations are required. Physical examination can provide general information about the defect, while imaging studies offer precise details about the local defect and help detect any associated lesions. Since the causes of chest wall defects are complex, the selection of diagnostic tests should be tailored to the specific clinical situation.

5.Diagnosis and Differential Diagnosis

Diagnosis of chest wall defects is relatively easy. It first requires a detailed medical history, which often helps in diagnosing the defect. Secondary defects have clear causes, while primary defects have no obvious cause and are generally congenital, often detected in infancy or early childhood.

Before making a final diagnosis, defects associated with special conditions should be excluded, such as rib absence in Poland syndrome, rib absence in thoracic dysplasia syndrome, and defects in sternal clefts. Although defects exist in these diseases, they are considered special pathological changes of the disease and are not suitable for discussion as independent chest wall defects.

Chest wall defects themselves are complex. When diagnosing, detailed information about the lesion should be obtained as much as possible: first, clarify the cause of the defect; second, clarify the location of the defect; third, clarify which structures are missing; fourth, clarify the surrounding structures of the defect; fifth, clarify the structures on the surface of the defect. This information not only determines the specific nature of the defect but also decides the choice of Surgical method, so it must be understood as clearly as possible.

6.Surgery

(1) Indications

After a clear diagnosis of chest wall defects, the next issue is treatment [14]. Treatment of chest wall defects involves many practical factors related to the disease itself and often influenced by other factors beyond the disease, so there is usually no unified consensus. For example, thoracotomy via rib bed often requires removing a rib, which artificially creates a chest wall defect that is considered the major drawback of the Surgery. In today's era of minimally invasive concepts, such defects are almost unforgivable. However, from the Surgeon's perspective, choosing this Surgical approach implies acceptance of this defect's rationality, so no additional treatment is usually done for the defect postoperatively. From the chest wall Surgery perspective, this approach is unreasonable. If symptoms arise from the defect, treatment is definitely needed. Another example is the previously common thoracoplasty, where multiple ribs are removed to ensure complete chest wall collapse. This creates a large defect, but such defects are considered reasonable and require no further treatment.
Regarding some primary defects, treatment opinions are also inconsistent. For example, some bony chest wall defects may not affect respiration or cause symptoms, nor have obvious external deformity. Such cases may not require Surgery, but if the patient insists, Surgery becomes necessary.
Clinically, there are differing opinions on the treatment of some defects, but for certain defects, treatment consensus exists. These defects include: ① Skin defects. Skin defects, or deep defects that include skin loss, present with obvious wounds. If left untreated, these defects will severely impact the patient's life and therefore must be eliminated through appropriate methods. ② Defects with paradoxical respiration affecting respiratory function. When a chest wall defect occurs, local softening of the chest wall may lead to paradoxical respiration. The presence of such breathing counteracts the effectiveness of respiratory effort. If too severe, respiratory function will be impaired, posing a serious threat to the patient's health and thus requiring treatment. ③ Complete full-thickness chest wall defects. These defects are equivalent to the removal of a portion of the chest wall, with intrathoracic organs directly exposed to the body surface. The negative pressure within the thoracic cavity is lost, and respiratory movements are severely affected. In cases of acute defects, the patient's condition becomes critical and requires emergency treatment. In chronic defects, a layer of fibrous tissue may form on the lung surface for protection. Although the patient may still be able to breathe, it is extremely painful and still requires appropriate management.

(2) Nature of the Surgery

The treatment of defects generally requires Surgical intervention. As a type of chest wall Surgery, defect repair also involves two main aspects: first, disease treatment; second, reconstruction [15]. The defect itself is a typical chest wall Surgical disease, so treatment of the disease is the primary objective. From the nature of the condition, a defect represents the loss of chest wall structures; therefore, reconstruction is a key component of the Surgery. Simple defects usually do not involve deformities, so the main focus of reconstruction is structural restoration.

Broadly speaking, the entire treatment process for chest wall defects falls under disease treatment. However, to emphasize the reconstructive aspect, only the Surgical actions directly addressing the lesion such as removal of diseased structures are considered treatment of the disease. Such procedures are seen in Surgeries for certain secondary defects. For example, in defects secondary to infection, the removal of infected tissue reflects the therapeutic aspect of the Surgery.

The reconstructive aspect is the most essential attribute of defect Surgery, as only reconstruction can ultimately eliminate the defect. However, in some special defect Surgeries, due to the difficulty and specific requirements of reconstruction, it may be necessary to perform lesion removal without reconstruction. In such cases, disease treatment becomes the sole attribute of the Surgery. These procedures are often relatively extreme, and significant structural and cosmetic issues of the chest wall may remain postoperatively. Nevertheless, there may be no alternative in order to treat the disease. This situation is seen in some Surgeries for chest wall defects caused by chronic lesions. Even if serious postoperative deformities occur, as long as the defect can be closed and the skin heals, the Surgery is still considered successful.

reconstruction Surgery for chest wall defects includes three basic components: bony structure reconstruction, soft tissue reconstruction, and skin reconstruction [15]. Since different defects involve different missing components, the reconstruction procedures can vary significantly. A simple skin defect only requires skin reconstruction. A defect involving only the bony structure may require only bony reconstruction. Defects involving both skin and soft tissue require reconstruction of both. If the bony structure is also involved, all three components must be reconstructed.

(3) Basic Principles of Surgery

For skin and soft tissue defects, if the area is small, direct suturing can be performed. This is an effective method to eliminate small defects. Due to the good elasticity of the skin, the postoperative appearance may not show obvious abnormalities. However, if the defect area is large, flap repair is required. Flaps can come from the surrounding defect area or other areas of the chest wall. If these flaps are insufficient for the Surgical needs, pedicled flaps or free flaps from other parts of the body can be considered.

Bony structure defects require reconstruction using autologous materials or artificial materials. The related materials and Surgical techniques are consistent with those used in chest wall. The reconstruction procedures for tumors are generally similar, so they will not be repeated here. It is important to note that reconstruction of chest wall defects is not entirely the same as reconstruction after simple chest wall tumor resection. After tumor removal, reconstruction can be performed immediately. However, for some special chest wall defects, appropriate preparation is necessary before reconstruction Surgery. For example, defects secondary to chest wall infections carries an infection focus; immediate reconstruction may easily lead to Surgical failure [16]. To avoid failure, infection must first be controlled, and chest wall reconstruction should be performed electively.

The essence of reconstruction is the restoration of the chest wall structure. Theoretically, the more completely these structures are restored and the closer they resemble the original structure, the better the outcome [14,15]. To achieve this, three basic requirements must be met: ①Structural restoration should be as close to the original as possible. The only way to achieve this is to replace the defect with an identical structure, which is clearly impossible. Clinically used materials either come from other parts of the body or are artificial. These materials differ significantly from the original structures. To make the Surgical outcome as perfect as possible, these materials must closely approximate the original structure.②Functional restoration should be as close to the original as possible. The chest wall structures all have specific functions. Good reconstruction outcomes depend heavily on restoring function. For example, in bony structure reconstruction, the materials used must have both sufficient hardness and flexibility. If the material is too soft, local softening may occur, and in severe cases, paradoxical respiration may persist. Such reconstruction clearly fails to meet the objective, so hardness is especially important. However, materials cannot be too hard either, as overly rigid materials cause loss of chest wall elasticity and can make the patient feel extreme discomfort locally. ③The appearance should be as aesthetically pleasing as possible. This is one of the most important requirements for reconstruction Surgery. Many chest wall defects severely damage appearance, and curing the disease is certainly the primary goal. However, if aesthetic considerations are fully taken into account, the Surgery will demonstrate a higher level of skill.

In summary, chest wall defects are a relatively complex thoracic Surgical disease. They can exist independently, present as a manifestation of other diseases, or occur during Surgeries for certain chest wall conditions. Therefore, analysis must be based on the specific situation, and the most appropriate treatment should be determined according to the clinical needs.

REFERENCES

[1] Wang, W. L. 2021. "Thoracic Wall Surgery: Basic Structure and Function of the Chest Wall." *Jinri Toutiao*, October 31.
[2] Wang, W. L. 2021. "Basic Concepts of Chest Wall Defects." *Thoracic Deformity Surgery Expert*, May 2.
[3] Williams, A. P., R. Marayati, and E. A. Beierle. 2019. "Pentalogy of Cantrell." *Seminars in Pediatric Surgery* 28 (2): 106–110.
[4] Hanafi, H. R., and Z. A. Zakaria. 2017. "Prenatal Diagnosis of Thoracoschisis and Review of Literature." *Case Reports in Obstetrics and Gynecology* 2017: 9821213.
[5] Rajput, A. K., V. Vardhan, and K. E. Rajan. 2000. "A Persistent Transpleural Fistulous Communication between Lung and Chest Wall." *Medical Journal of Armed Forces India* 56 (3): 259–261.
[6] Sandler, G., and A. Hayes-Jordan. 2018. "Chest Wall Reconstruction after Tumor Resection." *Seminars in Pediatric Surgery* 27 (3): 200–206.
[7] Pate, J. W. 1989. "Chest Wall Injuries." *Surgical Clinics of North America* 69 (1): 59–70.
[8] Vairinho, A., A. Al Hindi, M. Revol, et al. 2018. "Reconstruction of an Anterior Chest Wall Radionecrosis Defect by a Contralateral Latissimus Dorsi Flap: A Case Report." *Annales de Chirurgie Plastique Esthétique* 63 (2): 182–186.
[9] Rouanet, P., J. M. Fabre, V. Tica, et al. 1995. "Chest Wall Reconstruction for Radionecrosis after Breast Carcinoma Therapy." *Annals of Plastic Surgery* 34 (5): 465–470.
[10] Urschel, H. C. 2000. "Poland's Syndrome." *Thoracic Surgery Clinics of North America* 10 (2): 393–403.
[11] Campbell, R. M., and M. D. Smith. 2007. "Thoracic Insufficiency Syndrome and Thoracic Scoliosis." *Journal of Bone and Joint Surgery (American Volume)* 89 (Suppl 1): 108–122.
[12] Fokin, A. A. 2000. "Cleft Sternum and Sternal Foramen." *Thoracic Surgery Clinics of North America* 10 (2): 261–276.
[13] Wang, W. L. 2020. "The Harms of Massive Chest Wall Defects." *Expert in Thoracic Deformity Surgery*, February 21.
[14] Wang, W. L. 2018. "Repair and Reconstruction of Chest Wall Defects." *Expert in Thoracic Deformity Surgery*, October 9.
[15] Wang, W. L. 2021. "Thoracic Surgery: Shaping and Reconstruction." *Jinri Toutiao*, October 31.
[16] Torto, F. L., G. Turriziani, C. Donato, et al. 2020. "Deep Sternal Wound Infection following Cardiac Surgery: A Comparison of the Monolateral with the Bilateral Pectoralis Major Flaps." *International Wound Journal* 17 (3): 683–69.

Primary chest wall defects refer to the localized absence of chest wall structures without a clear cause [1]. The missing components can be any one of the three basic structures of the chest wall. Clinically, defects in bony structures are common, while isolated skin or soft tissue defects are extremely rare. In some special cases, defects involving all three structures may occur simultaneously. This situation can be seen in Cantrell's pentalogy [2] and an extremely rare deformity called (thoracoschisis) [3-5]. Cantrell pentalogy involves a full-thickness chest wall defect, with the heart herniating through the defect to the body surface. Thoracoschisis is similar to Cantrell pentalogy but generally does not involve cardiac malformations; instead, it is mainly associated with herniation of abdominal viscera. Abdominal organs can herniate through the chest wall defect in thoracoschisis, forming an extremely severe deformity. Cantrell pentalogy has been described in the sternal cleft chapter and will not be repeated here. Thoracoschisis is extremely rare and is considered part of the (limb-body wall complex deformity). Due to the complexity of the condition and its multidisciplinary involvement, it will not be discussed in detail here. This section focuses on defects of the chest wall bony structures.

1. Basic Concepts

The chest wall is composed of skin, soft tissue, and bony structures. The bony structures refer to the thorax, which consists of three components: ribs, costal cartilage, and sternum. A defect can form if any part or structure of the thorax is missing. Primary chest wall defects are generally divided into two types: independent chest wall defects and associated defects. The former refers to defects that exist alone without other diseases and represent true defects; the latter occur as part of other conditions and are not considered independent defects.

Primary bony chest wall defects are relatively rare. In the past, this type of defect received little attention, and there are no related clinical reports; therefore, its incidence is unknown. We have encountered such defects clinically, but the number of cases is relatively small, and no specific incidence statistics have been conducted. The defect can occur alone in the ribs, costal cartilage, or sternum, or it can involve multiple bony structures simultaneously. The defect can be located in any part of the thorax, with the soft tissue and skin remaining intact.

2. Pathogenesis

The pathogenesis of primary chest wall bony structure defects is unclear. Since most cases are congenital, the mechanism is complex. Referring to the pathogenesis of Poland syndrome, it may be related to localized blood supply during the fetal period [6]. The development of any structure requires nutrients. During the fetal period, the blood supply to certain structures is affected for various reasons, the nutrients required for development will be insufficient, leading to maldevelopment or absence of those structures. If these structures are the bony components of the chest wall, defects may form. Additionally, the pathogenesis of the sternal cleft can be referenced; some defects may be related to specific embryonic developmental disturbances [7]. For example, if the fusion of the sternum is disrupted, defects may occur. Besides these two possible explanations, there may be other more complex factors, but the exact mechanisms remain unclear.

3. Pathological Changes

Primary bony chest wall defects can occur in different locations. When located on the anterior chest wall, the defect may involve the sternum, costal cartilages, and ribs. Defects on the lateral and posterior chest walls involve only the ribs. The defect may present in various shapes, with the edges either surrounded by continuous bony structures forming a complete border or showing residual bone stumps left by the bony absence. The defect area is filled with soft tissue, which is generally weak, and the surface may be covered by other chest wall tissues; soft tissue developmental abnormalities may also be present. The skin over the defect is intact, but the appearance may show a depression due to the localized defect. This situation can occur in any type of defect. If there is a localized defect at the lower end of the sternum, it can form a pectus excavatum, which is a special type of pectus excavatum distinct from the common type.

4. Hazards

The bony structure of the chest wall is the fundamental framework of the thoracic cage. Once a defect occurs in the bony structure, it will first affect the integrity and stability of the thoracic cage, ultimately impacting its various physiological functions. Furthermore, changes in the thoracic cage can affect the stability of the spine, thereby further amplifying the impact of the defect.

The main hazards of bony chest wall defects include the following [8,9]: ① Flail chest and paradoxical respiration: Due to the absence of bony support, local softening of the chest wall may occur. Small defects are usually not severely harmful and have minimal impact on respiratory function. However, if the defect is extensive and not covered by strong soft tissue, significant paradoxical breathing may occur, inevitably impairing respiratory function. ② Chest wall collapse and reduced thoracic volume: Following a defect, the loss of local bony support can lead to soft tissue and skin collapsing inward under the influence of negative intrathoracic pressure. This collapse not only affects the thoracic contour but may also reduce thoracic volume, directly impairing respiratory function. ③ Loss of protective capacity due to absence of bony structures: One of the critical functions of the chest wall is to protect the intrathoracic organs. When the bony structure is missing, this protective role is compromised. This is particularly dangerous when the sternum is involved, as the heart and mediastinal structures lie directly beneath soft tissue, making the heart more vulnerable to injury. ④ Loss of thoracic stability and spinal deformity: The bony chest wall is a symmetrical and integrated structure. Balanced forces on both sides of the spine are essential for maintaining its normal shape. When a defect occurs, thoracic stability is compromised, and the spine may be subjected to uneven forces, leading to deformities such as scoliosis. This is especially true when the defect involves ribs adjacent to the spine, eliminating their supportive function and directly contributing to spinal curvature. ⑤ Variations in soft tissue attachment points, affecting related functions. Under normal circumstances, the soft tissues of the chest wall, especially the muscles, are attached to stable bony structures, which is essential for their function. If the corresponding bony structures are missing, the muscle attachment points will be altered or even lost, inevitably impairing their related functions. ⑥ Alteration in chest wall shape, resulting in visible deformity. The normal shape of the thoracic cage relies on the integrity and coordination of all its components. If part of the structure is missing, the overall integrity is compromised, inevitably affecting the chest wall's shape. In addition to localized collapse mentioned earlier, secondary structural changes may occur, leading to complex thoracic deformities.

Based on the above analysis, it can be seen that once a defect occurs in the bony structure of the chest wall, various thoracic functions may be affected. Therefore, such defects often cause significant harm. This kind of harm differs from that of other chest wall diseases and can sometimes be even more severe.

5. Clinical Manifestations

After the loss of the bony structure of the chest wall, multiple adverse effects may occur. These effects can manifest through various clinical symptoms. The appearance of symptoms is related to several specific factors: Firstly, the extent of the defect. Small defects usually do not produce obvious symptoms. If the defect is extensive, the earliest manifestations are typically flail chest and paradoxical respiration, leading to a series of respiratory symptoms. Such defects may also affect other systems, such as the circulatory system, resulting in corresponding symptoms. Secondly, the location of the defect. In males, the anterior chest wall has less overlying soft tissue, so a bony defect here easily leads to chest wall softening and obvious paradoxical breathing, with more severe symptoms. In females, the presence of breast tissue may mask paradoxical breathing, resulting in milder symptoms. Defects in the lateral chest wall also have less soft tissue coverage and tend to show more obvious symptoms. If the defect is located on the back, the overlying thick tissues and the scapula help mask paradoxical movement, making symptoms less apparent. Thirdly, the affected structure. Beneath the ribs lies the lung, so defects in this area can have a greater impact on respiration. Beneath the sternum lies the mediastinum, including the heart and great vessels; if a defect occurs here, these structures lie just beneath the skin. With the loss of protective bone, cardiac displacement may occur. Since defects in this area may directly connect to both pleural cavities, both lungs may be affected simultaneously.

In summary, mild chest wall bony structure defects may present without any symptoms. However, as the severity of the defect increases, various obvious symptoms may gradually appear. These symptoms may originate from the respiratory system or the circulatory system. The appearance of symptoms indicates that the defect is relatively severe and requires active treatment.

The local signs of chest wall bony structure defects are generally quite evident, and may include a clearly floating chest wall and paradoxical respiration. If the defect is located in the anterior chest wall, visible cardiac pulsations may be observed. Palpation can detect the defect and the surrounding structures. The edges may feel smooth and continuous, or bony remnants may be palpable.

6. Examination

Clearly determine the defect's location, size, surrounding structures, and surface features. X-ray examination can roughly reveal the shape of the defect, but the imaging quality varies depending on the defect's location. Defects near the midline of the anterior chest wall have poor visibility due to overlap with the cardiac silhouette. Defects on the lateral chest wall are poorly shown on the frontal view, and overlap with the heart on the lateral view also results in suboptimal imaging. CT scans can display the shape of the defect from different angles, but since these are not three-dimensional images, they are not very intuitive. The ideal examination is a three-dimensional reconstructed image, which shows all the details of the defect and is a very useful diagnostic tool.

7. Diagnosis and Differential Diagnosis

Key diagnostic points for primary chest wall bony structure defects include the following aspects: ① It must be confirmed that the defect is a primary lesion with no clear cause, not secondary to trauma, Surgery, or other underlying chest wall diseases; ② The chest wall skin is intact, with no skin defects; ③ There is a localized absence of bony structure causing a defect in the chest wall; ④ Other congenital diseases such as Poland syndrome [10], thoracic dysplasia syndrome [11], and sternal cleft [12] must be excluded.

In addition to the above key points, the diagnosis of primary chest wall bony structure defects also requires clarification of the following information:① Location of the defect: This refers not only to the position on the thorax but more importantly to the specific location on the chest wall. The thorax location determines the content of reconstruction, while the chest wall location determines the Surgical approach details. ② Contents of the defect: It is essential to clearly identify which structures are missing, as different structures require different Surgical methods. Only by understanding the exact missing structures can the Surgery be targeted effectively to achieve good outcomes. ③ Surrounding structures of the defect: This information helps not only with the placement and fixation of reconstructive materials but also assists in the preparation of some special materials. ④ Surface structures of the defect: The surface anatomy determines the Surgical approach. If no important structures are present on the surface, the ideal approach is naturally through the area closest to the defect. However, if important structures such as the scapula or, in females, the mammary gland are present, the Surgical route must be designed to avoid these structures. The differential diagnosis of primary chest wall bony structure defects mainly involves distinguishing them from other types of bony structure defects. First, it is necessary to differentiate from bony structure defects caused by other primary chest wall Surgical diseases. Second, it is important to distinguish from various types of secondary chest wall bony structure defects. Since the treatment methods for defects of different natures vary significantly, careful differentiation is essential.

8.Surgery

(1) Indications for Surgery

Primary chest wall bony structure defects can be managed with three main approaches: no treatment, conservative treatment, or Surgical treatment. Some bony defects, although clearly present, may be hidden in location, causing neither cosmetic issues nor symptoms. Such defects pose no harm to the patient and can be safely ignored without any intervention. Other defects may cause mild symptoms but do not significantly affect the function of vital organs. In these cases, if the patient does not desire Surgery, symptomatic treatment alone can be considered. However, for defects that are extensive and cause significant damage. For obvious defects, active Surgical treatment is generally necessary to prevent serious harm to the body.

For patients with severe defects, the decision to perform Surgery is relatively straightforward. However, for those with mild symptoms, the choice often depends on subjective factors. Some patients with minor or even no symptoms and inconspicuous defects may opt out of Surgery, yet some still desire Surgical intervention. Conversely, patients with relatively severe defects might refuse Surgery along with their families. Additionally, the Surgeon's own subjective factors can influence this decision. Some doctors who are not skilled in defect repair might hesitate to admit their limitations and may advise patients against Surgery that is actually necessary. These situations are similar to those encountered in chest wall deformity treatment, highlighting the unique nature of this condition. This unique nature gives the Surgical decision two missions: first, to cure the disease, and second, to achieve aesthetic reconstruction. These dual missions represent the fundamental goals of all chest wall Surgeries.

(2) Surgery

The Surgery for primary chest wall bony structure defects mainly involves reconstruction, with the goal of restoring the integrity of the thoracic cage [13,14]. From the perspective of operative details, reconstruction can be divided into two types: functional reconstruction and structural reconstruction. The former does not require restoring the normal structure of the thoracic cage but focuses on eliminating the defect and alleviating symptoms. Structural reconstruction is a more advanced form that aims to restore the detailed structure of the thoracic cage as much as possible, making its shape as close to normal as possible.

Functional reconstruction is relatively simple and involves directly repairing the defect using appropriate materials, without the need to consider the intricate details of the defect. This method has been commonly used in the past. Materials such as titanium mesh, acrylic, bone cement, and polyester fabric can be used to directly cover and repair the defect. By eliminating the defect, this approach also addresses local flail chest and paradoxical respiration, thereby achieving the Surgical goals.

Structural reconstruction not only aims to eliminate the defect but also to restore the normal structure of the thorax, thus placing higher demands on both the reconstruction materials and techniques. For defects involving ribs and costal cartilages, materials that closely resemble these structures in shape can be chosen, such as Matrix RIB [15], which is considered an ideal reconstruction material [16]. For defects involving the sternum, digitally manufactured materials that better approximate the shape of the sternum and surrounding structures can be selected if conditions permit (Figure 4-2-1). If digital materials are unavailable, other materials can still achieve good results, with the key being the reconstruction technique (Figure 4-2-2). reconstruction techniques involve several important aspects, including the choice of incision, exposure of the defect, trimming, placement, and fixation of the materials, all of which require careful attention.

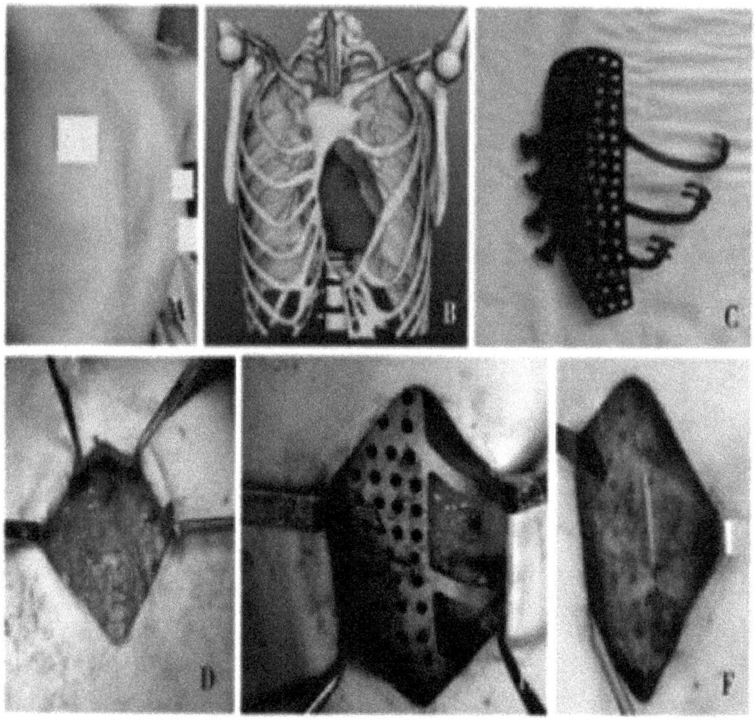

Figure 4-2-1: Digital Material
Reconstruction Surgery for Primary Chest Wall Defect (A. External appearance of the patient with primary chest wall defect, showing a slight local depression at the defect site; (B. 3D image showing the location of the defect, involving most of the sternum and multiple left-side costal o cartilages and ribs; C. Personalized digital material designed based on the defect information; D. Surgical exposure of the defect area; E. Placement and secure fixation of the digital material into the defect; F. Closure of the incision after covering with a fibrous membrane

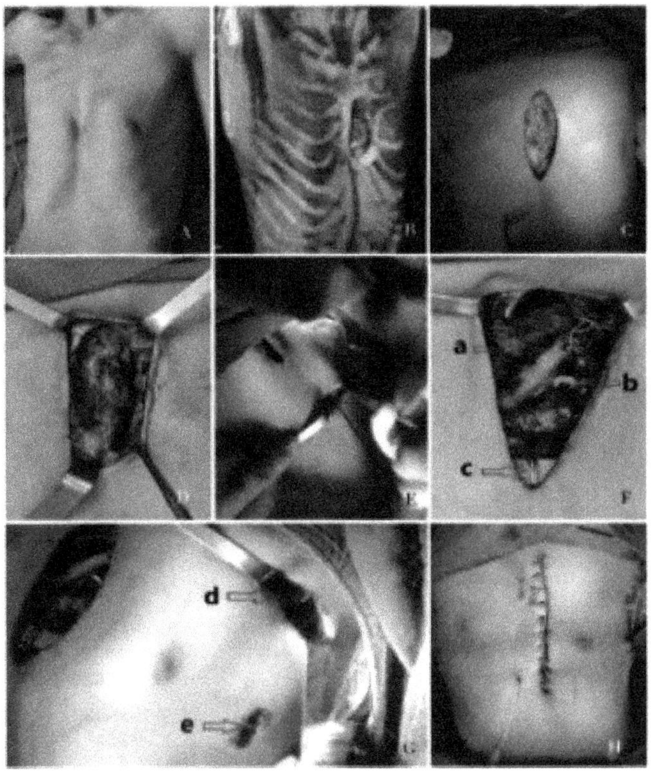

Figure 4-2-2: Reconstruction Surgery Using Autologous Rib, Matrix RIB, and Steel Plate (A. Patient with primary chest wall defect and complex deformity of the anterior chest wall; B. 3D reconstruction image showing the defect location, involving the sternum and multiple costal cartilages and ribs on the left chest wall; C. Skin incision made anterior to the defect; D. Exposure of the defect site;(E. Incision on the left chest wall exposing ribs, placement of steel plate and fixation wires; (F. Harvesting of an autologous rib from the right chest wall for reconstruction, combined with Matrix RIB to repair the defect, along with the use of a shaping steel plate for chest wall deformity correction. a. Autologous rib. Matrix RIB; c. Shaping steel plate; G. Showing the left edge of the defect and fixation sites of the reconstruction materials. d. Matrix RIB fixed at the left edge of the defect; e. Fixation site of the shaping steel plate; H. Appearance of the chest wall after closure of the incision)

From the nature of the Surgery, reconstruction belongs to the category of plastic Surgery. Given this attribute, full consideration must be given to the overall shape issue [17]. This issue involves not only the shape of the thorax but also the overall appearance of the chest wall. Therefore, in the specific Surgical procedure, besides completing the reconstruction of the bony structures, attention must also be paid to the soft tissue and skin. Simple bony structure defects generally do not involve defects of the skin and soft tissue. However, because a skin incision is required and the reconstruction materials need to be placed beneath the soft tissue, proper management of the incision and the soft tissue in the operative field is essential. Only in this way can an ideal aesthetic outcome be achieved.

9. Prognosis

Primary chest wall bony structure defects are usually singular in nature, and the Surgical goals are clear. Current materials and techniques can adequately meet the needs of reconstruction, resulting in a relatively high success rate for Surgery. The Surgical outcome is greatly influenced by the choice of materials and the Surgical technique. If both are effectively combined during the procedure, good Surgical results can generally be achieved.

REFERENCES

[1] Wang, W. L. 2021. "Basic Concepts of Chest Wall Defects." *Thoracic Deformity Surgery Expert*, May 27.

[2] Williams, A. P., R. Marayati, and E. A. Beierle. 2019. "Pentalogy of Cantrell." *Seminars in Pediatric Surgery* 28 (2): 106–110.

[3] Ardicli, B., A. Karaman, A. Ozyazici, et al. 2017. "Isolated Thoracoschisis: Case Report." *Turkish Journal of Pediatrics* 59 (2): 217–220.

[4] Hanafi, H. R., and Z. A. Zakaria. 2017. "Prenatal Diagnosis of Thoracoschisis and Review of Literature." *Case Reports in Obstetrics and Gynecology* 2017: 9821213.

[5] Vujovic, D., A. Sretenovic, M. Raicevic, et al. 2017. "Thoracoschisis Associated with Limb Body Wall Complex." *APSP Journal of Case Reports* 8 (3): 19.

[6] Vazirnia, A., and P. R. Cohen. 2015. "Poland's Syndrome: A Concise Review of the Clinical Features Highlighting Associated Dermatologic Manifestations." *American Journal of Clinical Dermatology* 16 (4): 295–301.

[7] Ashok Raja, J., G. Mathevan, K. Mathiatrasan, et al. 2014. "Closing the Cleft over a Throbbing Heart: Neonatal Sternal Cleft." *BMJ Case Reports* 2014: bcr2014204529.

[8] Wang, W. L. 2020. "Harms of Large Chest Wall Defects." *Thoracic Deformity Surgery Expert*, February 21.

[9] Wang, W. L. 2018. "Harms of Rib Loss." *Thoracic Deformity Surgery Expert*, December 5.

[10] Charlier, P., S. Deo, F. M. Galassi, et al. 2019. "Poland Syndrome before Alfred Poland: The Oldest Medical Description (Paris, France, 1803)." *Surgical and Radiologic Anatomy* 41 (10): 1117–1118.

[11] Campbell, R. M. 2013. "VEPTR: Past Experience and the Future of VEPTR Principles." *European Spine Journal* 22 (Suppl 2): 106–117.

[12] Wang, W. L. 2021. "Sternal Cleft and Chest Wall Defects." *Thoracic Deformity Surgery Expert*, October 3.

[13] Wang, W. L. 2020. "Reconstruction Issues of Chest Wall Defects." *Thoracic Deformity Surgery Expert*, May 9.

[14] Wang, W. L. 2018. "Repair and Reconstruction of Chest Wall Defects." *Thoracic Deformity Surgery Expert*, October 9.

[15] Wang, W. L. 2021. "Technical Issues in Chest Wall Reconstruction Using MatrixRIB." *Thoracic Deformity Surgery Expert*, March 22.

[16] Wang, W. L. 2020. "New-Generation Chest Wall Reconstruction Technology: Digital Material Chest Wall Reconstruction." *Thoracic Deformity Surgery Expert*, September 7.

[17] Wang, W. L. 2021. "Thoracic Surgery: Shaping and Reconstruction." *Toutiao (Jinri Toutiao)*, October 31.

Section 3

SECONDARY CHEST WALL DEFECT

Compared to primary chest wall defects, secondary chest wall defects are a more common type of defect. Secondary chest wall defects always have a clear cause, which is the main distinction from primary defects [1]. Secondary defects may exist independently, but due to their underlying causes, they are often associated with other conditions or arise during the treatment of other diseases. These defects can be either temporary or permanent. As a result, the situations involving secondary chest wall defects are generally much more complex than those of primary defects.

1. Causes of Secondary Chest Wall Defects

Common clinical causes of chest wall defects include the following aspects:

(1) Trauma

Trauma can lead to the loss of various chest wall structures, resulting in different forms and degrees of defects ranging from the skin to soft tissue and bony structures. This type of defect is commonly encountered in clinical practice [2]. The related content is discussed in the relevant chapters on chest wall trauma and will not be repeated here.

(2) Surgical Resection

When a chest wall infection occurs, necrosis of various tissue structures within the infectious focus may develop. These necrotic tissues can undergo liquefaction and eventually be discharged through a rupture in the skin surface. In such cases, the infectious lesion itself constitutes a defect [3]. Due to the involvement of numerous infection-related aspects, this type of defect is discussed in the chapter on chest wall infections.

(3) Surgery

Surgery on the chest wall or within the thoracic cavity is the most common cause of chest wall defects. There are various types of Surgeries, and each may lead to the loss of chest wall structures through different mechanisms, resulting in an actual defect. Clinically, these Surgeries include the following: ①Certain specialized plastic or orthopaedic repair Surgeries [4]. To repair defects in other parts of the body, it is often necessary to remove one or more ribs or costal cartilages from the chest wall to use as graft materials. After these structures are removed, reconstruction is generally not performed at the donor site, resulting in localized chest wall defects. This is a commonly encountered secondary defect in clinical practice. ②Lesion resection Surgeries for certain thoracic wall diseases [5]. In general, after lesion removal, reconstruction should be carried out according to standard procedures.

Reconstruction, however, due to various limitations, if reconstruction cannot be performed during Surgery, a chest wall defect will remain postoperatively (Figure 4-3-1). This situation can occur after chest wall tumor resection. Since such Surgeries often involve reconstruction, secondary defects of this type are relatively uncommon. Chest wall infections after Surgery can also leave defects, but due to the presence of infection, reconstruction is generally not suitable. Therefore, defects are often present after such procedures. of course, some authors choose to proceed with reconstruction regardless of infection. If no recurrence of infection occurs postoperatively, then no defect will remain. However, if infection recurs, the reconstruction material must be completely removed; this will once again result in a chest wall defect. ③ Extended radical mastectomy for breast cancer [6]. This type of Surgery involves not only the removal of the breast tumor and breast tissue but also the deep pectoralis major and minor muscles, as well as parts of the ribs and costal cartilage. In breast Surgery, reconstruction of the bony structures of the chest wall is generally not performed during the procedure, which results in a chest wall defect. Strictly speaking, the nature of the defect left by this Surgery is similar to that seen after tumor resection of other chest wall regions. Since breast Surgery is an independent specialty, breast Surgeons often have a particular perspective on chest wall reconstruction. However, if the patient develops complications due to the chest wall defect postoperatively and requires further treatment, it becomes a straightforward chest wall defect issue, one that needs to be addressed by thoracic wall Surgeons. ④Thoracotomy via the costal bed [1]. In the past, one common thoracic Surgical approach involved entering the thoracic cavity through the costal bed, which required the removal of a rib and its costal cartilage. During closure, reconstruction of the removed rib was not performed, leaving behind a postoperative chest wall defect. Before the widespread adoption of minimally invasive thoracic Surgery, this incision was very common. Few questioned its rationale or saw the need to reconstruct the rib defect. In recent years, as open Surgeries have become less frequent, such cases of postoperative defects have also become increasingly rare. When compared with minimally invasive incisions, this approach is clearly not ideal. The resulting defect is, even more clearly, something that must be reconstructed.⑤ Thoracoplasty [7]. In treating pulmonary tuberculosis or chronic lung abscesses, when the lesion was persistent and difficult to cure, Surgeons would intentionally remove parts of the bony chest wall to allow the chest wall to collapse and compress the lesion, ultimately sealing it off to achieve therapeutic goals. This Surgery came at the cost of destroying the structure and shape of the thoracic cage. While it had a clear therapeutic effect, the damage was significant, and it is now rarely used. Occasionally, patients who underwent this Surgery many years ago may still be encountered clinically. Such cases essentially involve large-area chest wall defects. If these defects later cause problems, further treatment becomes necessary. ⑥ Failed chest wall reconstruction Surgeries. Following an initial reconstruction, some patients develop complications that prevent the reconstruction materials from remaining in the body, necessitating their removal. Once the materials are taken out after removal, the chest wall will be left with a significant defect. The previously mentioned cases of failed Surgery due to chest wall infection fall into this category. This situation can also occur after Surgery for chest wall tumors. If the Surgery fails due to infection or other reasons, the reconstruction materials must be removed, resulting in a new defect.

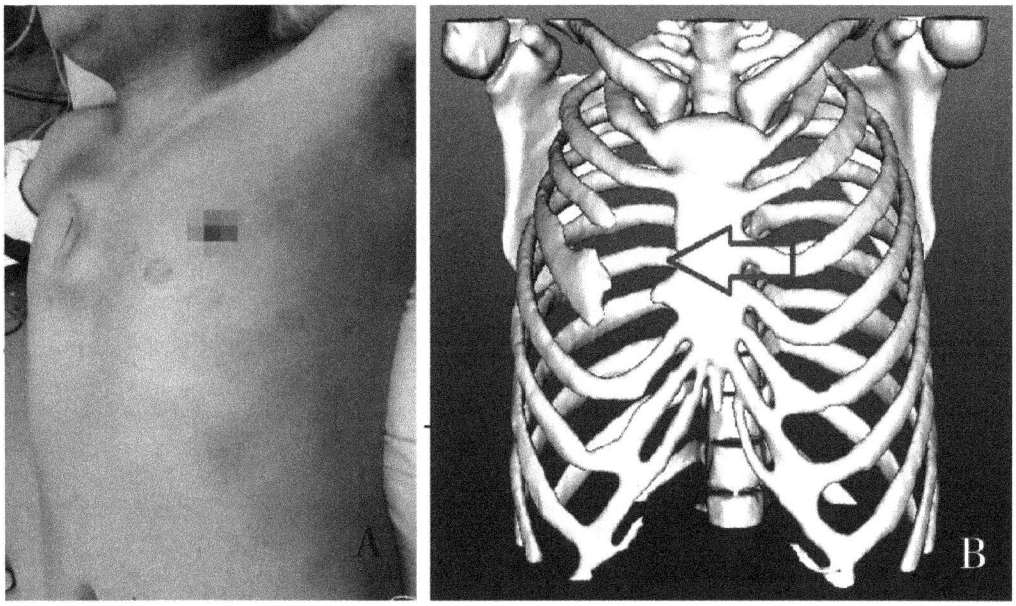

Figure 4-3-1 Chest wall defect left after Surgery (A. The patient underwent Surgery due to a localized lesion of the costal cartilage. The affected costal cartilage was removed, but no reconstruction was performed, resulting in a secondary chest wall defect; B. A 3D reconstruction of the chest wall shows the absence of the right 2,3 costal cartilages, with a clearly visible localized defect.)

(4) Other Treatments

After breast cancer resection, many patients undergo local radiotherapy, which can cause necrosis of the local skin and deeper structures, ultimately resulting in chest wall defects [8]. This type of defect is extremely severe and challenging, and it will be discussed in detail in the following chapters.

From the causes of secondary chest wall defects, it is evident that, aside from trauma, most secondary chest wall defects are related to medical interventions. In most cases, these defects result from the removal of chest wall structures without subsequent reconstruction. If reconstruction cannot be performed due to objective limitations, it can be understandable. However, some failures to perform reconstruction are entirely due to human factors, and such outcomes are regrettable.

2. Pathological Features

The pathological characteristics of secondary chest wall defects are closely related to their causes. Ribs or costal cartilages removed during plastic Surgery or orthopaedic Surgery are generally limited in scope and located in relatively fixed positions, such as the costal arch or certain specific ribs or costal cartilages. After such Surgeries, the resulting defect tends to be localized, with the defect area corresponding exactly to the site where the bony structures were removed [4]. Defects left after chest wall tumor resection are generally more complex. The tumor's location, the extent of invasion, Surgical principles, and techniques vary, resulting in considerable differences in postoperative defects [9]. Defects following anterior chest wall tumor resection are typically larger, potentially involving the sternum and bilateral costal cartilages, and in more severe cases, both sides' ribs may be affected. Defects following lateral chest wall tumor resection usually involve only the ribs or costal cartilages and generally do not affect the sternum. Defects after chest wall infection are quite complex because the extent of the infectious lesion is often uncertain, leading to considerable variability in the shape and size of postoperative defects. Chest wall defects following thoracotomy via the costal bed are generally located deep within the incision scar. The length is usually limited to the scope of one rib and sometimes includes the costal cartilage, resulting in a narrow and elongated defect. Defects following thoracoplasty have an indeterminate shape. Due to large-scale loss of bony structures and the overall collapse of the chest wall, the defect's shape cannot be accurately described, but it is definitely an extremely severe defect [7]. Defects resulting from the removal of materials after failed chest wall reconstruction are also relatively complex. The extent and shape of the defect mainly depend on the area excised during the first Surgery. If the first Surgery fails and a wider excision of the wound is necessary, the defect will be significantly larger than the initial one.

3. Clinical Manifestations

Secondary chest wall defects are complex, and their clinical manifestations are correspondingly diverse [10-12]. These defects initially present with symptoms related to the primary disease. Once a defect develops, the symptoms often become noticeably more severe than before. The symptoms of the primary disease are specific and vary significantly depending on the underlying condition. In addition to these specific clinical manifestations, a series of nonspecific symptoms may also appear. These nonspecific symptoms are mainly related to the direct damage that the defect causes to the thoracic cage. Mild defects may produce no symptoms, while severe defects can cause a variety of different symptoms. Each defect may present with either specific or nonspecific signs. Secondary defects following trauma often present with obvious wounds, where various injuries to the chest wall structures can be seen within the wound. Postoperative secondary defects, except those resulting from failed Surgeries, generally do not have open skin wounds; the appearance usually shows only localized scarring. When the defect is large, abnormal respiration and paradoxical chest wall movement may occur. If the defect is located in the precordial area, visible cardiac pulsation may be observed.

4. Examinations

In addition to a simple physical examination, secondary chest wall defects require various related imaging studies. X-ray examination is the most basic test and can provide general information about the defect. CT scanning is the most important, as it can reveal detailed information about the defect itself and the surrounding structures. Even more importantly, it can also assess the primary disease, making it a very valuable diagnostic tool.Three-dimensional reconstruction can provide more comprehensive information and should be performed whenever possible if the conditions allow.

5. Diagnosis

The diagnosis of secondary chest wall defects is relatively straightforward. Given a confirmed cause, if clear symptoms and signs are present along with examination results, secondary chest wall defects can be definitively diagnosed. When the defect is evident, almost all defects can be traced to a cause, falling under the category of secondary defects, except for primary defects. Therefore, differential diagnosis is generally unnecessary. The main task is to accurately understand the cause of the defect and gather as much additional information as possible, which will assist in guiding the treatment of the defect.

6.Surgery

(1) Surgical Indications

Once secondary chest wall defects are diagnosed, the next step is treatment. When the defect is minor, patients generally have no obvious symptoms or signs. If the patient has no specific complaints about the defect, treatment may not be necessary. However, if the defect is large and the patient has significant symptoms or concerns about appearance, active treatment should be pursued. Treatment can be divided into conservative treatment and Surgical treatment. Conservative treatment mainly focuses on symptomatic relief and is used to eliminate symptoms. This type of treatment has no effect on the appearance or the defect itself. If conservative treatment is ineffective or if the patient wishes to completely eliminate the defect, Surgical treatment can be considered.
Surgery for defects is similar to Surgery for deformities. The Surgical indication can be decided by the physician, but in many cases, the doctor's decision may not be fully understood by the patient. Therefore, the best approach is to let the patient decide. If the patient feels the defect is unsightly or uncomfortable, and symptoms cannot be relieved by conservative methods, Surgery is

recommended. If the patient neither feels the defect is unsightly nor uncomfortable, Surgery is not necessary.

(2) Nature of Surgery

The nature of Surgery for secondary chest wall defects also falls into two categories: therapeutic and reconstructive. In fact, for defect reconstruction Surgeries, these two purposes are essentially unified. This is because the defect itself is both a pathological condition and a structural deformity, allowing both goals to be achieved through a single Surgical procedure.

(3) Preoperative Preparation

Due to the presence of underlying primary diseases, the treatment of secondary chest wall defects is often complex. To ensure the success of Surgery, thorough preoperative preparation is essential. One of the most important aspects of preparation is addressing the primary disease. If the defect is caused by trauma, trauma management and stabilization must be completed first. If the cause is infection, infection control measures must be implemented beforehand. If the defect results from previous Surgeries, preparation should be tailored according to the specific circumstances of the prior procedures. In addition to managing the primary disease, special preoperative preparations are needed, generally covering two main areas: material preparation and technical preparation. The main Surgical task in treating these defects is reconstruction, particularly of the bony structures. However, unlike primary bone defects, secondary chest wall defects often involve skin and soft tissue damage as well, which must be carefully evaluated and addressed. This is the key difference compared to simple primary bony structure defects. Technical preparation refers to preoperative planning of Surgical details, including the choice and placement of incisions, flap management, and other intraoperative considerations. All these elements must be carefully planned in advance [13-15].

(4) Surgical Principles

The causes of secondary chest wall defects vary, and the specific pathological conditions differ significantly. As a result, the Surgical approaches are diverse and cannot follow a fixed model. However, the general principles of management remain consistent [11–15]: ①The primary lesion must be thoroughly addressed. Most secondary chest wall defects occur following Surgery for a primary disease. Before undertaking reconstruction, it is essential to ensure that the primary lesion has been completely eradicated. If the lesion remains, not only is reconstruction meaningless, but it may also lead to Surgical failure. For example, in the case of an infectious lesion, some oppose reconstruction during the initial Surgery due to concerns that the presence infection may interfere with the retention of foreign materials. If infection is still present during the second Surgery, the same problems encountered in the first operation may arise again.

Under such conditions, Surgery is clearly inappropriate. Therefore, before proceeding with reconstruction, the infectious focus must be completely eliminated. Otherwise, the Surgery. Reoperation can be performed. For secondary defects following tumor resection, the key intraoperative focus is to ensure that no residual tumor tissue remains around the defect. If such tissue is still present, it must be completely removed; otherwise, the Surgery is meaningless. ② Structural reconstruction should be prioritized. Structural reconstruction aims to fully restore the integrity of the thoracic cage, taking detailed anatomical structures into account to maximize the restoration of the chest wall's original shape. Functional reconstruction, on the other hand, focuses only on closing the defect without regard to detail, which may result in postoperative deformities. Structural reconstruction is the ideal approach and should be implemented whenever possible. If, for various reasons, structural reconstruction is not feasible, then functional reconstruction must be carefully considered and carried out (Figure 4-3-2). ③ Soft tissue reconstruction should also be addressed. Secondary chest wall defects often involve the loss of multiple tissue types, among which soft tissue loss is significant. To ensure good Surgical outcomes, soft tissue reconstruction should be performed alongside bony reconstruction whenever possible (Figure 4-3-3). ④ Aesthetic outcomes should be fully considered. One of the goals of reconstructive Surgery is to restore the normal appearance of the chest wall. During the Surgical procedure, constant attention should be paid to the overall appearance of the chest wall to achieve a normal or even aesthetically pleasing postoperative result.

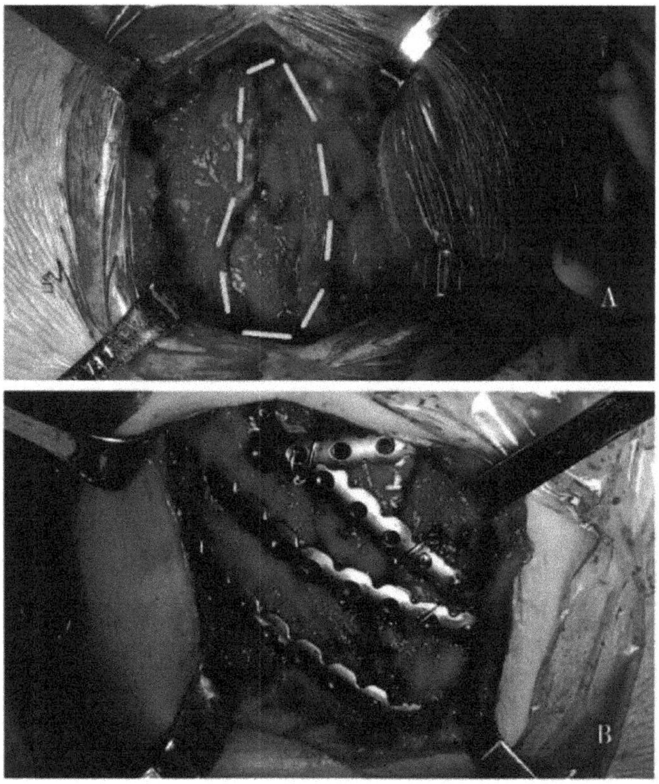

Figure 4-3-2 Functional reconstruction using Matrix RIB. The patient underwent resection of the 1, 2, 3 costal cartilages on the right side. Because the remaining portion of the 1st rib is located deep and is adjacent to the subclavian vessels and nerves, structural reconstruction of this rib was not feasible. Therefore, functional reconstruction was performed using Matrix RIB. The purpose of the reconstruction was to eliminate the local defect left by the resection of the 1st costal cartilage. (A. Exposure of the chest wall defect site; B. reconstruction of the deformed area using Matrix RIB.)

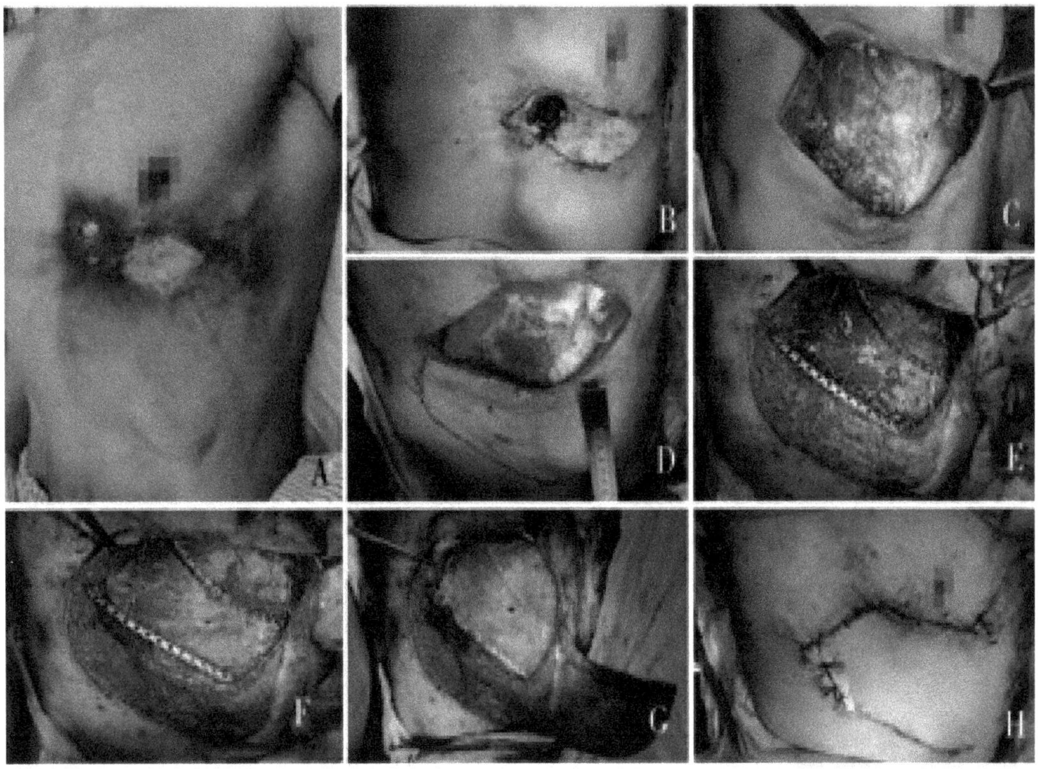

Figure 4-3-3 reconstructingtive Surgery for full-thickness secondary chest wall defect (A. Full- thickness defect of the left chest wall, with a small skin ulceration directly communicating with mediastinal structures, surrounded by obvious chronic lesions. B. An elliptical skin incision was made around the lesion to remove all diseased skin and tissue. C. Necrotic ribs were resected, exposing the left thoracic cavity. D. An abdominal wall flap was designed in preparation for wound closure. E. The bony structure was reconstructed using Matrix RIB. F, G. A fibrous membrane was used as a lining on both the inner and outer surfaces of the Marigraph. The abdominal wall flap was transferred to the wound, covering the defect and sutured to the surrounding skin)

(4) Key Surgical Points

In the specific Surgical procedures for secondary chest wall defect repair, several technical points need attention [11-15]: ① Incision Implementation. For defects secondary to previous Surgeries, it is best to select the incision at the scar of the first Surgery. For defects after tumor or infection Surgeries, the incision needs to be designed according to the specific characteristics of the lesion. Considering the necessity of soft tissue reconstruction, especially the possible use of flaps, the Surgical incision design must meet both the needs of bony structure reconstruction and soft tissue reconstruction. Besides these points, general factors in incision design such as trauma, exposure, and aesthetics must also be fully considered. Only by comprehensively taking all factors into account can the most satisfactory incision be designed. ②

Exposure of the Defect. If the skin incision design is ideal, after the incision is made, the defect should be precisely within the incision, making exposure convenient and not very difficult. However, some defects are severely deformed, such as those after thoracoplasty, where not only is it difficult to identify the edges, but the shape is completely distorted. In such cases, exposure of the defect will be very challenging. Regardless of the difficulty, the defect must be fully exposed to lay the foundation for satisfactory reconstruction. ③ Shaping of Materials. Although chest wall defects manifest as the loss of chest wall structures, in many cases, they lead to overall abnormal chest wall shape. If only the defect itself is reconstructed without holistic consideration, postoperative chest wall deformity may still persist. To achieve better results, it is necessary to design the shape of the reconstructive materials and, within feasible limits, to adjust the Surgical.
posterior thoracic shape, to achieve the most satisfactory result. ④Fixation of Materials. The reconstructive materials need to be firmly fixed to the bony structures to ensure stability. However, since materials are rarely custom-designed specifically for the defect, achieving good fixation requires reasonable design based on the characteristics of the materials and the surrounding structures of the defect, so that the materials can ultimately be securely fixed. ⑤Soft Tissue reconstruction. Soft tissue reconstruction has two main purposes: one is to cover the bony reconstruction materials with soft tissue; the other is to maintain the chest wall's appearance to ultimately achieve a more aesthetic shape. The most direct source of soft tissue is the surrounding soft tissues in the Surgical field, mainly muscle tissue. If there is insufficient soft tissue locally, tissue transfer from more distant sites can be considered. In this case, various muscle flaps or musculocutaneous flaps serve as excellent reconstructive materials. ⑥ Management of Skin Incision. If the skin incision is designed properly, postoperative skin suturing generally does not present difficulties. However, for some reconstructive Surgeries such as those with obvious local bulging after bony reconstruction suturing the skin incision can be quite challenging. In such cases, one can consider freeing the skin as much as possible around the incision to increase skin mobility before attempting closure again. If suturing remains unsuccessful, the use of flaps can be considered to manage the closure.

7. Prognosis

Patients with secondary chest wall defects often have a history of one or more injuries, making the pathology more complex and treatment more challenging a significant test of the Surgeon's skills. However, regardless of the type of secondary lesion, as long as treatment is carried out strictly according to the principles, good outcomes can generally be achieved. Conversely, if management is improper, the Surgery may fail again. This situation is similar to secondary defects caused by previous Surgical failures. In such cases, the condition becomes even more complicated, and treatment poses greater challenges.

REFERENCES

[1] Wang, W. L. 2021. "Basic Concepts of Chest Wall Defects." *Expert on Thoracic Deformity Surgery*, May 27.
[2] Pate, J. W. 1989. "Chest Wall Injuries." *Surgical Clinics of North America* 69 (1): 59–70.
[3] Brown, R. B., and J. Trenton. 1952. "Chronic Abscesses and Sinuses of the Chest Wall: The Treatment of Costal Chondritis and Sternal Osteomyelitis." *Annals of Surgery* 135 (1): 44–51.
[4] Lee, L. N., and K. D. Boahene. 2013. "A Novel Technique for Sculpting Costal Cartilage in Microtia Repair and Rhinoplasty." *JAMA Facial Plastic Surgery* 15 (5): 349–351.
[5] Spindler, N., S. Kade, U. Spiegl, et al. 2019. "Deep Sternal Wound Infection: Latissimus Dorsi Flap Is a Reliable Option for Reconstruction of the Thoracic Wall." *BMC Surgery* 19: 173.
[6] Jones, C., and R. Lancaster. 2018. "Evolution of Operative Technique for Mastectomy." *Surgical Clinics of North America* 98 (4): 835–844.
[7] Samson, P. C., and J. David, et al. 1950. "Upper Lobe Lobectomy and Concomitant Thoracoplasty in Pulmonary Tuberculosis: A Preliminary Report." *California Medicine* 73 (6): 547–549.
[8] Rouanet, P., J. M. Fabre, V. Tica, et al. 1995. "Chest Wall Reconstruction for Radionecrosis after Breast Carcinoma Therapy." *Annals of Plastic Surgery* 34 (5): 465–470.
[9] Hazel, K., and M. J. Weyant. 2015. "Chest Wall Resection and Reconstruction: Management of Complications." *Thoracic Surgery Clinics* 25 (4): 517–521.
[10] Wang, W. L. 2020. "The Hazards of Massive Chest Wall Defects." *Expert on Thoracic Deformity Surgery*, February 21.
[11] Wang, W. L. 2021. "Principles for Managing Skin Ulceration after Radiotherapy for Breast Cancer." *Expert on Thoracic Deformity Surgery*, January 13.
[12] Wang, W. L. 2019. "Matrix-Rib Chest Wall Reconstruction: Chest Wall Ulceration 20 Years after Breast Cancer Radiotherapy." *Expert on Thoracic Deformity Surgery*, April 12.
[13] Wang, W. L. 2019. "Digital Materials: Repair and Reconstruction Surgery for Large Chest Wall Defects after Breast Cancer Radiotherapy." *Expert on Thoracic Deformity Surgery*, September 27.
[14] Wang, W. L. 2017. "Design of Skin Incisions in Thoracic Reconstruction Surgery." *Expert on Thoracic Deformity Surgery*, March 30.
[15] Wang, W. L. 2018. "Repair and Reconstruction of Chest Wall Defects." *Expert on Thoracic Deformity Surgery*, October 9.

The breast is an important organ located on the chest wall. According to anatomical classification, it should fall within the scope of chest wall Surgery. However, breast specialty Surgery has a long history and has developed quite maturely, so it is no longer appropriate to place it under chest wall Surgery. Nevertheless, even though it is not a single specialty, due to the natural anatomical connection, breast diseases cannot be completely separated from chest wall Surgery [1]. Breast cancer is a malignant tumor occurring in the breast. Because of its high malignancy, it often invades the surrounding tissues. When the invasion exceeds the breast tissue itself, it becomes a subject of chest wall Surgery, inevitably creating a connection between the two specialties. Additionally, during radiotherapy for breast cancer patients, the radiation cannot be confined solely to the breast, causing the chest wall to also be irradiated [2]. Radiation inevitably causes some related complications to occur on the chest wall, which consequently become part of chest wall Surgical treatment.

1. Basic Concepts

Essentially, breast cancer is more like a malignant tumor of the chest wall and should be discussed in the chapter on chest wall tumors. However, as mentioned above, since breast Surgery has become completely independent, it is obviously inappropriate to include breast cancer in chest wall Surgery discussions. Therefore, only issues related to chest wall Surgery can be addressed. There are many issues linking breast cancer to chest wall Surgery. First is the direct invasion of the tumor. If breast cancer invades deeply, it can directly reach the chest wall muscles or even invade the ribs. If it invades laterally, more chest wall structures may be affected. Thus, the presence of tumor invasion closely ties breast cancer to chest wall Surgery. Second is the issue of tumor metastasis. Breast cancer can metastasize through various pathways, with metastases that can be either near or distant. Since the chest wall is the closest structure to the breast, it can also become a site of tumor metastasis. Once breast cancer metastasizes to the chest wall, the two become naturally linked. Third is the issue of tumor resection. Simply removing the tumor during breast cancer Surgery is often unsafe; in most cases, the surrounding structures must also be removed. These structures happen to be part of the chest wall. Whether performing radical mastectomy or extended radical mastectomy, partial removal of the chest wall structures is required [1].

This Surgical approach connects the two specialties. Fourth is the issue of postoperative adjuvant therapy. As mentioned earlier, when radiotherapy is applied locally to the lesion site postoperatively, the chest wall inevitably becomes part of the radiation field, thereby indirectly linking breast cancer and chest wall Surgery [2].

From the above analysis, it can be seen that although breast cancer is not a disease of chest wall Surgery, the natural anatomical relationship makes it impossible for breast cancer to exist independently without involving the chest wall. Therefore, certain aspects of chest wall Surgery cannot be ignored in the treatment of breast cancer patients. Many tasks related to the issues mentioned above will be discussed in other chapters; here, the focus is primarily on the problem of chest wall defects.

There are two types of chest wall defects related to breast cancer: the first type is defects caused by untreated breast cancer, which is the initial and the second type is defects resulting from Surgery for breast cancer. The formation of the first type of defect is related to local necrosis, liquefaction, and shedding of tumor tissue, which is mostly seen in advanced-stage breast cancer. This situation is now very rare. However, even if such cases are encountered clinically, patients would primarily be treated by breast Surgeons, so this type of defect still falls under the scope of breast Surgery. Although chest wall Surgeons have the capability to handle such defects, it is not appropriate for them to be involved too early. The second type of defect occurs after breast cancer Surgery. Strictly speaking, by this point, the breast itself is no longer an issue, so it is more appropriate for chest wall Surgeons, rather than breast Surgeons, to manage these defects. This section focuses on defects occurring after breast cancer Surgery.

Chest wall defects after breast cancer Surgery can occur in two situations: ① Chest wall defects caused by tumor recurrence after breast cancer Surgery; ② Chest wall defects caused by radiotherapy following breast cancer Surgery (Figure 4-4-1). Breast cancer is a malignant tumor, and some patients may experience recurrence after Surgery. When the tumor recurs, it may invade surrounding and deeper tissues. Because local blood supply is compromised after the first Surgery, severe tumor proliferation may lead to necrosis due to poor blood flow. After tissue necrosis, local tissue may slough off, eventually forming ulcers and defects. These defects can involve the skin and soft tissues but often affect bony structures, thus creating secondary chest wall defects this is the first situation. The second situation involves defects caused by radiotherapy after breast cancer Surgery [3-5]. Many patients receive radiotherapy after Surgery, which helps consolidate treatment efficacy and thoroughly kill cancer cells. However, radiotherapy often leads to a common complication: chronic local ulcers and chest wall defects. Since the blood supply to the chest wall after breast cancer Surgery is already poor, radiation may further damage blood flow and directly cause necrosis of soft tissue and bone. When all these factors combine, local chest wall ulcers may develop, fail

to heal, and eventually result in chest wall defects.
The first situation is necrosis and defect caused by tumor recurrence, while the second situation is necrosis and defect caused by radiation damage. Although the outcomes of the two situations are similar, their pathogenesis and pathological features of the defects are different. The lesion in the first situation The lesson in the first situation is relatively superficial and mainly located in the soft tissue. Although the bony structures may be involved, there is not necessarily a structural defect, and the area surrounding the lesion is often entirely composed of tumor tissue. In contrast, the lesion in the second situation is deeper and more extensive, with obvious involvement of bony structures, but typically there is no tumor tissue around the lesion. This is the most significant difference between the two. Once the defect forms, the area is exposed on the body surface, making it highly susceptible to infection, which further worsens the local lesion.

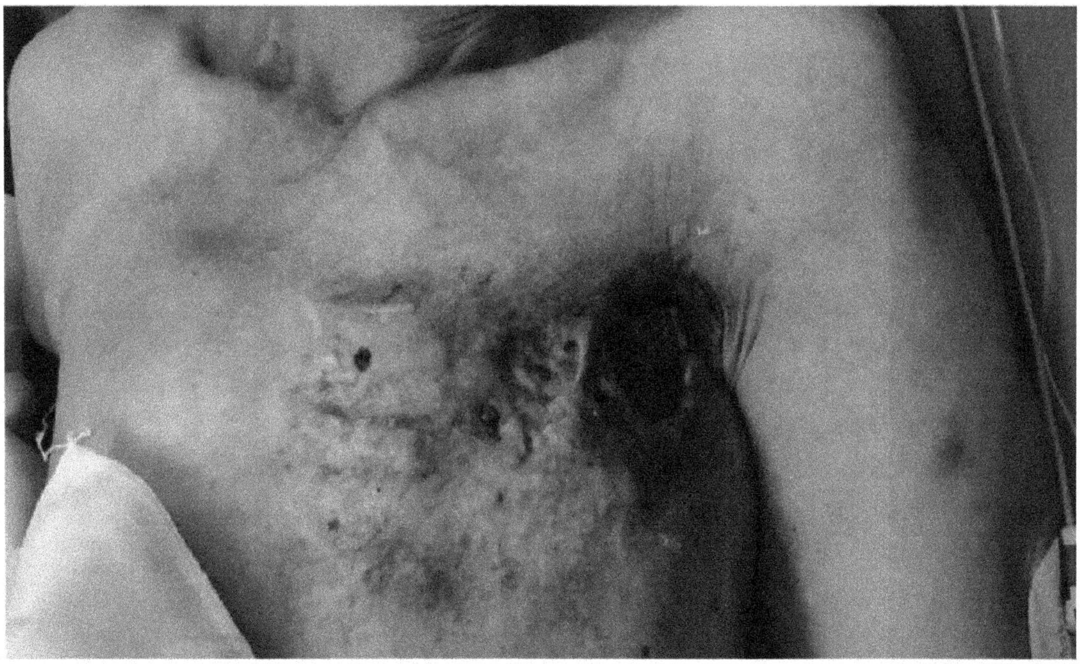

Figure 4-4-1 Defect caused by radiotherapy after breast cancer Surgery (The defect penetrates the full thickness of the chest wall, reaching deep into the thoracic cavity, with extensive necrosis of the surrounding skin and chest wall tissues).

2. Harm

Breast cancer itself is a malignant tumor, and if it recurs, the harm is very serious [6]. If chest wall defects occur on this basis, the harm becomes even more severe. At this point, the damage is not only caused by the malignant tumor itself but also includes a series of new harms resulting from the chest wall defect. These harms can cause extremely serious impacts on the patient's physical and mental health. After breast cancer radiotherapy, if the tumor is completely eliminated, it is a great blessing for the patient. However, if a chest wall defect develops, it will bring additional harm. The harm caused by chest wall defects involves multiple aspects. The skin ulceration on the surface often causes patients great suffering, severely affecting their quality of life and causing significant health impacts [4,5]. If the defect penetrates the full thickness of the chest wall, the harm is even more severe, with the most serious cases potentially endangering the patient's life.

3. Clinical Manifestations

After breast cancer is complicated by chest wall defects, patients may present with various clinical symptoms. The most common symptom is localized pain, which is usually dull and well localized. If the defect involves the full thickness of the chest wall, respiratory symptoms may appear. The defect typically shows clear local signs. In cases where the defect is caused by breast cancer recurrence, there is often a visible tumor mass centered in the defect area, with surface ulceration containing necrotic tissue. When the defect is large, deeper bony structures may be exposed, or there may be direct communication with the thoracic cavity. In defects caused by radiotherapy, no recurrent tumor is found around the defect, but the surrounding skin often shows extensive radiation damage with poor blood circulation and possible pigmentation changes. These defects can be superficial or deep and may have secretions or necrotic tissue. Such defects can also penetrate the full thickness of the chest wall, directly exposing the thoracic cavity. When the defect is not fully penetrated, paradoxical breathing may occur; if fully penetrated, air can move in and out of the thoracic cavity.

4. Examination

Postoperative chest wall defects following breast cancer Surgery are relatively straightforward to examine. The initial step involves physical examination for direct observation of the defect. Subsequently, imaging studies are performed for detailed assessment. CT scanning is the fundamental imaging modality, providing detailed visualization of the lesion and surrounding structures. Three-dimensional reconstruction from CT data not only clearly demonstrates bony structures but also displays adjacent tissues, making it an ideal diagnostic tool (Figure 4-4-2).

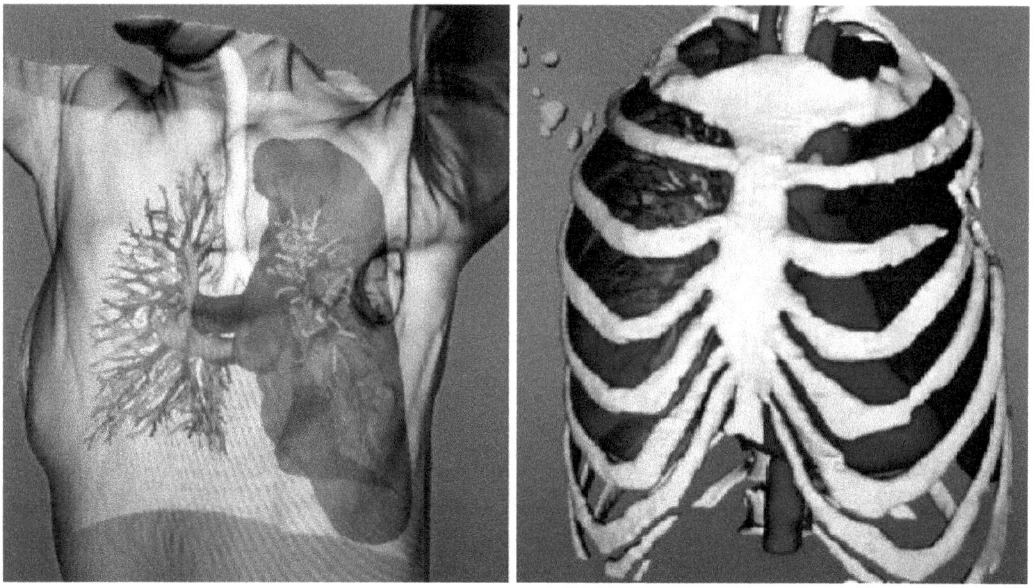
Figure 4-4-2: Three-Dimensional reconstruction Scan of Chest Wall Defect (Shows defects in both bony structures and soft tissues)

5. Diagnosis

The diagnosis of chest wall defects following breast cancer Surgery is relatively straightforward. Key diagnostic points include: a history of breast cancer Surgery, followed by skin ulceration, tissue necrosis, and ultimately the formation of a defect at the original lesion site. Based on these criteria, the diagnosis can generally be confirmed.

The main differential diagnosis to consider is chest wall infections and similar conditions. Such diseases typically lack a history of breast cancer, are localized, and generally do not exhibit invasive growth.

After the diagnosis of a post-mastectomy defect is established, the following key issues must be clarified: ① Presence of Tumor Recurrence: Chest wall defects can result from either tumor recurrence or radiation therapy. Although both may occur after breast cancer Surgery, the presence of a recurrent tumor is not always guaranteed. This distinction must be clarified before Surgery, as it directly influences the treatment approach. ② Presence of Tumor Tissue Around the Lesion: Treatment of the defect involves not only the defect site itself but also the surrounding structures. Therefore, it is essential to determine whether tumor tissue is present in adjacent areas, as this will directly impact the scope of Surgical resection. ③ Presence of Infection Within the Lesion: While reconstruction is the primary focus of treating a defect, the presence of infection significantly affects the type and method of reconstruction. If there is a confirmed infection, osseous reconstruction cannot be performed simultaneously, which is almost considered a contraindication to Surgery. If infection is ruled out, reconstruction of the bony structure can proceed immediately.④ Extent of Lesion Involvement: The extent to which the lesion has spread determines the range of Surgical resection required. This is a key factor in making Surgical decisions and must be clearly identified preoperatively.⑤ Degree of Bony Structure Destruction: One of the essential components of reconstruction is restoring the bony structure. The degree of bony involvement must be assessed before Surgery to effectively guide the Surgical plan. All of these factors are directly related to Surgical procedures. If not clarified preoperatively, the Surgery may be performed blindly and is unlikely to yield satisfactory results.

6. Surgery

(1) Surgical Indications

Simple recurrence of breast cancer does not necessarily require Surgical treatment. However, once a chest wall defect occurs, Surgery becomes essential not only to eliminate the tumor, but also to address the defect. Chest wall defects caused by postoperative radiotherapy can severely impact a patient's physical and mental health, and thus also require Surgical intervention. The main contraindications for surgery include: ①Poor overall health of the patient, making them unable to tolerate Surgery; ②Extensive metastasis of breast cancer, rendering local tumor resection of limited value; ③Excessively large defect area with no suitable skin flaps available for coverage.

(2) Surgical Methods

(i) Chest Wall Defects Caused by Tumor Recurrence Breast Cancer Surgery

When a chest wall defect forms due to recurrent breast cancer, it indicates several critical issues:① Recurrent breast cancer: This is an undeniable reality. Confirming the recurrence is of decisive importance in making Surgical decisions. ② Serious condition: The occurrence of local necrosis and defect formation after tumor recurrence indicates that the local disease is severe and requires thorough and careful management. ③ Loss of chest wall structure: The structural integrity of the chest wall has been compromised, necessitating Surgical repair and reconstruction.

From the above three questions, it can be seen that once the tumor recurs after breast cancer Surgery, it will cause great harm to the human body, so Surgery must be performed as soon as possible. The basic principles of Surgery are: ① Complete removal of the recurrent tumor; ② Complete removal of the lesion; ③ Reconstruction of the chest wall structure.

In Surgeries for simple chest wall tumors, where infection is not present, reconstruction of the bony structure can be performed directly, followed by reconstruction of the skin and soft tissues. However, in cases where chest wall defects result from recurrent breast cancer, a sterile Surgical field cannot be guaranteed. If artificial materials are used for bony reconstruction in such a setting, they become foreign bodies in an already contaminated field. The presence of these foreign materials can interfere with wound healing. Therefore, the use of artificial materials for reconstructing the bony structure is generally not recommended in such cases. Instead, the defect should be filled directly with soft tissue, followed by the reconstruction of the skin and soft tissue layers. Soft tissues have good blood supply and natural antibacterial properties, which help mitigate the disadvantages posed by infection. This approach not only ensures that the defect receives the necessary reconstruction but also promotes proper healing of the skin incision. This strategy is crucial for the successful treatment of chest wall defects.

During the actual Surgical procedure, specific soft tissues can be selected to fill the bony structural defect first. These soft tissues may be sourced from the greater omentum or from surrounding muscle flaps [7]. If the muscle flap is sufficiently large, it can not only fill the bony defect, but also assist in repairing the local soft tissue defect. In this type of defect repair Surgery, skin defects are generally present. If the area of the skin defect is not too large, it can typically be directly closed by mobilizing nearby skin or using local advancement flaps. If the skin defect is large, the surrounding skin flaps can be fully mobilized and directly stretched to achieve closure. If direct closure is difficult, flap reconstruction is necessary. Flaps are first selected from nearby areas; if these do not meet the Surgical requirements, flaps from more distant regions are considered. For very large defects, local flaps are generally insufficient for reconstruction, so free flaps or pedicled flaps from distant sites may be used.

(ii) Chest Wall Defects Caused by Postoperative Radiotherapy

After breast cancer, chest wall defects caused by postoperative radiotherapy following breast cancer Surgery are the most common type of secondary defects. Patients typically receive radiotherapy after breast cancer Surgery, after which they gradually develop skin ulceration, necrosis, and breakdown. The defect progressively deepens, eventually involving the bony structures, which may lead to bone necrosis and shedding, resulting in a full-thickness defect [8,9]. Because the defect area has undergone radiotherapy, there is generally no tumor tissue around the defect, but tissue necrosis is pronounced. Therefore, when performing Surgery for this type of defect, it is essential to first remove the necrotic tissue as thoroughly as possible before proceeding with further operative steps.

During reconstruction, if the wound is clean and there are no obvious signs of infection, the use of artificial materials for reconstruction can be considered. Artificial materials may include options such as MatrixRIB (Figure 4-4-3) or custom-designed digital implants (Figure 4-4-4). After the artificial material is placed, it must be covered with soft tissue to complete the soft tissue reconstruction (Figure 4-4-5). If there are clear signs of infection, the use of artificial materials is not recommended. In such cases, the defect should be filled solely with soft tissue. The source of the soft tissue is similar to that used in chest wall defect Surgeries following tumor recurrence.

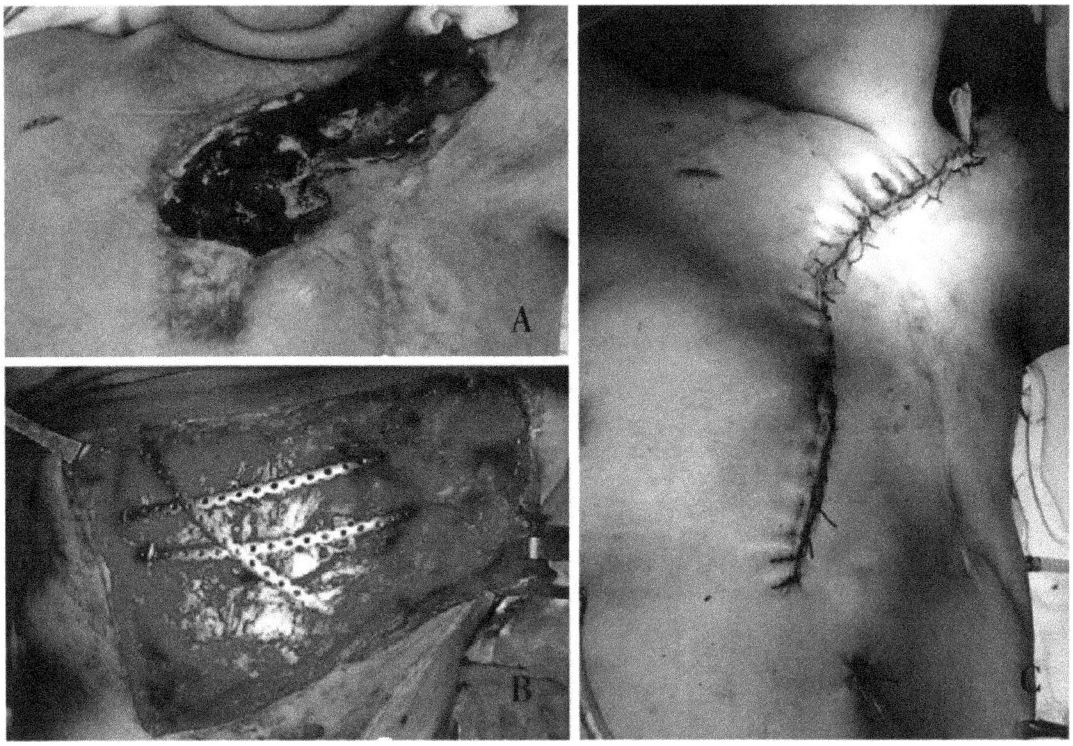

Figure 4-4-3 Chest Wall reconstruction Using MatrixRIB. (A. Large chest wall defect caused by postoperative radiotherapy after breast cancer Surgery. B. After removing all necrotic tissue, the bony structure is reconstructed with MatrixRIB, then covered with surrounding soft tissue, and the skin is directly sutured. C. Postoperative appearance of the chest wall)

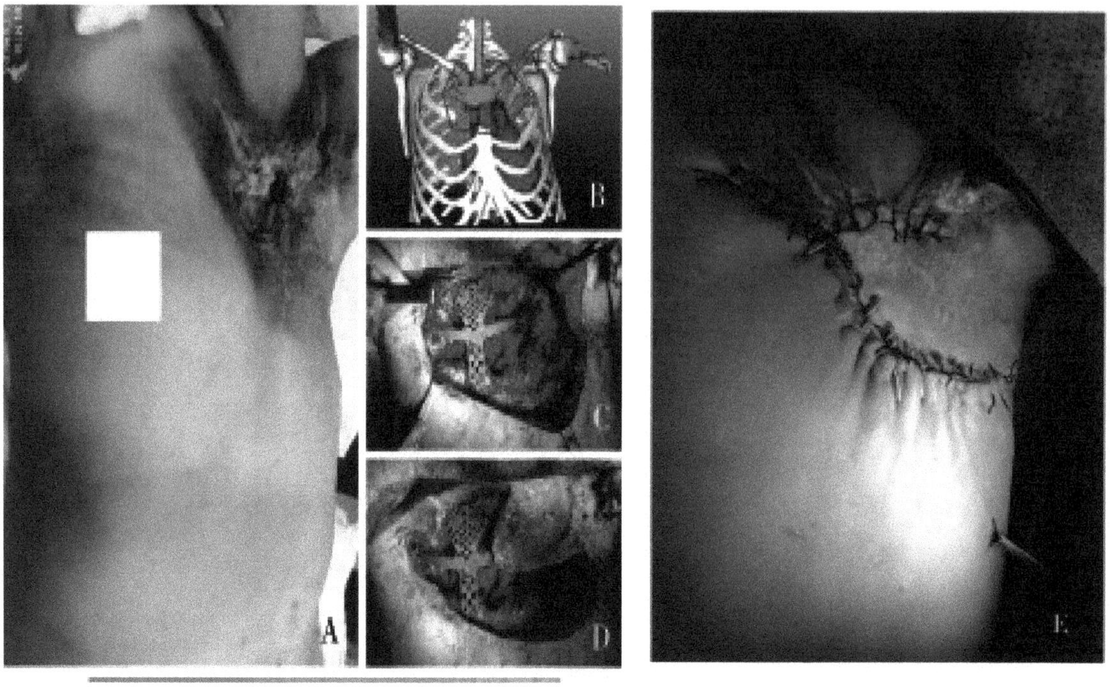

Figure 4-4-4 Chest wall reconstruction using prosthetic (digital) materials (A. Large chest wall defect caused by post-radiotherapy after breast cancer Surgery, involving the full thickness of the chest wall and extending to the mediastinum; B. 3D reconstruction image showing the extent of the lesion; C. reconstruction of the bony chest wall structure using prosthetic material; D. Coverage of the prosthetic material with surrounding tissue flaps to close the incision; E. Postoperative appearance of the chest wall)

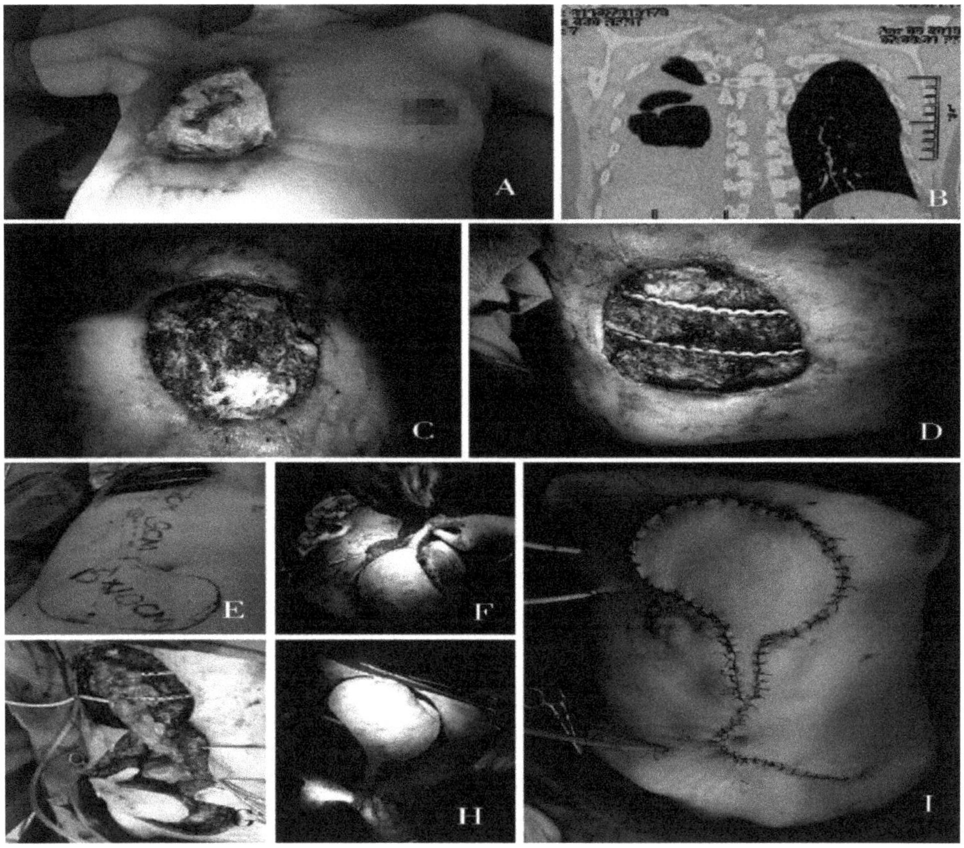

Figure 4-4-5 Large Chest Wall Defect Caused by Postoperative Radiotherapy for Breast Cancer: reconstruction Using Matrix RIB for Bony Structures, and Rectus Abdominis Flap with Omentum for Soft Tissue Repair. (A. Massive full-thickness chest wall defect on the right side caused by radiotherapy following breast cancer Surgery, involving extensive necrosis; B. CT reveals associated lesions within the thoracic cavity and pleural thickening, with obvious pathological changes; C. Debridement is performed, necrotic tissue removed, and the anterior segments of the right 5, 6 ribs with costal cartilage excised to expose fresh tissue; D. Matrix RIB is used to reconstruct the bony chest wall structure; E. Design of the rectus abdominis flap; F. Harvesting of the rectus abdominis flap; G. Accessing the abdominal cavity, the greater omentum is mobilized and pulled to cover the chest wound; H. The rectus abdominis flap is transposed and sutured into the defect; I. Postoperative appearance of the chest wall and abdominal wall.)

Reoperation for postoperative defects after breast cancer Surgery often faces a particular challenge: infection within the lesion. If an infection is present, artificial materials cannot be used for bony structure reconstruction, which becomes the greatest limitation of such Surgeries. This significantly affects the overall outcome of the procedure.

After such procedures, bony defects of the chest wall may still remain, categorizing them as secondary defects that still require Surgical intervention. Looking at the full course of treatment for these types of defects, the process essentially becomes a two-stage Surgery: Stage one focuses on eliminating the soft tissue and skin defects, as well as clearing the infected area. Stage two is performed later, once infection has been controlled, and is aimed specifically at the reconstruction of the bony structure.

This second-stage Surgery is conducted in a sterile field and typically does not involve major skin or soft tissue defects, significantly increasing the success rate. Breast cancer is a malignant tumor, and patients often undergo great suffering during the initial resection Surgery. Once a defect occurs, the patient faces even greater distress. However, if a follow-up Surgery can thoroughly remove the lesion, prevent tumor recurrence, and close the skin defect, the patient's quality of life can be greatly improved and their suffering eliminated. Therefore, such Surgeries are of critical importance to patients. Whenever conditions permit, Surgical completion should be pursued as fully as possible.

7.Prognosis

Chest wall defects following breast cancer Surgery often involve three fundamental chest wall Surgical conditions: chest wall tumors, chest wall infections, and chest wall defects. This chapter focuses primarily on the issue of chest wall defects, with only a discussion of the defect-related problems. Because chest wall tumors and infections are also involved, treatment is often very complex. To evaluate treatment outcomes, it is necessary to use the treatment standards for all three conditions in a comprehensive manner. In other words, the evaluation should not be based solely on the results of defect treatment but must also consider the effectiveness of tumor and infection management.

Chest wall defects after breast cancer Surgery are a very challenging clinical problem. They pose a significant challenge not only to thoracic Surgeons but also to breast Surgeons. The vast majority of doctors do not have the expertise to manage such conditions. Due to the complexity of the Surgery, the risk of Surgical failure is also very high. Many patients undergo multiple Surgeries without achieving defect healing and eventually have to give up on Surgical treatment. However, no matter how difficult these defects are, the condition is not truly incurable. As long as the basic Surgical principles are carefully followed in precision, the defect can ultimately be completely treated.

REFERENCES

[1] Libson, S., and M. Lippman. 2014. "A Review of Clinical Aspects of Breast Cancer." *International Review of Psychiatry* 26 (1): 4–15.

[2] Rouanet, P., J. M. Fabre, V. Tica, et al. 1995. "Chest Wall Reconstruction for

Radionecrosis after Breast Carcinoma Therapy." *Annals of Plastic Surgery* 34 (5): 465–470.
[3] Wang, W. L. 2021. "Principles for Managing Skin Breakdown after Radiotherapy for Breast Cancer." *Thoracic Deformity Surgery Experts*, January 13.
[4] Wang, W. L. 2019. "Matrix-Rib Chest Wall Reconstruction: 20 Years of Chest Wall Ulceration after Radiotherapy for Breast Cancer." *Thoracic Deformity Surgery Experts*, April 12.
[5] Wang, W. L. 2019. "Digital Materials: Repair and Reconstruction Surgery for Massive Chest Wall Defects after Breast Cancer Radiotherapy." *Thoracic Deformity Surgery Experts*, September 27.
[6] Wapnir, I. L., and A. Khan. 2019. "Current Strategies for the Management of Locoregional Breast Cancer Recurrence." *Oncology (Williston Park)* 33 (1): 19–25.
[7] Huang, Boxiang, Yongfeng Li, Jia Li, et al. 2013. "Pedicled Omental Transplant Combined with Pectoralis Major Myocutaneous Flap for Treatment of Radiation-Induced Sternal Osteomyelitis: Two Cases." *Guangdong Medical Journal* 34 (6): 826.
[8] Ha, J. H., S. O. Park, H. Chang, et al. 2018. "Optimal Reconstruction Method for Large Radionecrosis following Breast Cancer Treatment: Utility of Free Transverse Rectus Abdominis Myocutaneous Flap Using Contralateral Internal Mammary Artery as Recipient." *Annals of Plastic Surgery* 81 (5): 584–590.
[9] Fosnot, J., J. P. Fischer, J. M. Smartt, et al. 2011. "Does Previous Chest Wall Irradiation Increase Vascular Complications in Free Autologous Breast Reconstruction?" *Plastic and Reconstructive Surgery* 127 (2): 496–504.

CHAPTER 5

CHEST WALL TRAUMA

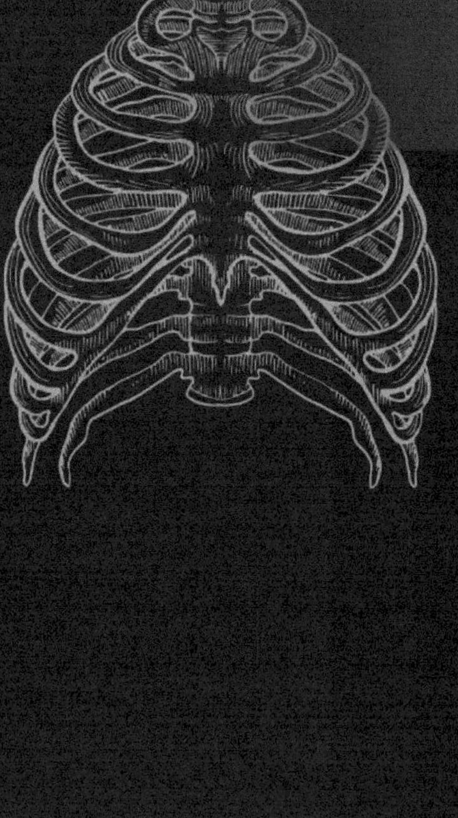

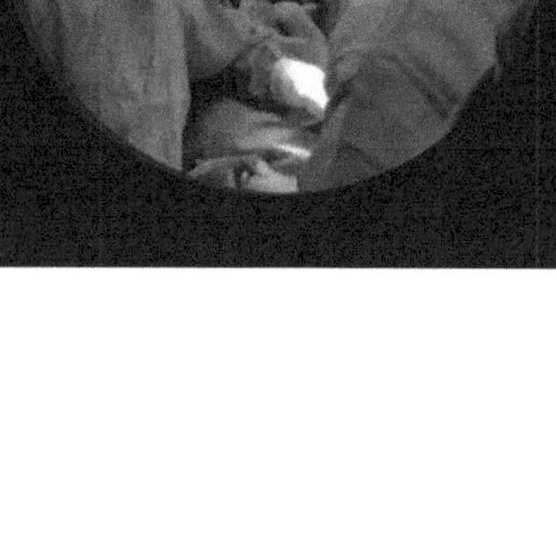

Section 1

OVERVIEW OF CHEST WALL TRAUMA

Chest wall trauma is a treatment item in traditional thoracic Surgery and is part of thoracic trauma. The focus of thoracic trauma treatment is generally on damage to the viscera in the chest cavity, and simple chest wall trauma is not taken seriously. For a long time, there has been almost only one item related to chest wall trauma, namely rib fractures, and other items are rarely mentioned. However, in reality, chest wall trauma is not limited to this [1,2]. The chest wall has a wide range and many structures. In addition to the ribs, there are many other structures. Therefore, the research on trauma cannot only focus on the ribs, but also must see the possibility of damage to other structures. The main reason why only the ribs were focused on in the past should be related to the positioning of chest wall diseases in the entire thoracic Surgery. Since the focus of thoracic Surgery work has always been on the inside of the chest cavity, not many people have paid attention to chest wall diseases. The most common chest wall trauma is rib fractures, so the ribs have become the most concerned structure. When chest wall Surgery regards chest wall trauma as a major treatment item for research, the situation will change a lot. The breadth and depth of research are very different from the era of thoracic Surgery. Breadth refers to the fact that more chest wall trauma is being paid attention to, and depth refers to the further deepening of the research content. This is the obvious difference between chest wall Surgery research on trauma and thoracic Surgery research.

1.Basic Concepts

Chest wall trauma refers to structural damage to the chest wall resulting from various violent forces. This concept involves two core elements: Cause of injury, Structural damage, there are multiple causes of injury, typically referring to mechanical external forces. When the force applied to the chest wall exceeds a certain threshold, it can cause structural failure, resulting in chest wall trauma. External force is the initiating factor of the trauma, while structural damage is the outcome. This damage can manifest in various forms, but its essence is the disruption of tissue continuity at different structural levels of the chest wall. Among the five primary conditions treated in chest wall Surgery, trauma is a particularly unique case. Strictly speaking, trauma is not a disease, but rather an injury and there are clear distinctions between the two. Cause: Trauma typically has a clear, identifiable cause, whereas diseases often do not have a specific or immediate cause. Onset: Trauma occurs suddenly and rapidly, while diseases usually develop gradually over a longer period. Outcome: The consequences of trauma are often severe and immediate, potentially life-threatening without urgent care. In contrast, the outcomes of diseases are usually less abrupt, and delay in treatment may not result in immediate danger. Due to these distinct differences, categorizing chest wall trauma as one of the basic "diseases" of chest wall Surgery is inaccurate. A more precise description is that chest wall trauma is a fundamental category of cases treated in chest wall Surgery.

Chest wall trauma has the following characteristics [1]: ①. Uncertainty: This feature manifests in many specific aspects and involves nearly every aspect of chest wall trauma. The time of trauma is uncertain, the location is uncertain, the injured area is uncertain, the severity is uncertain, the nature of the injury is uncertain, the physical signs are uncertain, the clinical manifestations are uncertain, and the prognosis is uncertain. Uncertainty implies a high degree of randomness, which is the greatest characteristic of trauma. Because so many uncertain factors are involved, trauma management must not be rigid or standardized. Flexibility is essential, and only by adapting treatment to the specific trauma situation can good outcomes be achieved. ② Urgency Trauma typically occurs suddenly and acutely, often causing irreversible outcomes within a very short time. This means trauma care must be performed without delay every second counts. Failure to act quickly can result in deterioration or even death. ③ Destructiveness All injuries or illnesses are destructive to some degree, but trauma tends to cause more severe and obvious damage. The destructiveness is often visible, such as in bruises, lacerations, or crush injuries, with clear structural deformities. When damage is severe, it can impair or endanger vital organ function, potentially resulting in fatal consequences. ④ Complexity Trauma is often the result of complex mechanisms of injury and produces complex clinical conditions. Each trauma case varies based on individual context. Therefore, expert evaluation and management are crucial; otherwise, treatment outcomes may be compromised. ⑤ Composite Nature The chest wall is not a standalone structure. It comprises many different tissues and anatomical components, and it is intimately connected with surrounding structures. This means chest wall trauma frequently involves multiple systems, reflecting its composite nature. This composite nature manifests in two main ways: First, the chest wall itself consists of skin, soft tissues, bones, and more delicate structures such as blood vessels and nerves. Second, the injury may extend to adjacent structures, such as: Intrathoracic organs (lungs, heart), which are the most common concurrent injuries. Upper abdominal organ, Bony structures around the chest (scapula, clavicle, thoracic vertebrae). When these surrounding structures are also damaged, the trauma is no longer a simple chest wall injury, but becomes a complex or compound trauma. It is important to note that, in traditional thoracic Surgery, chest wall trauma accompanied by intrathoracic injuries is still classified as "chest trauma." However, in chest wall Surgery, such cases are viewed as true compound injuries, not isolated chest wall injuries. This shift from simple to compound trauma does not necessarily mean that multiple specialists are required. In emergency trauma care, the chest wall Surgeon bears the responsibility and duty to manage these complex injuries as much as possible independently.

Given that chest wall Surgery includes aspects of orthopaedic Surgery, chest wall Surgeons often have technical advantages when managing complex traumatic injuries skills, they must be proficient in. From the above analysis, it is evident that chest wall trauma is a very unique "type of condition", involving many specific issues. However, traditional thoracic Surgery has not paid close attention to these problems, which clearly hinders the effective treatment of chest wall trauma. Chest wall Surgery is a brand-new specialty, with concepts and techniques that are completely different from those of traditional thoracic Surgery. Therefore, when chest wall trauma is managed by chest wall Surgeons, the outcomes can be entirely different and often significantly improved.

Chest wall Surgery has two fundamental attributes: chest wall orthopaedics and chest wall plastic Surgery [3]. This means that chest wall Surgeons must not only focus on the basic aspects of the chest wall, but also pay attention to orthopaedic and plastic Surgery aspects. If we consider that chest wall Surgery originated from traditional thoracic Surgery, then in reality, the work of chest wall Surgeons spans three specialties: thoracic Surgery, orthopaedics, and plastic Surgery. One key aspect of chest wall trauma is skeletal injury, and the most specialized doctors for dealing with bones are, of course, orthopaedic Surgeons. However, in traditional thoracic Surgery practice, these issues were handled by thoracic Surgeons. This approach is open to discussion.

This is open to discussion. It is easy to imagine that if rib or sternum fractures were handled by orthopaedic specialists, the outcomes would certainly be different. Chest wall Surgeons possess the professional qualities of orthopaedic doctors. Therefore, when chest wall fractures are managed by chest wall Surgeons, the treatment is naturally more appropriate and refined than when handled by traditional thoracic Surgeons. Similarly, chest wall trauma also involves many aspects of plastic Surgery. In the past, thoracic Surgeons mainly focused on life-saving measures and paid little attention to reconstructive or aesthetic concerns, an understandable approach. However, once the principles of plastic Surgery are integrated, the treatment outcomes improve significantly. This work, originally belonging to plastic Surgeons, now also falls within the scope of chest wall Surgeons, because the concept of reconstruction and aesthetics is deeply rooted in all aspects of chest wall Surgery. This is one of the key differences between chest wall Surgery and traditional thoracic Surgery.

2. Causative Factors

In theory, any external factor, when strong enough and directly acting on the chest wall, can cause structural damage to the chest wall, leading to chest wall trauma. There are many types of external factors, which can generally be categorized into two types: physical and chemical [1]. Due to the complexity of chemical factors, they will not be discussed for now. Physical factors may include mechanical, electrical, optical, and radioactive elements all of which can cause chest wall injuries. In clinical practice, the most commonly encountered are mechanical factors. Based on this, chest wall injuries can be classified into various specific types such as blunt trauma, sharp trauma, gunshot wounds, firearm injuries, crush injuries, falls, impact injuries, collision injuries, and blast injuries. These causative factors differ in nature and mode of action, resulting in different outcomes. However, from the perspective of fundamental physical principles, there are commonalities among them. The basic mechanism by which physical factors cause injury is essentially a collision between external objects and the human body. The mechanics and outcomes of such collisions can be studied through classical Newtonian mechanics and applied mechanics. These studies are of great significance for understanding and treating trauma.

3. Pathology and Pathophysiology

Pathological changes refer to alterations in various structural layers. When chest wall trauma occurs, under the influence of various external factors, all the structures of the chest wall undergo significant changes. These changes manifest from the outer layers to the inner layers and can present in different forms. When external factors act on the chest wall, the first part to come into contact with the injuring factor is the skin.

Theoretically, the skin should be the first structure to be damaged. However, due to the varying magnitude of external force and the different properties of the internal components of the chest wall, different outcomes can occur, resulting in so-called closed injuries and open injuries [1,3].

In closed injuries, the skin remains intact. The damage can affect soft tissues or bones underneath without breaking the skin. In open injuries, the skin is breached with a wound, and the injury extends from the outside inward, potentially reaching the bones or even the thoracic cavity. When the external force is not strong enough to break the skin but sufficient to damage the underlying structures, a closed chest wall injury occurs. However, if the force is strong enough to exceed the skin's tolerance, then all structures may sustain damage, resulting in what is known as an open chest wall injury.

Closed chest wall injuries involve intact skin, but the underlying soft tissues may suffer various degrees of compression or impact, potentially leading to local hematomas or edema. The bones might show no obvious changes. However, if the force is strong enough, different degrees of fractures may occur, ranging from a single fracture to multiple fractures affecting various areas. Open chest wall injuries are characterized by a visible break in the skin. All structures along the wound path are likely to sustain severe damage, including structural rupture. If blood vessels or nerves pass through the wound, they may also be damaged. Open injuries can also involve bone fractures, which may occur in a single rib or involve multiple bones and locations.

Open injuries can manifest in various forms depending on the nature of the trauma, and are typically categorized as contusions, lacerated contusions, and lacerations. Each of these injuries can range in severity. However, the most serious form of injury is not among these three, but rather a tissue defect [1]. When the injury is severe enough, parts of the chest wall structures may be lost, resulting in a defect. This is considered one of the most severe types of trauma. If the defect is limited to the skin or soft tissue, it remains localized. However, if the entire thickness of the chest wall is lost, the pleural cavity becomes exposed, leading to an open chest injury. Such a condition clearly goes beyond typical chest wall trauma. If the defect is extensive and accompanied by significant blood loss, it can: Seriously impair respiratory function, potentially leading to circulatory system complications.

When chest wall trauma occurs, the human body exhibits two types of responses: local response and systemic response. 1. Local Response: This is a direct continuation of the trauma and may include local bleeding, swelling, and exudation. If not promptly managed, it may lead to infection of the wound. 2. Systemic Response: Divided into two main components: ① Stress Response: The body reacts rapidly to cope with the crisis. Key physiological changes include: Sympathetic nervous system activation, Release of pituitary and adrenal cortex hormones, Resulting in: Elevated blood glucose, Increased blood pressure, Faster heart rate, Rapid breathing.

These are part of the body's self-protection mechanisms. Psychological reactions (emotional shifts, defensive behaviours, coping responses) may also occur and can exacerbate physiological stress. ② Organ Dysfunction: When the trauma is severe, major organ function may become impaired, potentially leading to organ failure. This may occur early but more commonly appears later, depending on the functional reserves of the organs. In the early stage, organs may compensate, but with further injury, dysfunction becomes evident. The organs most closely related to chest wall trauma are: The heart, The lungs, The kidneys.

4. Clinical manifestations

When chest wall trauma occurs, the human body often presents with obvious symptoms, originating from both local and systemic sources [1,3]. 1. Local Symptoms: Pain is the most prominent local sign: In open injuries, pain is well localized, mostly near the wound. In closed injuries, since the skin remains intact, pain may be less precisely localized, but typically corresponds with the area of internal injury. The location and nature of pain can aid in assessing the underlying structures that may be damaged. Presence of additional pain in other areas (e.g., abdomen, back, or shoulders) may indicate associated injuries, such as involvement of internal organs or the spine. 2. Systemic Symptoms:

Primarily related to organ dysfunction, especially respiratory impairment. Chest wall trauma can cause: Dyspnea, reduced ventilation, in severe cases, hypoxemia or even respiratory failure. Other systemic signs may include: Restlessness or altered consciousness, Abnormal blood pressure or heart rate, Hemorrhagic shock in cases of significant blood loss.

Early symptoms include respiratory issues, along with other systemic symptoms such as fever, irritability, anxiety, and fatigue. If shock occurs due to bleeding, symptoms such as delirium and coma may also appear.

The signs of chest wall trauma can also be categorized into local and systemic signs. Local signs mainly include redness, swelling, bruising, and lacerations at the site of injury. Skin contusions may present with obvious wounds over a large area but do not involve deeper structures. Lacerations may show visible tears with blood oozing from the wound. If the tear is large, deeper structures of the chest wall may be exposed. When various forms of chest wall defects occur, internal structures of the chest wall may be exposed through the defect, which may directly communicate with the thoracic cavity. Air leakage may be observed at the site, along with paradoxical respiratory movements

.

5. Examination

Physical examination is the most basic form of assessment and allows for a preliminary understanding of the trauma. Based on this, additional examinations should be conducted according to the severity of the injury to further clarify detailed information about the trauma.

The most fundamental examination is X-ray imaging, which is convenient, quick, and highly effective for evaluating the bony structures of the chest wall [1]. Therefore, it is generally considered the first-choice examination [1]. Based on the X-ray findings, further imaging studies such as CT scans may be considered to provide more detailed information [1,5–7]. In addition to these two imaging methods, if there is a suspicion of injury to other parts of the body, such as the heart, an echocardiogram (ultrasound of the heart) may be performed. Through these examinations, it is possible to gather the most comprehensive information about the injury and achieve the most accurate diagnosis.

It is particularly important to highlight the examination of costal cartilage, as X-rays cannot visualize costal cartilage, making injuries to this structure difficult to detect. In such cases, ultrasound examination can be considered a simple and effective method. Ultrasound can provide highly accurate descriptions of lesions in both ribs and costal cartilage, and should be performed when there is suspicion of such issues.

The main limitation of ultrasound is that clinicians cannot directly view three-dimensional images of the ribs or costal cartilage. Even if radiologists provide two-dimensional images, they cannot clearly show the relationship between the cartilage and surrounding structures, which hinders clinical judgment. In such

cases, marking the suspicious site on the body surface is the simplest and most practical approach. If conditions permit, intraoperative ultrasound can also be used to assist Surgery and provide more accurate guidance.
When conducting evaluations, the more examination methods used, the more beneficial it is for diagnosing trauma. However, trauma is distinct from most other diseases in that it is often urgent and life-threatening. If the patient's condition allows, step-by-step examinations are appropriate. But if the injury is severe and emergency intervention is needed, unnecessary tests should be avoided, and the patient should be taken directly to the operating room to avoid delays in treatment. In such situations, physical examination becomes critically important and can almost determine the patient's outcome.

6.Treatment

The treatment of chest wall trauma consists of two main parts: the first is conservative treatment, and the second is Surgical treatment [1]. Conservative treatment primarily The focus should be on mild injuries, such as general skin contusions or certain less severe closed injuries. All open injuries and closed injuries involving the deep and vital structures of the chest wall require Surgical treatment.
Thoracic wall trauma Surgery is a type of thoracic wall Surgical procedure, and thus it fundamentally retains two essential characteristics: one is therapeutic, and the other is reconstructive. Although trauma itself is not a disease and therefore, in theory, should not involve treatment in the conventional sense, broadly speaking, trauma care is essentially a form of treatment. Therefore, it can be described as both therapeutic and reconstructive. In traditional thoracic trauma Surgery, the focus has been solely on treatment, while the reconstructive aspect has often been neglected. This clearly reflects the difference between two approaches to trauma care. Let me know if you want this adapted for academic, clinical, or plain language use.
The timing of Surgery for chest wall trauma must be determined based on the patient's actual condition [6,8,9]. It may range from the most urgent emergency Surgery to scheduled or elective procedures [1]. The specific type of injury should dictate the appropriate Surgical approach.

(1) Emergency Surgery

When thoracic wall trauma occurs and the injury is extremely severe, with impaired function of vital organs and life-threatening conditions, emergency Surgery is required. In such cases, every second counts the harmful factors must be eliminated as quickly as possible, and the function of vital organs restored. This is the basic guarantee for the success of the Surgery. Situations requiring emergency Surgery often involve massive bleeding or severe respiratory distress. In cases of extensive thoracic wall defects or acute and severe damage to heart and lung function, there are no conservative treatment options available, so early Surgical intervention is essential.

(2) Scheduled (Time-Limited) Surgery

Some injuries may not be life-threatening but are quite evident and can cause both physical and psychological harm to the patient. If conservative treatment cannot eliminate the harm, Surgical intervention becomes necessary. In such cases, Surgery does not need to be performed immediately but must be completed within a certain time frame and should not be excessively delayed. This is known as scheduled or time-limited Surgery. This approach allows time to manage the trauma more effectively. During the waiting period, thorough preoperative preparation must be carried out to achieve better Surgical outcomes. Typical examples of such Surgeries include treatment of rib fractures, sternal fractures, or other multiple injuries that fall under the category of scheduled Surgery.

(3) Elective Surgery

If the patient's injury is evident and meets the indications for Surgery, but does not pose an immediate threat to life, sufficient preoperative preparation can be made, and Surgery can be performed at a suitable time. This type of Surgery is known as elective Surgery. Some procedures involving the repair and reconstruction of defects can be carried out as elective Surgeries.

7. Some Special Surgeries

(1) Surgeries for Chest Wall Trauma Combined with Intrathoracic Organ Injuries

Chest wall trauma is often accompanied by injuries to intrathoracic organs. The lungs and heart are the most commonly affected organs, while other organs such as the trachea and oesophagus can also be damaged in some severe cases [4,10]. Once these injuries occur, chest wall trauma often becomes very complex and serious. In such cases, it is necessary not only to address the chest wall injuries but also to treat the intrathoracic injuries. The focus of treatment at this stage is on intrathoracic damage, which is precisely the traditional scope of thoracic Surgery. Although chest wall Surgery is an independent discipline, it originates from thoracic Surgery, and therefore managing such trauma is not particularly difficult.

(2) Surgeries for Chest Wall Trauma Combined with Injuries to Other Parts of the Body

When chest wall trauma occurs, in addition to possible damage to intrathoracic structures, other parts of the body may also be injured [10]. For example, structures in the abdomen adjacent to the chest wall, as well as the spine, scapula, and clavicle, may all be involved. During the management of these injuries, if the chest wall Surgeon is not capable of handling the associated structural damage, they must collaborate with specialists from the relevant medical fields. Only through such interdisciplinary cooperation can successful trauma treatment be ensured.

8. Prognosis

The prognosis of chest wall trauma is influenced by many factors, which can generally be divided into two categories: objective factors and subjective factors [1]. Subjective factors are related to the patient's time of seeking medical attention, their tendency and access to care, and their attitude toward treatment. They are also influenced by the doctor's level of awareness and technical expertise. Objective factors mainly include two aspects: the severity of the trauma and the conditions for treatment. If the injured person can reach the hospital in time for treatment, and if the doctor can make full use of the available medical technology, a good outcome is usually achievable. However, if the trauma is extremely severe and treatment cannot proceed smoothly due to various reasons, a good result cannot be expected.

REFERENCES

[1] Wang, W. L. 2021. "Issues in the Treatment of Chest Wall Trauma." *Expert in Thoracic Deformity Surgery*, November 3.

[2] Caragounis, E. C., Y. Xiao, and H. Granhed. 2021. "Mechanism of Injury, Injury Patterns, and Associated Injuries in Patients Operated for Chest Wall Trauma." *European Journal of Trauma and Emergency Surgery* 47 (4): 929–938.

[3] Wang, W. L. 2021. "The Relationship between Chest Wall Surgery and Other Specialties." *Toutiao (Jinri Toutiao)*, November 2.

[4] Dogrul, B. N., I. Kiliccalan, E. S. Asci, et al. 2020. "Blunt Trauma-Related Chest Wall and Pulmonary Injuries: An Overview." *Chinese Journal of Traumatology* 23 (3): 125–138.

[5] Rodriguez, R. M., G. W. Hendey, and W. R. Mower. 2017. "Selective Chest Imaging for Blunt Trauma Patients: The National Emergency X-Radiography Utilization Studies (NEXUS-Chest Algorithm)." *American Journal of Emergency Medicine* 35 (1): 164–170.

[6] Palas, J., A. P. Matos, V. Mascarenhas, et al. 2014. "Multidetector Computed Tomography: Evaluation of Blunt Chest Trauma in Adults." *Radiology Research and Practice* 2014: 864369.

[7] Oikonomou, A., and P. Prassopoulos. 2011. "CT Imaging of Blunt Chest Trauma." *Insights into Imaging* 2 (3): 281–295.

[8] de Campos, J. R. M., and T. W. White. 2018. "Chest Wall Stabilization in Trauma Patients: Why, When, and How?" *Journal of Thoracic Disease* 10 (Suppl 8): S951–S962.

[9] Stolberg-Stolberg, J., J. C. Katthagen, T. Hillemeyer, et al. 2021. "Blunt Chest Trauma in Polytraumatized Patients: Predictive Factors for Urgent Thoracotomy." *Journal of Clinical Medicine* 10 (17): 3843.

[10] Besha, Y. M., F. Mertzlufft, H. W. Kottkamp, et al. 2020. "Analysis of Risk Factors in Thoracic Trauma Patients with a Comparison of a Modern Trauma Centre: A Monocentre Study." *World Journal of Emergency Surgery* 15: 45.

Section 2

MECHANISM OF INJURY OF CHEST WALL INJURY

Chest wall trauma refers to the damage to various structures and tissues of the chest wall caused by external injurious factors. Traditionally, thoracic Surgery research on chest wall trauma has focused primarily on the outcomes namely, the impact of structural damage on the human body and the corresponding treatment measures while paying little attention to the injury process itself. This focus aligns more with clinical specialties. However, this clearly represents a limitation in previous research. Understanding the injury process is actually very important, as it not only helps to clarify the detailed mechanisms causing the damage, but also aids in injury prevention and contributes to trauma treatment. Therefore, it is necessary to conduct further study on this topic.

There are many factors that cause chest wall trauma. Due to the variety of injured locations, structures, and tissues, the outcomes of such trauma are highly diverse. Studying the injury process thus presents a significant challenge. However, with careful observation, it is possible to identify fundamental patterns and establish reasonable physical models, which will aid in the study of the mechanisms of trauma.

1. The Mechanical Principles of Chest Wall Trauma

The process of trauma is often quite complex, and on the surface, it may seem difficult to find any patterns. However, if analyzed from a mechanical perspective, discovering these patterns is not difficult. In fact, all trauma processes can be regarded as a collision between two objects whether it is a sharp injury or a blunt injury, whether it is an impact, compression, fall, firearm injury, stabbing, or a strike, all trauma involves one object striking another. One of these objects is the external force or instrument applying the impact, and the other object is the human chest wall. The collision process between these two objects can be studied on two levels: 1. The first level focuses solely on the nature of the forces acting between the two objects, without considering changes in the shape of the objects under these forces. 2. The second level focuses on the internal changes within the objects, especially within the chest wall's internal structures, under the action of external forces. The first level pertains to classical Newtonian mechanics, while the second level relates to the mechanics of materials. Strictly speaking, the latter also falls under Newtonian mechanics.

When conducting the above research, several concepts must be clearly understood: First is external force, which is easy to comprehend. It refers to the force applied to the chest wall by an external injuring object. Second is stress, which can be viewed as a reactive force. It refers to the force generated by the chest wall in response to the external force, resisting it. External force and stress are an equal pair of forces but serve obviously different functions. The external force acts to damage the structure of the chest wall, causing various structural failures; stress, on the other hand, is the force that maintains the structure's original shape. As long as external force and stress remain balanced, the body's structure can avoid destructive changes. However, as the magnitude of the external force increases, the stress also gradually increases. The location where stress acts is within the finer internal structures of the chest wall.

If the internal structures cannot withstand the stress, injury will occur. This shows that, although trauma may appear to be directly caused by external force, this is not entirely true. The external force is merely a surface phenomenon that actually causes the injury is stress. It is the changes in stress that directly lead to the occurrence of damage.

In the study of fracture theory, there are theories related to stress fractures, which can effectively explain the mechanism of their occurrence [1,2]. Besides fractures, these theories are also applicable to injuries of other structures or tissues. This is especially true for chronic injuries, where such theories are even easier to understand.

In addition to stress fractures, there is another type of fracture in clinical practice known as traumatic fractures. These fractures occur more suddenly and rapidly, in contrast to the gradual development of stress fractures. However, if the entire injury process were artificially prolonged, there would be no essential difference between the two. Therefore, the principle of stress is also applicable to traumatic fractures. For the sake of easier explanation and better understanding, some have introduced alternative theories that seem more intuitive and rational. These theories originate from engineering mechanics and are based on three main concepts: 1. Point load, 2. Area load, and 3. Shear force. Whether the chest wall structure becomes damaged depends on two key factors: The magnitude of the external force, primarily the shear force; The load-bearing capacity of the structure itself. The magnitude of the shear force is directly related to the intensity of the external force, while the structural capacity depends on its inherent properties. These properties are evaluated through two indicators: Strength, and Stiffness. To understand strength, another concept must be clarified: strain, which refers to the amount of deformation a material experiences under external force. Within a certain range, stress and strain have a linear relationship. If the applied load continues to increase beyond what the structure can withstand, the material reaches a yield point, entering a non-elastic region. Continued loading will eventually lead to structural collapse. The maximum stress at this stage is called ultimate stress, which defines the structure's strength—its capacity to resist damage. Stiffness, on the other hand, refers to a structure's ability to resist elastic deformation. Strength and stiffness are two critical indicators of a structure's mechanical performance. Among the three main structural components of the chest wall: Bone has the lowest stiffness but the highest strength; Skin has the highest stiffness and moderate strength; Soft tissues have moderate stiffness and the lowest strength. Each structural component is composed of various elements, which differ in their stiffness and hardness. Therefore, their resistance to destruction also varies. When a particular form of destructive force acts on the chest wall, each structure responds according to its own tolerance to damage, leading to various types of injuries. When these injuries collectively manifest, they appear as the different clinical trauma types observed in practice.

2. Trauma Caused by Specific Injuring Factors

(1) Sharp Force Injuries

Sharp injury is one of the most common types of chest wall trauma. The most obvious feature of this injury is the large point load, which produces extremely strong shear force, thus forming the most intense local damage, that is, fracture. Clinically, this injury is called a laceration. When a laceration occurs, since the stress is released in the shortest time, there is almost no damage to the surrounding structures, and the real damage is limited to the wound. If there are no important structures in the wound, this injury will not be too serious. However, if there are important blood vessels or nerves, the consequences of the injury will be very serious [3,4]. However, the injury at this time is an additional injury after the laceration and has little to do with the direct injury.

Another feature of sharp injury is that the soft tissue is obviously damaged, while the bone structure is less damaged. This is the most common injury manifestation, but there are exceptions. If the injury is strong enough, the bones will also be injured, resulting in fractures.

(2) Firearm Injuries

Firearm injuries are a special type of trauma, most commonly seen during wartime and rarely encountered in peacetime. These injuries also involve extremely high point loads, but unlike sharp-force injuries, the wounding object travels at an extremely high speed and carries tremendous energy [4,5]. During the injury process, this energy is fully transferred to the chest wall. The immense energy propels the surrounding tissues along the wound track to move outward, away from the impact point. This movement happens very quickly. Due to the strength and stiffness of the structures involved, they attempt to return to their original shape and position in a short period. However, since the structural displacement has already occurred, damage is inevitable, though it may not be immediately visible to the naked eye. The range of injury from firearm wounds often extends well beyond the visible wound track, which is the most prominent feature of this type of injury.

(3) Blunt Force Injuries Blunt force injuries

Primarily results from strikes or impacts by blunt objects. Strictly speaking, all impact injuries, falls, and crushing injuries fall into this category, and they share a common characteristic: an increase in the area over which the force is applied [6]. Compared to sharp-force injuries, blunt injuries involve a larger contact area, and the resulting shear forces occur around the impacted region. For structures with lower rigidity, such as soft tissues, rupture generally does not occur. However, for more rigid structures, such as bones, fractures are more likely. This is the fundamental cause of many closed chest wall injuries and also the most significant distinction from sharp-force injuries. Nevertheless, in terms of the nature of the applied force, there is no essential difference between the two. The main difference lies in the magnitude of the force. A sharp object with very light force will not cause a laceration, just as a blunt object with extremely high force can cause a laceration not only in rigid bones but also in the skin. This shows that the damage caused by different objects to the chest wall is relative. In most cases, different types of objects may cause different types of injuries. However, if we extend the area of action and prolong the duration of the force, the nature of all injury processes is essentially the same—the only real difference lies in the degree of force applied.

(4) Injuries to Different Chest Wall Structures

The chest wall can be classified into three structural types: 1. Skin, 2. Soft tissues, and 3. Bony structures. In most cases, trauma affects the chest wall from the outside in, forming what is known as an open injury [7]. In other cases, trauma may directly damage internal chest wall structures without visible skin damage; this is referred to as a closed injury. These two types of injuries differ in nature, severity, and mechanism of occurrence.

For any kind of trauma, the causal force first acts on the skin, making it the first structure likely to be injured. However, skin is a special structure with unique strength and stiffness. These two properties make the skin more susceptible to sharp-force injuries, but also give it strong resistance to blunt-force impacts. In contrast, the deeper structures show the opposite characteristics.

For example, the bony structures of the chest wall differ significantly from the skin in terms of strength and stiffness. This means their ability to withstand injurious forces also differs greatly. Sharp objects have a small area of impact, and their damage primarily results from high point loads. Such loads typically do not cause harm to bones, which possess greater strength and stiffness, so in sharp-force injuries, the bones often remain undamaged.

However, in the case of blunt-force injuries, due to the significant differences in how bone and skin tolerate external forces, the damage varies. Within a certain range of force, it is often the bone, rather than the skin, that suffers structural damage first. This is the mechanism behind the formation of closed injuries.

Different structures have different properties, and the mechanisms of injury also differ accordingly. Even within the same type of structure, variations in the internal microstructure can lead to different injury outcomes. For example, although ribs and the sternum are both bones, they differ in many aspects. These differences may be reflected in basic physical characteristics such as location, shape, and size, and even more so in internal composition and structural details. These differences play a decisive role in the injury process.

The sternum is more robust than the ribs, and it is closely connected with surrounding structures such as the costal cartilage, costal arch, and clavicle, which gives it greater strength. In contrast, the ribs are significantly less strong. In addition to these factors, the ribs occupy a much larger area of the chest wall compared to the sternum, which increases the likelihood of injury. These factors explain why rib fractures are clinically much more common than sternal fractures. For each individual bone, the likelihood of injury to different parts also varies. This is influenced by several factors: First, it relates to the shape of the bone. According to theories in engineering mechanics, areas where the cross-section of an object changes abruptly or where the surface is rough or uneven tend to have stress concentration internally. These areas become mechanical weak points and are often the most prone to injury. For example, ribs are not uniformly cylindrical; they have irregular shapes. Their shape changes multiple times along their length, and these transition areas are more susceptible to damage. Second, it is associated with muscle protection. The chest wall contains a large number of muscles, which are part of its soft tissue. On the surface, it may seem that chest wall muscles have little to do with fractures, but that's not the case. Muscles help protect bones by absorbing external forces and also participate in resisting injury. Muscles and bones form an integrated unit, with bones becoming a part of this structural complex. As a result, the injury resistance of the whole unit increases, reducing the likelihood of bone fractures. The main muscles of the chest wall include the pectoralis major, pectoralis minor, serratus anterior, and latissimus dorsi, with the pectoralis major being the most significant. The relationship between the pectoralis major and the chest bones is similar to that between limb muscles and long bones of the limbs. Muscle tension can significantly increase the strength of the muscle-bone complex, thereby enhancing resistance to injury. Third, it depends on adjacent structures. The ribs run from top to bottom, and each rib has different relationships with nearby structures. The first rib lies beneath the clavicle, and its front side is covered by the pectoralis major fibres, making it a very concealed area and thus less likely to fracture. The upper ribs are covered on the back by the scapula and back muscles, serving as a protective shield, making fractures less likely there as well. The bottom two ribs lie deep within the back muscles, which also offer strong protection, so fractures there are relatively rare. This demonstrates that the presence of surrounding structures provides significant protection for bones.

(5) Consequences of Trauma

The result of trauma is structural damage, which can vary in severity. The mildest form of damage is internal and invisible to the naked eye, referred to as microtrauma. When microtrauma accumulates, it may lead to macroscopic damage visible to the eye. Macroscopic injuries come in various forms: extensive surface damage is called a contusion [6]; localized deep tissue injury is a laceration; when both are present, the condition is known as a contused laceration. Although these three types differ in nature, they do not directly reflect the severity of injury; an extensive contusion may be more serious than a minor laceration. For the same anatomical location, a contused laceration may appear more severe, but the most severe form of injury is the complete loss of local structure, known as a defect [7]. This occurs when a traumatic force completely destroys and separates part of the chest wall, resulting in visible structural loss.

Chest wall defects can occur in two main ways: Extreme blunt force, which exceeds the structural tolerance of the chest wall, leading to complete destruction and detachment of tissues; and Penetrating trauma, where all structures in a localized area are removed, even if the force is not maximal, resulting in a similarly severe defect.

Chest wall trauma represents an acute, structural injury to the chest wall and is difficult to compare with other thoracic Surgical conditions in terms of severity. Nevertheless, it often leads to serious consequences, demanding high vigilance and professional intervention by thoracic Surgeons following fundamental Surgical principles [8].

REFERENCES

[1] Robertson, G. A. J., and A. M. Wood. 2017. "Lower Limb Stress Fractures in Sport: Optimising Their Management and Outcome." *World Journal of Orthopedics* 8 (3): 242–255.

[2] Lee, J., and K. B. Fields. 2017. "Sternal Stress Fracture in a Middle-Aged Woman." *BMJ Case Reports* 2017: bcr2016218203.

[3] Greberski, K., P. Bugajski, and S. Rzymski, et al. 2015. "Penetrating Thoracic Injuries: Treatment of Two Patients after Suicide Attempts." *Kardiochirurgia i Torakochirurgia Polska* 12 (1): 62–64.

[4] de Melo, A. S. A., L. B. M. Moreira, F. M. C. Pessoa, et al. 2017. "Tomographic Aspects of Penetrating Thoracic Trauma: Injuries from Firearms and Other Weapons." *Radiologia Brasileira* 50 (6): 372–377.

[5] Kolling, D. B. E., L. Hackenberg, J. H. Rathjen, et al. 2021. "Penetrating Injuries in Germany: Epidemiology, Management, and Outcome Analysis Based on the TraumaRegister DGU®." *Scandinavian Journal of Trauma, Resuscitation and Emergency Medicine* 29: 80.

[6] Dogrul, B. N., I. Kiliccalan, E. S. Asci, et al. 2020. "Blunt Trauma-Related Chest Wall and Pulmonary Injuries: An Overview." *Chinese Journal of Traumatology* 23 (3):

125–138.
[7] Wang, W. L. 2021. "Treatment of Chest Wall Trauma." *Expert in Chest Deformity Surgery*, November 3.
[8] Hamilton, C., L. Barnett, A. Trop, et al. 2017. "Emergency Department Management of Patients with Rib Fracture Based on a Clinical Practice Guideline." *Trauma Surgery & Acute Care Open* 2 (1): e000133.

Chest wall trauma is a complex form of injury that can affect all the structures of the chest wall. Among these, the ribs are the most susceptible to damage [1]. This is closely related to the inherent characteristics and distribution pattern of the ribs. Rib fractures can occur as isolated injuries or as part of other types of chest wall trauma. Since many trauma-related issues involve the management of rib fractures, it is necessary to address them separately.

1. General Overview

Rib fracture is one of the most important topics in the study of chest trauma within traditional thoracic Surgery. Surgical treatment for rib fractures began relatively early and has matured over time. Due to the simplicity of the Surgical procedure and its relatively low risk, many primary-level healthcare facilities are capable of performing such operations. Given the urgency of treating chest trauma, most cases require prompt, local intervention. As a result, many patients receive initial care at local facilities, with fewer being transferred to large hospitals. In recent years, as thoracoscopic Surgery has become more widely adopted, many large hospitals have shifted their focus to intrathoracic procedures, placing less emphasis on chest wall Surgery. Consequently, the number of rib fracture Surgeries performed in large hospitals has further decreased. This lack of involvement from major hospitals has led to a shortage of research on rib fractures, which has negatively impacted academic progress in this field. Research on rib fractures has seen limited advancement in recent years. Some believe that the treatment of rib fractures has reached its limit, suggesting that further breakthroughs are unlikely. However, this view reflects a developmental bottleneck. All forms of progress are relative: rapid advancement often occurs before a bottleneck is encountered, after which progress slows. Nevertheless, this does not signify stagnation but rather a period of energy accumulation.

Once this energy reaches a critical point, the bottleneck may be broken, leading to new advancements. Current Bottlenecks in Rib Fracture Research At present, research into rib fractures faces several major bottlenecks, which can be summarized as follows:① Rigid Mindsets: Rib fractures have long been considered one of the most traditional forms of chest trauma in thoracic Surgery, with clinical practices established for many years. Because rib fractures are typically regarded as simple bone injuries, they have not received adequate attention. This lack of focus has allowed outdated concepts to dominate the field unchecked. ② Outdated Surgical Methods: As a typical type

of tubular bone, the Surgical approach to rib fractures primarily involves fixation. To date, there are essentially three traditional fixation methods used in clinical practice [2,3]: Intramedullary Fixation: Insertion of a fixation device into the medullary cavity of the rib. Encircling External Fixation: This involves the use of a special fixation plate that wraps around the rib. Clinically, two main materials are used: shape-memory alloys and titanium alloys. Plate-and-Screw External Fixation: This method is modelled after conventional bone fixation techniques, where a fixation plate is placed across the fracture site and secured with screws. Currently, these three traditional methods remain the standard in rib fracture Surgery, and no new fixation techniques have been designed or invented. Lack of Innovation in Surgical Access: Traditionally, all rib fracture fixation Surgeries have been performed through open procedures, which involve direct visual access to the fracture site. This conventional approach lacks novelty and does not incorporate advancements in minimally invasive techniques. Current Bottlenecks in Rib Fracture Research (Part II) ③ The Surgical approach lacks innovation. Traditional rib fracture fixation Surgeries have all employed open fixation, performed under direct vision as open procedures. In recent years, influenced by thoracoscopic Surgery, some have gradually attempted to fix rib
fractures under thoracoscopy [4,5]. Although such procedures can be technically completed, their actual significance remains in question. On the surface, thoracoscopic Surgeries may appear innovative, but in reality, they are more likely seen as trend-following and deviate from the fundamental principles of chest wall Surgery. ④ There has been no breakthrough in Surgical materials. Fracture fixation requires fixation materials, which are essential for completing the procedure. Over the years, various materials have been developed and applied clinically, but currently only a few are in regular use. While these materials are improvements over previous generations, they still have deficiencies and require further development. Unfortunately, current research and development efforts are clearly lagging, and some obvious flaws remain unresolved.

Rib fractures, by nature, fall within the domain of orthopaedics. Although thoracic Surgery has made significant advances, its focus is not on fracture research, so the existing problems in rib fracture research are understandable. One key aspect of chest wall Surgery is its orthopaedics component. Given this intrinsic orthopaedics nature, studying rib fractures offers clear advantages, providing both conceptual and technical support for future work.

2. Mechanism of Injury

Rib fractures can result from various causes, with the most common being external trauma such as falls, collisions, or blunt force impacts. From a mechanistic perspective, the occurrence of a rib fracture primarily depends on two key factors: The magnitude of the external force This refers to the intensity and direction of the traumatic impact applied to the chest wall. The rib's inherent load-bearing capacity

This includes the structural strength and flexibility of the rib, which can vary based on age, health condition, and anatomical characteristics. When the external force significantly exceeds the rib's natural ability to withstand it, a fracture occurs. Thus, rib fractures are the result of a mismatch between the destructive force applied and the rib's mechanical resilience. Mechanism of Injury: The magnitude of external destructive force depends on the specific type of trauma involved. However, this force is often a vague concept in practice, making it difficult to quantify solely by its absolute value. While external force is the primary determinant of whether a rib fracture will occur, the actual occurrence of a fracture also hinges significantly on the rib's intrinsic load-bearing capacity. Under normal circumstances, ribs possess a certain degree of strength and stiffness, providing them with considerable resistance against external impact. This is one of the reasons the thoracic cage serves as an effective protective structure for vital organs. However, because the human body contains multiple ribs each differing in location, size, and shape. The capacity to resist damage also varies among them. Some ribs or specific segments are more prone to fractures, while others rarely break, indicating that different ribs and different parts of the same rib have varied resistance to external trauma. In addition to anatomical differences, several clinical risk factors contribute to an increased likelihood of rib fractures. These include: ① Osteoporosis A condition characterized by changes in the internal structure of the rib, commonly seen in elderly individuals or those with certain underlying diseases. Weakened bone structure leads to reduced strength and stiffness, making the ribs more susceptible to fracture. ② Thin or slender ribs Normal ribs are not perfectly tubular but rather curved and irregular in shape. However, there is a general expectation of thickness or robustness. When, due to various reasons, the ribs become thinner either overall or in specific segments, their resistance to destructive force diminishes, making fractures more likely. ③ Deformities Structures with uniform shape and composition typically have even distribution of strength and stiffness, which helps prevent fractures. When deformities are present, local changes in physical properties can create weak points that are more vulnerable to injury. ④ Localized pathological changes Healthy ribs typically offer strong resistance to external damage. If a section of a rib is affected by disease, its mechanical properties are compromised, increasing the likelihood of fractures. In clinical practice, pathological fractures often occur from minimal trauma due to such weakened areas. In summary, rib fracture risk is influenced not only by the intensity and type of trauma but also by the biological and structural condition of the ribs themselves. This indicates that the rib structure itself has been severely damaged and cannot withstand the impact of external forces.

Rib fractures can exist independently, but because the chest wall structure is an organic whole and is closely connected with the thoracic cavity and surrounding organs, rib fractures are often combined with injuries to other structures [1,6,7]. The most common is the injury inside the chest cavity, which may include contusion, laceration, and laceration of the lungs, as well as damage to the heart and large blood vessels. The presence of combined injuries makes the clinical manifestations of rib fractures extremely complicated.

3.Clinical Manifestations

The main symptom of a simple rib fracture is localized pain, which may worsen during breathing, coughing, or movement. Due to the pain, patients might exhibit respiratory symptoms, such as shallow or laboured breathing. If the fracture is accompanied by lung injury, the respiratory symptoms will be more pronounced, potentially including shortness of breath, wheezing, or respiratory distress. In cases where the injury is associated with severe damage to the heart or major blood vessels, circulatory symptoms may also appear, such as hypotension, rapid heart rate, or signs of shock. When multiple ribs are fractured in multiple locations, it may result in a flail chest, a condition where a segment of the chest wall moves abnormally (paradoxical respiration) during breathing. This can significantly impair respiratory function and lead to symptoms of hypoxia such as cyanosis, restlessness, or confusion [1,6–8].

The main signs of rib fractures include local tenderness, palpable fracture ends, palpable separation of fracture ends when compressed, increased pain, floating of the chest wall and abnormal breathing in multiple fractures. If it is an open injury, various specific injuries of the wound can be seen.

4. Examination

Physical examination can roughly determine the location and extent of rib fractures. For further examination, X-ray examination can be the first choice [1]. Although X-ray examination is not accurate, it can show rib fractures in certain parts more clearly and has high value. CT examination can be considered when necessary. CT examination has a good exposure to fractures, but it is only effective for local areas and it is difficult to show the structure of the entire rib. Its biggest advantage is that it can show the damage to surrounding organs well [1,6]. The most advanced examination method at present is three-dimensional reconstruction examination. This examination can not only reveal the details of the fracture, but also reveal all information related to the operation. Its biggest disadvantage is that it is slow, the process is cumbersome, and it is difficult to obtain results immediately. For patients who need emergency Surgery, this examination is not very meaningful. In recent years, ultrasound examination has been paid attention to and can obtain better fracture information and has certain value (Figure 5-3-1).

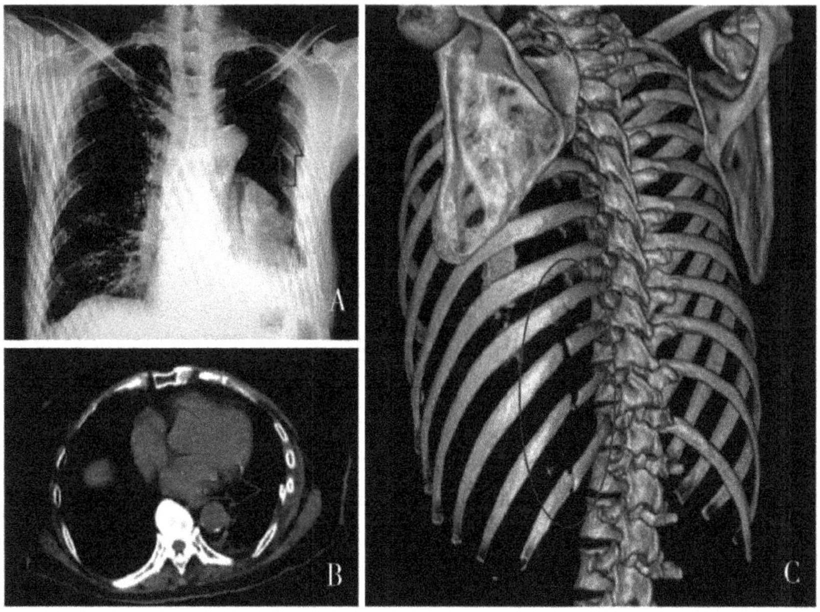

Figure 5-3-1 Imaging examination of rib fracture (A. X-ray image, which can show the fracture ends and their relationship with the entire thorax, making it easier to determine the location of the fractured rib, but sometimes the display is unclear; B. CT examination,which can show the local fracture and the damage in the thoracic cavity, but it is difficult to show the overall location of the rib; C. Three-dimensional reconstruction, which can clearly show the detailed information of the rib fracture)

5.Diagnosis

Rib fractures generally have a clear history of trauma, and the symptoms and signs are also relatively clear. If combined with imaging findings, diagnosis is not difficult. However, considering that rib fractures are often combined with other trauma, the following should be noted when diagnosing them: ① Clarify the location and number of fractures. The location and number directly determine the choice of treatment method and the specific operation details, and must be clarified before Surgery. Focus on clarifying two situations, namely single fracture in a single place and multiple fractures in multiple places. The former sometimes does not require Surgical treatment, while the latter involves the problem of floating chest wall, and the treatment principles are different from those of general fractures (Figure 5-3-2). ② Whether there is damage to other structures of the chest wall. The ribs are located in the chest wall and are closely integrated with other structures of the chest wall. If trauma can cause rib fractures, it is very likely to cause damage to other structures of the chest wall at the same time, so it needs to be clarified. Other structures that may be damaged include soft tissue, sternum, and costal cartilage. Soft tissue damage is not easy to find, and unless it is an open injury, it is difficult to determine whether such tissue is damaged. In trauma involving rib fractures, soft tissue damage is usually not very serious. If it is an open injury, it needs to be taken seriously. Injury to the sternum and costal cartilage often occurs with rib fractures. Since it involves issues of Surgical materials and Surgical methods, it is necessary to clarify before Surgery. ③ Whether there is any combined damage to the internal organs in the chest cavity. The chest wall structure is located on the outside of the chest cavity. Once such a structure is damaged, the internal organs in the chest cavity will not be spared. Therefore, rib fractures are often combined with damage to the internal structures of the chest cavity. Even if there is no damage to specific organs, it may be due to hemothorax, pneumoperitoneum, etc.

The appearance of chest trauma may affect the function of thoracic organs. Therefore, when diagnosing rib fractures, it is essential to assess the condition of the thoracic cavity simultaneously. If abnormalities are found, they must be addressed concurrently.④Presence of injuries in other parts of the body: Traumatic injuries are often complex. While they may be localized to the chest wall, more commonly, they involve multiple areas of the body. In the overall assessment of trauma, a rib fracture might be a minor issue compared to potentially life-threatening injuries elsewhere. If vital organs in other body regions are affected, those injuries must take priority over rib fractures. Hence, upon discovering a rib fracture, a comprehensive examination of the entire body is necessary to determine the best treatment approach.⑤Presence of functional impairment of vital organs: Rib fractures may be accompanied by damage to critical organ functions. Such injuries can be life-threatening and must be identified and managed promptly.

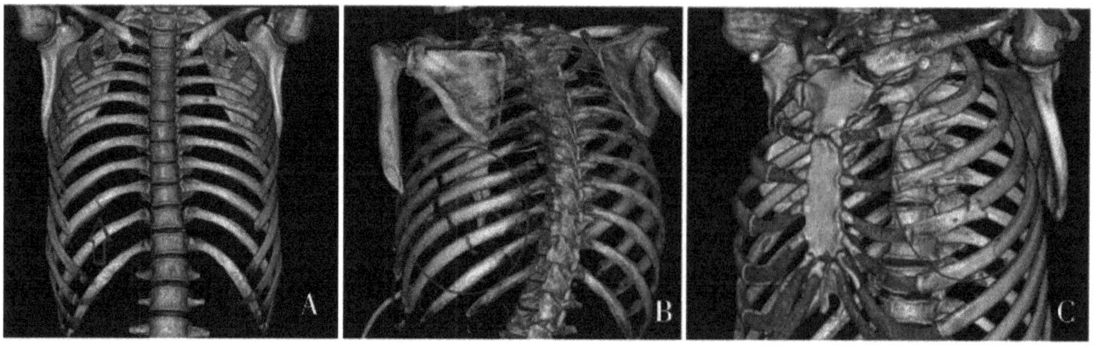

Figure 5-3-2 Location and number of rib fractures (A. Single rib fracture; B. Multiple rib fractures; C. Multiple rib fractures)

The harm caused by rib fractures themselves can range from mild to severe. However, because they may involve injuries to other areas, the specific situation is often very complex. Therefore, when diagnosing rib fractures, a comprehensive and macroscopic assessment and observation are necessary to enable scientific and appropriate treatment.

The main differential diagnosis for rib fractures is pathological fractures. Essentially, pathological fractures are also fractures and are not fundamentally different from traumatic fractures. However, the fractures discussed in this chapter pertain to chest wall trauma caused by injurious forces, which are clearly distinct from pathological fractures. The root cause of pathological fractures lies in primary diseases of the bone itself. Since the nature of these primary diseases differs from trauma, they fall under the category of other chest wall diseases. The primary diseases causing pathological fractures can include tumors or conditions such as osteomyelitis. These diseases typically have a long course, and fractures can occur without a clear traumatic cause. The fracture site may present with specific signs, and imaging examinations often reveal obvious lesions. In contrast, ordinary traumatic rib fractures do not show such clear pathological lesions.

6.Surgical Treatment

(1) Indications and Timing for Surgery

After the diagnosis of rib fracture, the next issue is treatment. There are two basic treatment methods [8]: one is conservative treatment. The second treatment method is Surgical fixation. Conservative treatment mainly involves symptomatic relief, with a particular focus on preventing complications. Some people use specially designed chest bands or adhesive tape for external fixation to promote fracture healing. These methods are relatively effective for mild rib fractures, but severe rib fractures are not suitable for conservative treatment. Surgical treatment of rib fractures primarily involves open reduction and internal fixation. However, there has long been controversy regarding the necessity of Surgery. In earlier times, fracture management was more conservative, and many experts were opposed to Surgery, especially for single, isolated rib fractures, for which conservative treatment was commonly recommended. With the development of various fixation materials, Surgery has gradually become the mainstream treatment. Regarding the choice of treatment method, some guidelines and expert consensus lists numerous detailed criteria. However, these items have limited practical significance. The most important principle is this: Except for simple rib fractures without obvious displacement of the fracture ends, all other types of rib fractures have indications for Surgery. The indications for Surgery are actually not complicated as long as conditions permit, Surgical intervention should be actively pursued. Currently, another controversial issue is the timing of Surgery [9], and there are also divergent views on this topic. The essence of this issue lies in the safety and effectiveness of the Surgery. For any type of trauma, early Surgery is certainly the best option. However, safety is the prerequisite for Surgery. If safety cannot be ensured, Surgery should not be performed prematurely.

Surgical treatment for simple rib fractures is straightforward and does not pose significant safety risks. However, since rib fractures are often accompanied by functional damage to other vital organs, the function of these vital organs must be prioritized when considering Surgery. If conditions permit, Surgery should naturally be performed as early as possible. If conditions do not allow, then a careful and scientific weighing of pros and cons is necessary. An important issue related to Surgical timing is the question of Surgery after the acute phase. If callus formation has already occurred at the fracture site especially if the area has stabilized and no longer moves with respiration or general activity then Surgery is no longer necessary.

(2) Surgical Principles

The basic principles of rib fracture Surgery are as follows: ① Secure fixation of the fractured ends; ② Restoration of rib continuity; ③ Correction of deformities; ④ Active management of associated injuries; ⑤ Prevention of complications.

The ultimate goal of rib fracture Surgery is the firm fixation of the fracture ends. However, this fixation must be strong and stable; if it fails to achieve that, the Surgery loses its value. Key considerations during Surgical fixation include: 1. Stability alone is not enough: In addition to secure fixation, the fracture ends must be well aligned to ensure proper healing and the restoration of rib continuity. 2. Avoid deformity: Fixation must follow the natural curvature of the rib. Any angulation or displacement can lead to malunion, which may deform the thoracic cage postoperatively. 3. Address associated injuries: Rib fractures are often accompanied by soft tissue, pleural, or organ damage. These must be properly managed during Surgery to avoid compromising the outcome or leading to further complications. 4. Prevent Surgical complications: Common issues include hemothorax or pneumothorax due to vascular damage during the procedure. These must be anticipated and managed effectively during the operation. In summary, solid fixation, anatomical alignment, comprehensive injury management, and complication control are the critical Surgical principles for optimal recovery and function after rib fracture Surgery.

(3) Surgical method

There are two basic approaches to rib fracture Surgery. The traditional approach is direct incision and fixation. In recent years, some people have begun to use thoracoscopy to assist in the fixation of rib fractures in the thoracic cavity [4,5,8]. Thoracoscopic Surgery has certain advantages, but not all

Rib fractures at these locations are all suitable for this technique. In most cases, direct open reduction and fixation remains the preferred Surgical method.

When performing open reduction and fixation Surgery, the primary consideration is the choice of incision. The fundamental principle is the "proximity principle," meaning the incision should be as close to the fracture site as possible. The closer the incision is to the fracture, the better the exposure and the easier the operation, allowing the incision to be made smaller. However, because there are important structures on the surface of the chest wall such as the breast and scapula, applying the proximity principle can sometimes be challenging. To successfully complete the Surgery, it is necessary to avoid these structures while still getting as close to the fracture site as possible to ensure adequate exposure and manoeuvrability. Besides important structures, another factor to consider is the cosmetic outcome of the chest wall Surgery. The essence of cosmetic concerns lies in the external shape of the chest wall. If the incision is made in a highly visible area, such as the upper anterior chest wall, the postoperative scar may affect appearance, so such locations should be avoided when possible. Instead, incisions should be placed in more concealed areas, while still respecting the proximity principle. The second principle in choosing the incision is to avoid important anatomical structures. The presence of the breast and scapula can obstruct exposure of certain fractures, so these structures should be avoided to prevent damage. Among the many structures of the chest wall, muscles are particularly important. Although muscles can be sutured after being cut, cutting muscle increases the risk of complications. Therefore, incisions should also avoid transecting major muscles whenever possible. For example, when the fracture is near the upper anterior chest wall close to the clavicular midline, a direct incision in this area might cut through the pectoralis major and minor muscles. Avoiding such muscles when possible is important. The third principle is to choose the smallest possible incision. This is a fundamental requirement in chest wall Surgery with plastic Surgery considerations. Unlike general thoracic Surgery, chest wall Surgery has an added emphasis on cosmetic results. Any Surgical approach must consider aesthetics, which depend on two factors: the overall shape of the chest wall and the postoperative scar. The incision directly affects the scar; thus, careful planning is required to achieve a good cosmetic outcome. Many factors influence scarring, with scar size being one of the most important. To obtain the best possible cosmetic result, the length of the incision should be minimized. This is a basic requirement for Surgical incisions.

After the incision is made, the next steps include exposing and fixing the fracture site. The exposure of the fracture can be achieved using different techniques. Fixation of the fracture requires specialized materials, and the specific procedures vary depending on the materials used. During the Surgery, the appropriate steps should be carried out according to the requirements of the chosen fixation materials (Figure 5-3-3). The fixation procedure for rib fractures itself is not technically very difficult; the key lies in managing certain special situations. These situations include: 1. Management of combined fractures involving the costal cartilage and sternum; 2. Management of associated injuries to intrathoracic organs; 3. Management of injuries located in distant areas outside the chest.

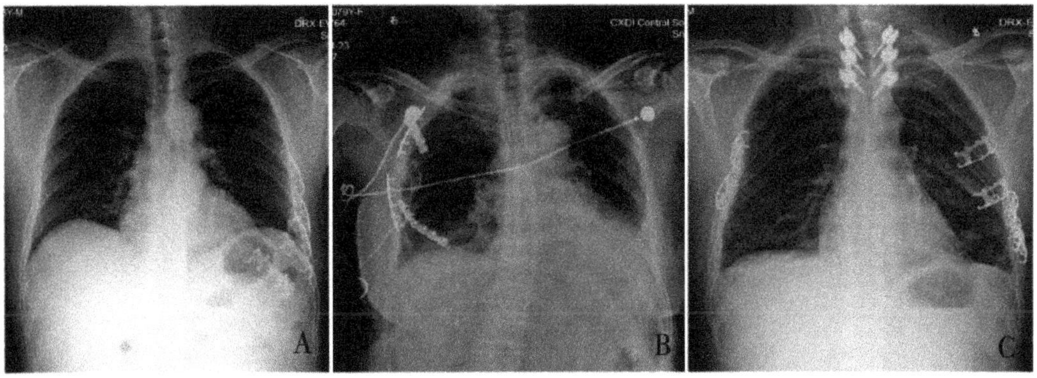

Figure 5-3-3 Fixation of rib fractures using different materials (A. Fixation of ribs using an embracing fixation plate; B. Fixation of ribs using MatrixRIB; C. Fixation of ribs using a memory alloy plate)

These special considerations must be addressed during Surgery, as their management directly affects the final Surgical outcome. The most challenging aspect of treating rib fractures is managing multiple fractures across several ribs, known as flail chest. Due to the complexity involved, this topic will be discussed in a separate chapter.

(4) Surgical complications

Rib fracture fixation Surgery itself is a Surgical operation, so some complications may occur. Complications include some common thoracic Surgery complications, such as pneumothorax, pleural effusion, etc., and may also include some special complications, such as fixation failure, etc. This is not only related to the Surgical technique, but also to the choice of materials. In addition, the patient's own factors are also one of the reasons for the failure of the operation. The patient's own factors may include the following aspects: ① Rib variation, local too thin, the material cannot be tightly fixed during fixation. Since the force cannot be fully applied, the fixation effect will inevitably be affected. ② The ribs are too fragile. Older patients may have osteoporosis, the ribs are soft, and the fixation cannot be too strong, which will also affect the fixation effect. ③ Improper movement of the patient in the early postoperative period affects the fit between the fixation plate and the rib fracture ends. These factors can have an adverse effect on the fixation effect and lead to Surgical failure.

Once the complications of rib fixation Surgery occur, they may cause great pain to the patient, so they must be properly handled. The general method used is re-fixation. However, if the ribs are severely injured and cannot be properly fixed, the most desperate measure is to reconstruct the bony structure of the chest wall. In essence, the essence of reconstruction is also fixation, but it is the fixation of the reconstruction material rather

than the fixation material. reconstruction has a wider scope and is a measure taken for extremely serious rib fractures.

7. Prognosis

Surgery for simple rib fractures is simple, and generally satisfactory results can be achieved after proper fixation. The most obvious sign is that the pain is reduced or disappears, local signs no longer exist, and other systemic symptoms are also significantly improved. Patients can get out of bed and resume normal work as soon as possible. This is the real meaning of Surgery. Multiple rib fractures are often more serious. In addition to the lesions of the ribs themselves, they are often combined with injuries to other structures. When implementing treatment, if you can start from the overall situation and make a systematic assessment and treatment of the trauma, you will also get good results. If it is not handled properly, it will affect the treatment effect, and unexpected complications or sequelae may even occur in the end.

Rib fractures are considered to be a relatively old type of trauma in traditional thoracic Surgery, and today's thoracic Surgeons rarely pay attention to it. Without attention, it is difficult to make new progress. However, small progress does not mean that there is no need for progress. In fact, there are still many issues surrounding rib fractures that need to be studied in depth, which is exactly what chest wall Surgery needs to do next.

REFERENCES

[1] Dogrul, B. N., I. Kiliccalan, E. S. Asci, et al. 2020. "Blunt Trauma-Related Chest Wall and Pulmonary Injuries: An Overview." *Chinese Journal of Traumatology* 23 (3): 125–138.

[2] Fokin, A. A., N. Hus, and J. Wycech, et al. 2020. "Surgical Stabilization of Rib Fractures: Indications, Techniques, and Pitfalls." *JBJS Essential Surgical Techniques* 10 (2): e0032.

[3] Zhang, Q., L. Song, S. Ning, et al. 2019. "Recent Advances in Rib Fracture Fixation." *Journal of Thoracic Disease* 11 (Suppl 8): S1070–S1077.

[4] Pieracci, F. M. 2019. "Completely Thoracoscopic Surgical Stabilization of Rib Fractures: Can It Be Done and Is It Worth It?" *Journal of Thoracic Disease* 11 (Suppl 8): S1061–S1069.

[5] Bauman, Z. M., R. Beard, and S. Cemaj. 2021. "When Less Is More: A Minimally Invasive, Intrathoracic Approach to Surgical Stabilization of Rib Fractures." *Trauma Case Reports* 32: 100452.

[6] Caragounis, E. C., Y. Xiao, and H. Granhed. 2021. "Mechanism of Injury, Injury Patterns, and Associated Injuries in Patients Operated for Chest Wall Trauma." *European Journal of Trauma and Emergency Surgery* 47 (4): 929–938.

[7] Kent, R., W. Woods, and O. Bostrom. 2008. "Fatality Risk and the Presence of Rib Fractures." *Annals of Advances in Automotive Medicine* 52: 73–84.

[8] He, Z., D. Zhang, H. Xiao, et al. 2019. "The Ideal Methods for the Management of Rib Fractures." *Journal of Thoracic Disease* 11 (Suppl 8): S1078–S1089.

[9] Prins, J. T. H., M. M. E. Wijffels, and F. M. Pieracci. 2021. "What Is the Optimal Timing to Perform Surgical Stabilization of Rib Fractures?" *Journal of Thoracic Disease* 13 (Suppl 1): S13–S25.

COSTAL CARTILAGE FRACTURES

Costal cartilage is an important component of the thorax and a type of bony structure of the chest wall. It may also fracture when subjected to external destructive forces. However, costal cartilage fractures are different from rib fractures and sternum fractures. Their diagnosis and treatment have their own characteristics, so they need to be discussed separately.

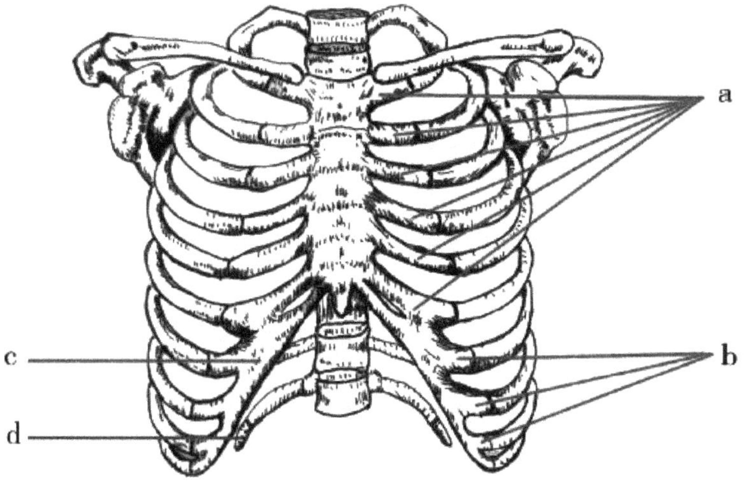

Figure 5-4-1: Classification of Costal Cartilage (a. Type A; b. Type B; c. Type C; d. Type D)

1.Structural characteristics of costal cartilage

Coastal cartilage is less popular, and because of this, few people really understand it. Most people imagine costal cartilage as the part where the ribs connect to the sternum. In fact, this view is not comprehensive. Costal cartilage in this form is just one form, not all costal cartilage. This form mainly exists at the connection

between the 1 - 6 ribs and the sternum. The connection between the other ribs and the sternum is not completed directly through the costal cartilage, but through another structure, which is the costal arch. The costal arch is the part in front of the 7-10 costal cartilage.

The parts connected to the ribs are independent of each other and fused at the front ends. The costal cartilages in these parts are not costal cartilages of standard shape, and strictly speaking, they are not costal arches, but should be part of the costal arches. In the section on costal arch deformities, the definition of the costal arch is described in detail. The coastal arch here is actually a narrow sense of the coastal arch. The 1 - 10 ribs have costal cartilages that are directly or indirectly connected to the sternum. The 11,12 ribs are floating ribs. Their front ends are not connected to the sternum, but they also have costal cartilages. However, the front ends of these costal cartilages are free and located in the tissues of the waist and back, and are not related to the sternum. It can be seen that there are four basic forms of costal cartilage (Figure 5-4-1): Type A, independent costal cartilage; Type B, partially independent costal cartilage; Type C, costal arch; Type D, costal cartilage free in the muscles of the waist and back. Because of the different forms of costal cartilage, the forms of lesions are also very different.

The posterior end of the costal cartilage is directly connected to the rib, with no joint present. The first costal cartilage forms a joint with the manubrium of the sternum, but it is immobile and is referred to as a synarthrosis. The 2-6 costal cartilages form amphiarthroses with the costal notches of the sternum, known as sternocostal joints. The 7 -10 costal cartilages are directly connected to the sternum, without forming joints.

The internal structure of the costal cartilage is different from that of the ribs and sternum, and this structural difference determines its distinct physical properties. Due to these differing physical characteristics, the ability to withstand external forces also varies. As a result, fractures in costal cartilage present different features compared to those in ribs or the sternum.

2. Mechanism of Costal Cartilage Fracture

Costal cartilage fracture is a relatively common type of fracture and often occurs together with rib or sternum fractures. Isolated costal cartilage fractures are less frequently seen [1,2]. The cause of costal cartilage fracture lies in the application of external force. When an external force acts on the costal cartilage either directly or indirectly and reaches a certain threshold, a fracture may occur. Compared to the ribs and sternum, costal cartilage possesses greater flexibility. In mechanical terms, this means it has higher elasticity or lower stiffness, making such structures generally less prone to fracture. However, when the external force reaches a sufficiently high intensity, a costal cartilage fracture becomes unavoidable, and such injuries can indeed occur.

The common sites of costal cartilage fractures generally correspond to the common sites of rib fractures, namely the costal cartilages connected to the 3-7 ribs. The costal arch has a broad range and is longer than the typical costal cartilages. Theoretically, this area should be more prone to fractures; however, in reality, such fractures are relatively rare. The main reason lies in its unique position and structure. The costal arch itself is highly elastic, with a free middle portion that lacks rigid structural constraints, which increases its range of motion. Greater mobility means better elasticity and cushioning ability. When subjected to external forces, it provides better cushioning, which allows local stress to be effectively released. Therefore, structural fractures are less likely to occur. of course, the external forces referred to here mainly mean those in blunt injuries. If the trauma is caused by a sharp object and directly affects the costal arch, the cushioning effect will have little significance. The sharp object can directly injure the costal arch, causing it to be severed and resulting in an actual fracture.

Isolated costal cartilage fractures are uncommon, which is related to the special position and characteristics of the costal cartilage itself. The 1-6 costal cartilages are located precisely between the ribs and the sternum. Although ribs are long tubular bony structures, they possess good overall elasticity and can provide some cushioning against external forces. One end of the costal cartilage is connected to the sternum, which itself has limited elasticity, but this does not affect the elasticity at the other end where it connects to the ribs. Because of this special positional characteristic, the costal cartilage receives good cushioning when subjected to external force. This cushioning results in a relatively low incidence of costal cartilage fractures. However, similar to the costal arch, when the costal cartilage is locally injured by a sharp object, the situation is completely different; the sharp object can directly injure the costal cartilage and cause a fracture.

Typical costal cartilage fractures can only occur in the middle of the costal cartilage, where both ends of the fracture are costal cartilage. However, fractures commonly seen in clinical practice are not like this; they occur at the junctions between the costal cartilage and other structures, such as the connection between the costal cartilage and the rib or between the costal cartilage and the sternum. According to reference [3,4], these fractures are theoretically not typical costal cartilage fractures, nor can they be classified as rib fractures or sternum fractures. But for convenience of description, we consider them as costal cartilage fractures. According to principles of material mechanics, these two sites are the most prone to fractures, mainly because the physical properties of costal cartilage differ from those of ribs and sternum. Fractures at these two sites differ from typical costal cartilage fractures and require special techniques for treatment.

3.Hazards

After an isolated costal cartilage fracture, the degree of harm depends on several factors. If the fracture is confined to the anterior chest wall specifically the 1-7 costal cartilages and there are no obvious complications, the risk is generally low. Due to the stabilizing presence of the superior and inferior ribs as well as the sternum, costal cartilage fractures typically do not result in displacement of the fracture ends and therefore do not lead to serious consequences. However, if multiple coastal cartilage fractures occur without accompanying rib fractures, the main risk arises from complications [4]. One such complication may be injury to surrounding blood vessels, particularly the internal thoracic artery, which is a major nearby vessel. If this artery is damaged, it can lead to severe haemorrhage. Even in these cases, the fractures generally do not involve major dislocation. Non-displaced costal cartilage fractures tend to pose less danger. But if displacement occurs, it may lead to serious outcomes [3]. When the fracture results from open trauma, there may be additional damage to adjacent structures, increasing the overall severity. In most cases, costal cartilage fractures are accompanied by fractures of surrounding structures, complicating the situation and requiring special attention.

Fractures of the 8-10 costal cartilages or costal arch are less common. Since there are fewer vital structures in that region of the chest wall, such injuries usually do not pose a major threat. However, because this area provides greater buffering capacity, a fracture here indicates that the patient has been subjected to significant external force. Such force may also injure other nearby structures, particularly upper abdominal organs like the liver or spleen. If these organs are damaged, the consequences can be very serious.

4. Clinical Manifestations

After a costal cartilage fracture occurs, the main symptom is pain, which can worsen with breathing movements or coughing. There is localized tenderness at the fracture site, and palpation may reveal the fracture ends. In cases of multiple costal cartilage fractures, localized chest wall flail motion may be observed, although the area generally does not soften. True flail chest and paradoxical breathing typically occur only when accompanied by rib fractures [3]. Lower costal cartilage fractures may be associated with costal arch fractures, in which case the detached costal arch may be palpated, with obvious fracture ends and significant mobility. Closed costal cartilage fractures may be accompanied by injuries to other structures, while open fractures can be localized or involve a wider range of damage

.

5. Examination

The basic method for diagnosing costal cartilage fractures is physical examination. However, if more detailed information is needed, imaging studies are required. Since cartilage tissue is not visible on X-ray, X-rays cannot detect costal cartilage fractures. Ultrasound has a certain value, but its ability to visualize costal cartilage fractures is limited [5]. CT (Computed Tomography) scans can clearly show the fracture site and surrounding details, making it a relatively practical diagnostic tool. The best method is 3D reconstruction imaging, which not only shows signs of costal cartilage fracture but also provides a detailed view of the chest wall and the entire thoracic area. This makes it a very valuable examination, although it does have its own limitations.

6. Diagnosis

Diagnosing a costal cartilage fracture is not difficult. Based on the mechanism of injury, main clinical symptoms, and examination results, a diagnosis can be easily made. However, to provide valuable guidance for treatment, three key issues must be clarified: ① Whether it is a simple costal cartilage fracture: Since such fractures are often accompanied by fractures of other bony structures, it is essential to rule out the possibility of other fractures before confirming the diagnosis of costal cartilage fracture. ② Injury status of the ribs and sternum: If the costal cartilage fracture is combined with rib and sternum fractures, the exact nature of these fractures must be diagnosed, as it directly affects the Surgical strategy. ③ Presence of combined injuries in other areas: If there are additional injuries beyond the costal cartilage, such as to thoracic organs, abdominal organs, or nearby structures like the scapula, clavicle, or thoracic vertebrae, they must also be diagnosed. These injuries similarly impact Surgical planning and must be clearly identified.

7. Surgery

(1) Surgery indication

Single-site costal cartilage fractures, if uncomplicated, can generally be treated conservatively. However, when there is severe local injury, significant complications, or associated damage to nearby structures, Surgical treatment becomes necessary. Indications for Surgical treatment of costal cartilage fractures include the following: ① Multiple costal cartilage fractures: Even in the absence of complications, such fractures compromise the stability of the thoracic cage and affect its function. Surgery is required to restore thoracic stability. ② Costal cartilage fractures combined with rib or sternum fractures: This represents multiple fractures involving bony structures, which can lead to an unstable chest wall or flail chest. Surgical stabilization is essential. ③ Fractures involving the costal arch: These are serious fractures that significantly impact the lower part of the thoracic cage, causing major functional impairment and severe pain. Surgery is necessary to restore structure and relieve symptoms. ④ Costal cartilage fractures with intrathoracic organ injury: Damage to internal thoracic organs often requires emergency Surgery. In such cases, the associated cartilage fractures should be repaired during the same Surgical procedure. ⑤ Costal cartilage fractures resulting from open trauma: Open injuries are always Surgical emergencies. If costal cartilage fractures are present, Surgical treatment is unavoidable. ⑥ Comminated costal cartilage fractures: These involve the cartilage breaking into multiple pieces. Even if thoracic stability is not significantly affected, the fragmented cartilage poses a risk and must be Surgically removed or fixed.⑦ Costal cartilage fractures with major vascular injury: Vascular damage leads to bleeding. If bleeding is severe, Surgery must be performed promptly to control haemorrhage and repair the fracture.

(2) Surgery

There are many methods for fixing costal cartilage fractures, which can generally be classified into three types: ① Direct suture fixation. ② Fixation using encircling plates. ③Fixation using the matrix RIB system [1,4]. Direct suture fixation typically involves using sutures to stitch together the two fractured ends of the costal cartilage.

The method is relatively simple but offers poor fixation results. When suturing a single site of costal cartilage fracture, the outcome is generally satisfactory. However, if suturing is applied to multiple sites or multiple costal cartilages, the fixation effect may not be ideal. The encircling fixation plate is a type of material originally designed for rib fracture fixation, which requires compression on the rib for effective stabilization. When this material is used for costal cartilage fixation, excessive compression may crush the cartilage, so the pressure must be moderate, and the fixation cannot be extremely firm. Matrix RIB is also a material used for rib fixation. The standard method involves inserting screws into the ribs on both sides of the fracture. However, the cartilaginous structure of the costal cartilage is fragile, and inserting screws can easily shatter it, leading to fixation failure. In conclusion, each of the three fixation methods has its own characteristics and specific requirements for the fixation site. Therefore, appropriate techniques must be carefully applied based on the actual clinical situation.

For the convenience of Surgical operation, we divide costal cartilage fractures into five basic forms (Figure 5-4-2): Type I, fracture at the sternocostal joint; Type II, fracture in the middle of the costal cartilage; Type III, fracture at the junction of the rib and costal cartilage; Type IV, fracture at the junction of the costal cartilage and the costal arch; Type V, fracture of the costal arch. The five forms of fractures are obviously different, and the specific fixation methods are also different.

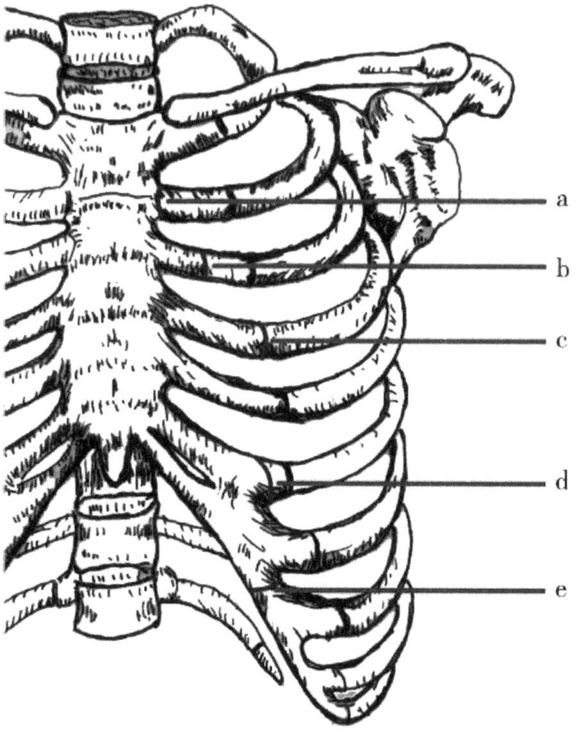

Figure 5-4-1: Classification of Costal Cartilage (a. Type A; b. Type B; c. Type C; d. Type D)

Type I Costal Cartilage Fracture occurs at the costosternal junction, and this type is quite unique. Since one side of the fracture lacks residual costal cartilage, it is not suitable to use various types of encircling fixation plates. Additionally, because the sternum is very hard, suturing is difficult, ordinary sutures cannot easily penetrate it, making standard suture fixation impractical. However, steel wires with needles can easily pass through both the sternum and costal cartilage, so this method of suturing can be considered a viable option. Apart from that, matrix RIB fixation can also be considered. One end of the plate can be secured to the surface of the sternum, and the other end can span the fracture and be fixed to the residual end of the costal cartilage on the opposite side. If there is concern that direct fixation to the cartilage may not be stable, a longer plate may be used to completely cover the costal cartilage and be directly fixed onto the rib instead. This usually results in satisfactory stability.

Type II Costal Cartilage Fracture occurs in the middle portion of the costal cartilage. All three fixation methods can be applied to this type of fracture: 1. Direct suturing is the simplest method and can be used for stabilization. 2. Encircling fixation plates can also be used; however, the stability of fixation may not always be satisfactory. 3. When using Matrix RIB for fixation, it is best to choose a longer plate that spans the entire length of the costal cartilage. One end should be fixed to the sternum, the other to the rib, and additional reinforcement can be applied on both sides of the fracture site along the costal cartilage.

Type III costal cartilage fracture occurs at the junction between the rib and the costal cartilage. Due to the hard bone texture at the rib end, even using needle-equipped steel wires makes suturing difficult or ineffective, so suture fixation is not recommended. Encircling fixation plates can be used; however, the fixation on the cartilage side may not be sufficiently secure. The most ideal fixation method remains the use of a Matrix RIB plate. The recommended approach is to span the entire costal cartilage, with: one end fixed to the rib, and

the other end fixed to the sternum. This method ensures strong and reliable stabilization of the fracture.
Type IV costal cartilage fracture occurs at the junction between the costal cartilage and the costal arch. Since both ends of the fracture are cartilage tissue, direct suturing can be considered as a fixation method. However, because the costal arch and costal cartilage are not aligned in the same direction, using an encircling fixation plate is difficult and often ineffective. In this situation, Matrix RIB fixation remains a viable option. The specific approach includes: First, place a Matrix RIB plate on the surface of the costal arch and fix it directly to the costal arch itself. Then, use another Matrix RIB plate to stabilize the fracture: One end is fixed to the rib at the distal end of the costal cartilage fracture. The other end is fixed onto the previously placed Matrix RIB plate on the coastal arch. This integrated fixation technique reflects the concept of chest wall reconstruction and offers enhanced stability and anatomical alignment.
Type V costochondral fracture is a costal arch fracture, which is different from all other costochondral fractures. The rib itself is relatively thick, with a straight edge on one side and a costochondral edge on the other side. The connection is of varying widths and is extremely irregular. Considering that the fracture ends are all cartilage, they can be sutured directly or fixed directly with a Matrix RIB plate, but are not suitable for fixation with an embracing fixation plate.
The five types of costal cartilage fractures described above essentially cover all forms of isolated costal cartilage fractures. These classifications refer specifically to pure costal cartilage fractures. It is important to note that in clinical practice, pure costal cartilage fractures are relatively uncommon. In most cases, they are combined with fractures of other bony structures. Therefore, in order to achieve satisfactory fixation of all fractures, it is necessary to make decisions based on the specific circumstances of each case (Figure 5-4-3).

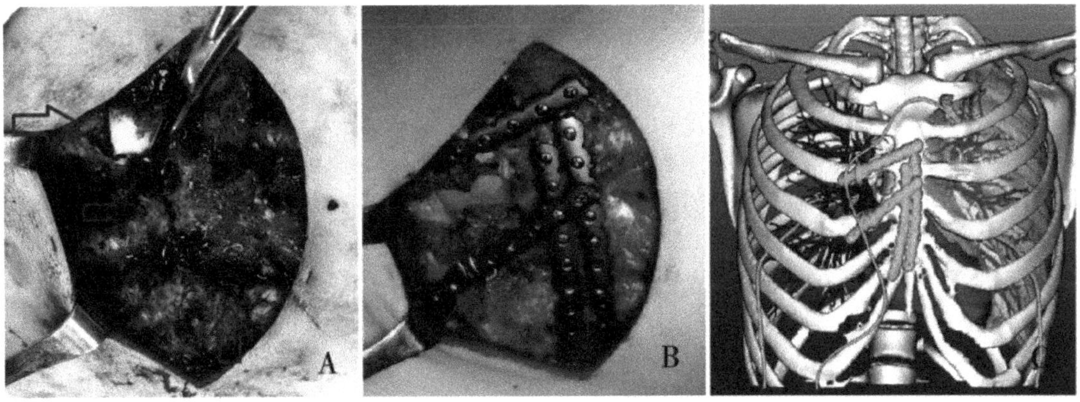

Figure 5-4-3: Fractures of the right 3, 4 costal cartilages combined with a fracture of the lower end of the sternum.

In all fracture fixation Surgeries, the key issue is the selection of fixation materials. As the above analysis shows, encircling fixation plates cannot meet the needs of all fixation procedures. In contrast, Matrix RIB proves to be effective across every type of fracture and can therefore be considered the preferred material. Especially when the specific location and structure of the fracture are not clearly identified, it is even more important to have such materials prepared to accommodate the requirements of various fracture fixations.

8.Prognosis

The fixation Surgery of costal cartilage fracture is relatively easy. Even if it is combined with fractures of other bone structures, as long as the material is selected appropriately and the fixation is performed according to the basic principles, good results can generally be obtained. However, like all other types of fractures, costal cartilage fractures are often combined with injuries in the chest cavity or other parts of the body, which makes the overall injury very uncertain. However, no matter how complicated the injury is, the basic treatment principles are relatively fixed. As long as the treatment is carried out strictly in accordance with these principles, the final effect will be relatively satisfactory.

REFERENCES

[1] El-Akkawi, A. I., F. V. De Paoli, G. Andersen, et al. 2019. "A Case of Severe Flail Chest with Several Dislocated Sternochondral Fractures." *International Journal of Surgery Case Reports* 65: 52–56.

[2] McAdams, T. R., J. F. Deimel, J. Ferguson, et al. 2016. "Chondral Rib Fractures in Professional American Football: Two Cases and Current Practice Patterns among NFL Team Physicians." *Orthopaedic Journal of Sports Medicine* 4 (2): 2325967115627623.

[3] Mohamed, S., A. Osman, A. Patel, et al. 2020. "Delayed Cardiac Tamponade following Blunt Chest Trauma due to Disruption of Fourth Costal Cartilage with Posterior Dislocation." *Trauma Case Reports* 29: 100340.

[4] Prins, J. T. H., and M. M. E. Wijffels. 2021. "Operative Treatment of Multiple Costochondral Dislocations in a Patient with Severe Rib Fractures and a Flail Chest following Trauma." *BMJ Case Reports* 14 (3): e239511.

[5] Mattox, R., K. E. Reckelhoff, A. B. Welk, et al. 2014. "Sonography of Occult Rib and Costal Cartilage Fractures: A Case Series." *Journal of Chiropractic Medicine* 13 (2): 139–143.

Section 5

STERNAL FRACTURES

Sternal fracture is a relatively rare chest wall injury. Among all fractures in the human body, sternal fractures account for less than 0.5% [1]. In chest wall trauma, the proportion is relatively high, though no accurate data is available. Multiple factors can cause sternal fractures. The most common scenario is traffic accidents, where the injured are often drivers who sustain injury due to compression from the steering wheel [1,2]. Other causes can also lead to sternal fractures, such as falls, crush injuries, and blunt impacts, which are also relatively common causes. The sternum is an important structural component of the thoracic cage. A fracture of the sternum can affect the shape and function of the entire thoracic cage, and thus, it must be given sufficient attention.

1. Mechanism

The sternum is located in the midline of the anterior chest wall and is a major structure of the thoracic cage. Since all ribs are directly or indirectly attached to the sternum, it serves as the primary load-bearing structure of the thorax. The sternum itself is relatively sturdy and strong, making it the strongest bone of the anterior chest wall. This characteristic gives it a high resistance to damage. However, because the sternum occupies a central and relatively large area on the anterior chest wall, it is more prone to injury. When external force exceeds the sternal threshold of resistance, a fracture may occur. This force typically originates from the front, which is the main mechanism causing sternal fractures [2]. The sides of the sternum are shielded by costal cartilage and ribs, so lateral forces generally do not directly cause sternal fractures. Because the sternum is stronger than other bony structures, when a fracture occurs, surrounding structures are often also injured. Therefore, isolated sternal fractures are relatively rare. In other words, once the sternum is damaged, nearby structures and organs are very likely to be injured as well. Clinically, it is common to see sternal fractures accompanied by: multiple rib fractures, costal cartilage fractures, injury to the heart and major vessels, lung injuries, and tracheal injuries, etc. When these conditions occur, the severity and complexity of the injury increase significantly [1-3].

2.Pathological Characteristics

Sternal fractures primarily occur in the body of the sternum, followed by fractures of the manubrium. Fractures of the sternal angle and xiphoid process are extremely rare [1]. Most fractures are isolated, but in cases of severe trauma, multiple fractures or even combined fractures may occur. The common sites of fracture are influenced by many factors, with the surface area of each part being a major factor. The most severely injured areas are typically those directly subjected to external force. Fractures may present as simple separations, but in more serious cases, displacement may occur either anteriorly or posteriorly [1]. The most severe scenario is partial loss of the sternum, known as a traumatic secondary sternal defect.

3. Hazards

After a sternal fracture occurs, the main hazards fall into two categories [1-3]: 1. The direct damage to the sternum itself, and 2. Impact on thoracic function. The sternal damage mainly stems from the fractured ends affecting surrounding structures, which can cause injury to nearby blood vessels, resulting in localized bleeding, or damage to other vital structures and organs, leading to corresponding complications. The impact on thoracic function primarily involves the appearance of the chest wall and its effect on respiratory and other physiological functions. A simple sternal fracture does not necessarily cause visible deformity. However, if there is displacement of the fracture ends, or if multiple fractures occur, localized depression or other deformities may be seen. Because breathing movements can cause intense local pain, the patient's respiration may be affected, which directly reflects the impact on organ function.

4. Clinical Symptoms

The main symptom of a sternal fracture is pain [4]. The pain is well localized, occurring near the fracture site, and it tends to worsen with breathing or physical movement. Due to the pain, patients may be reluctant to breathe deeply, which can lead to respiratory symptoms. If there is an associated lung injury, the respiratory symptoms may become even more pronounced. If the heart is compressed, or there is bleeding or blood loss from other causes, signs of circulatory system failure may also appear. Since sternal fractures usually result from strong external forces, patients often have combined injuries to surrounding structures, and may exhibit symptoms related to these additional injuries.

In terms of physical signs, sternal fractures typically present with prominent local signs. The fracture ends of the sternum can often be palpated, with marked tenderness at the site, and local movement may be detected. When there are accompanying rib cartilage or rib fractures, multiple fracture ends over a broader area may be palpable. If local chest wall softening occurs, it may lead to chest wall flail and paradoxical respiration. When there is an associated lung injury, corresponding pulmonary signs may be present. If the heart or great vessels are damaged, corresponding cardiovascular signs may also be observed.

5. Examination

The first step in the examination of sternal fractures is physical examination. For simple sternal fractures, especially for thin patients, physical examination can basically determine the location and nature of the fracture. Because of the soft tissue covering the front of the sternum, obese patients can only find tenderness sometimes, and other physical signs are difficult to find. X-ray examination is the first choice for further examination. In the frontal film, it is difficult to find the fracture site due to the overlap of the sternum and spine (Figure 5-5-1A). The lateral film examination effect is ideal, and the approximate location of the fracture end can also be seen (Figure 5-5-1B). CT examination is very helpful for diagnosis. It can not only show the location of the fracture end, but also examine the condition of the entire chest, which is very helpful in excluding chest mergers (Figure 5-5-1C, D) [4]. Ultrasound examination is a new method that has emerged in recent years [5]. It can describe the condition of the fracture end very clearly and can be used as an option for sternal fracture examination. The only regret is that it cannot provide more intuitive images like X-rays. This requires gradual adaptation for Surgeons who are accustomed to looking at X-rays. With the continuous advancement of technology, the equipment for ultrasound examination has been improved.

With continuous technological advancements, ultrasound equipment is now available for intraoperative use. Such equipment is highly helpful for intraoperative localization, especially when performing certain minimally invasive procedures, making intraoperative ultrasound a valuable examination. The most direct clinical display is 3D reconstruction, which involves three-dimensional imaging of all thoracic structures, including the sternum (Figure 5-5-1E). This type of examination not only reveals the details of the fracture but also provides all the information needed for Surgery. However, the biggest issue with this type of examination is the time factor since emergency Surgery, its practicality still needs improvement. Results cannot be produced in the shortest possible time, and many patients with sternal fractures require

The local examination of sternal fracture is not too difficult, but because other structural injuries are often combined, the combined injuries must be examined at the same time during the examination. This aspect of the examination mainly includes three items: ① The damage to the costal cartilage and ribs around the sternal fracture. Since the fixation of ribs or costal cartilage requires special materials and instruments, if there is no preparation before the operation and the damage is found temporarily during the operation, it will affect the fixation during the operation. Therefore, it is necessary to clarify whether these parts are damaged before the operation so as to make corresponding preparations. The most easily missed diagnosis in clinical practice is the costal cartilage fracture. Since the costal cartilage cannot be displayed during X-ray examination, if only X-ray examination is performed before the operation without other examinations, it may cause a missed diagnosis.

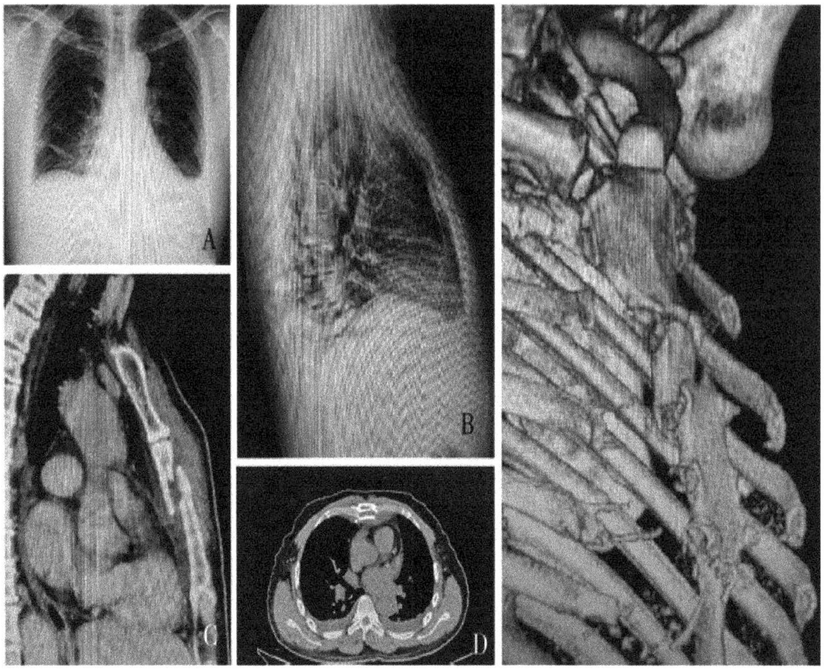

Figure 5-5-1 Imaging examination of sternal fracture (A. X-ray anteroposterior film. The sternal shadow overlaps with the mediastinum, making it difficult to show the sternal fracture. B. X-ray lateral film. The sternal shadow is located in the front and can show the local sternal fracture. C. CT sagittal image. It can clearly show the local sternal fracture and related information of the mediastinum. D. CT cross-sectional image. It can show some information about the sternal fracture. E. Three-dimensional reconstruction image. It can show a three- dimensional image of the local sternal fracture)

To avoid missing a costal cartilage fracture, special attention should be given to examining the condition of the costal cartilage near the ends of the sternal fracture. Performing CT and ultrasound examinations can easily detect costal cartilage fractures. ② The condition of intrathoracic organs. When thoracic organs are involved, their injuries are often more serious than the sternal fracture itself and must be prioritized during Surgery. If only the sternal fracture is considered while intrathoracic injuries are overlooked, and these are discovered unexpectedly during Surgery, it will complicate Surgical management.③ Associated injuries to other parts of the body. Sternal fractures may be accompanied by injuries elsewhere in the body, and the treatment of those injuries may also affect the management of the sternal fracture. Therefore, a thorough preoperative examination of the entire body must be completed to ensure that no associated injuries are missed.

6. Diagnosis

The diagnosis of an isolated sternal fracture is relatively straightforward. A preliminary diagnosis can be made based on the history of trauma, symptoms, and physical signs, while imaging studies can help confirm the diagnosis. Since sternal fractures are often accompanied by injuries to surrounding structures and other parts of the body, a thorough screening for associated injuries must be conducted during diagnosis to avoid missing any concurrent damage. Overall, the key point in diagnosing a sternal fracture does not lie in identifying the fracture itself, but in ruling out associated injuries. This is essential to avoid missed diagnoses.

7. Treatment

(1) Conservative Treatment

Once the diagnosis of sternal fracture is confirmed, the next issue is treatment. There are many opinions on the treatment of sternal fracture, and it is difficult to unify different opinions. In the past, some people were not enthusiastic about Surgical treatment, believing that conservative treatment could be used in most cases [2,4]. On the contrary, others advocated active Surgery. Objectively speaking, the decision on treatment should be weighed from many aspects. If conservative treatment can effectively eliminate symptoms, promote fracture healing, and avoid complications, it is, of course, a good choice. If such measures are ineffective, Surgery must be chosen without hesitation. The indications for conservative treatment are as follows: ① The fracture ends are well aligned, with no displacement, and do not shift with breathing or movement. Although there is an actual fracture, there is no significant harm. Fixation in such cases would not improve the alignment of the fracture ends and could instead cause additional injury due to Surgery. Therefore, Surgical treatment is not meaningful and is not recommended. Sternal fractures where the patient did not seek medical attention promptly and the fracture has already healed with displacement. In such cases, examination may reveal a clear sternal fracture with poor alignment and obvious displacement of the fracture ends, but both sides of the fracture have already become fixed. The purpose of sternal fracture Surgery is fixation, and if the fracture has already stabilized on its own, Surgery is unnecessary. Performing Surgery in such cases would involve breaking the formed callus, causing further injury. ③ A simple sternal fracture that does not compromise thoracic stability but is accompanied by severe injuries in other parts of the body. Such injuries may involve areas like the brain. Since the positioning for cranial Surgery is not suitable for simultaneous sternal fracture Surgery, and additional Surgery may pose further risks to the patient, conservative treatment of the simple.

Sternal fracture may be considered without Surgical intervention. Conservative treatment measures mainly include necessary symptomatic treatment, supportive Conservative treatment measures mainly include necessary symptomatic treatment, supportive care, and rehabilitation therapy. For patients who are not suitable for conservative.

Patients who are being treated require Surgical treatment.

(2) Surgical Treatment

In addition to the above-mentioned cases of conservative treatment, most cases of thoracic spine require Surgical treatment. Surgical treatment has a very good reason: ① Thoracic spine is the most important structure of the chest. The stability of the chest skeleton is the key to maintaining the body's weight balance. Because all the soft tissues and skeletal structures of the chest are directly or indirectly attached to the chest, some of the thoracic force is also indirectly loaded on the chest. Inevitably, change will bring many problems to the human body. Poor alignment results in severely compromised load-bearing capacity, which will inevitably have a serious impact on the human body. Therefore, Surgical fixation is necessary. ② The sternum is the core structure of the thoracic cage. If the sternum itself is unstable, it may affect the stability of the entire thoracic cage, thereby causing a series of problems. Therefore, once a fracture occurs, it must be addressed. ③ After a sternal fracture, the fractured ends move with respiratory motion. If not treated, the patient will experience significant pain, making it necessary to fix the fracture ends. ④ Sternal fractures are often accompanied by injuries to surrounding structures. If these injuries are not treated in a timely manner, their harm may be even more severe than that of the sternal fracture itself. ⑤Even if a sternal fracture is a simple fracture, due to the presence of many important surrounding structures and organs, if it is not fixed in time, the fracture ends may continue to damage nearby structures, leading to further injuries. Therefore, it is necessary to intervene to prevent such complications. In summary, for sternal fractures, as long as the fracture is not a simple, clean break, Surgical intervention should be actively pursued.

The basic principles of sternal fracture Surgery are: ① Proper fixation of the fracture ends; ② Active management of associated injuries; ③ Effective prevention of complications.

The fixation of sternal fractures has a long history, with the first fixation Surgery performed by McKim in 1943[2]. Over the course of extensive clinical practice, various methods have been used. In the early years, there were no specialized fixation devices, and fixation methods were diverse. The most common method was direct fixation with steel wires. Because the cortex of the sternum is hard and difficult to suture through, steel wire fixation was trembly challenging and the fixation results were not always satisfactory. With the development of fixation techniques, many specialized materials for sternal fixation have been introduced in clinical practice. Materials have been developed [6-9]. These materials use different principles for fixation, but the results are not always satisfactory. The main reason is that the designs are overly idealized and do not take into account the characteristics of the internal structure. Common problems include the following: ①Designs are too rigid. The materials use hard, straight plates that do not consider the curvature of the sternum surface. Such designs make it difficult for the material to fit closely to the sternum. Even if a certain fixation effect is achieved, the material may lift up locally in some areas, which is not conducive to incision suturing.② Many materials are too thick, focusing only on fixation strength while neglecting the special characteristics of the location. Since there is little soft tissue on the surface of the sternum and poor blood supply, overly thick materials not only affect postoperative healing but also cause the foreign body to protrude visibly on the surface, which is unsightly and prone to injury, causing discomfort to the patient. ③Some materials achieve fixation by clamping the sternum from both sides. However, because the clamping positions often do not align well with the intercostal spaces, this frequently causes difficulties during Surgery and affects the Surgical outcome. If the fixation materials are unsatisfactory, the Surgical outcome will be compromised.

If the fixation material is not satisfactory, the effect of the operation will be compromised. Therefore, the design and selection of materials are important factors in determining the effect of the operation. We have used a variety of materials to perform sternal fracture Surgery. In comparison, we believe that MatrixRIB is considered a relatively ideal fixation material [2,4]. The specific method is (Figure 5-5-2): First, make an incision along the midline of the anterior chest wall. The incision should extend sufficiently beyond both ends of the fracture site. After exposing the fracture site, carefully dissect along the bony structures of the chest wall on both sides. Remove any accumulated blood and surrounding hematoma at the fracture ends. Align the sternal fracture ends, then fix them using 2 - 3 MatrixRIB plates crossing the fracture site. Secure 2 - 3 screws on each side of the fracture ends. After fixation, use the soft tissue within the incision to cover the MatrixRIB plates as much as possible, then close the skin incision. If there are concomitant costal cartilage or rib fractures during the Surgery, MatrixRIB can be used to fix those as well.
MatrixRIB is a material designed for rib fractures, but if used in sternum fractures, satisfactory results can also be achieved. Its main advantages are as follows: ①The thickness of MatrixRIB material is moderate, with sufficient strength to meet the needs of fixation, but not too thick, which does not affect healing and appearance after Surgery, and is not easy to be bumped; ② MatrixRIB can be shaped at will. The shape of the plate can be adjusted according to the surface of the sternum before fixation, which can ensure that the plate fits tightly with the sternum, not only ensuring the fixation effect, but also preventing the plate from partially tilting; ③ MatrixRIB is fixed with screws, which can span the anterior and posterior cortices of the sternum at the same time, and the fixation is quite firm, which can ensure a good fixation effect; ④ MatrixRIB only needs to be fixed on the surface of the sternum, and there is no need to consider the shape problem too much, which makes the operation simpler and the effect easier to control; ⑤ MatrixRIB itself can meet the fixation needs of rib fractures and costal cartilage fractures. If fractures in

these parts are combined, fixation can be implemented at the same time, which makes the material preparation simpler; ⑥ MatrixRIB can remain in the body for life and does not need to be removed by Surgery again, which will reduce the cost and pain of patients due to plate removal.

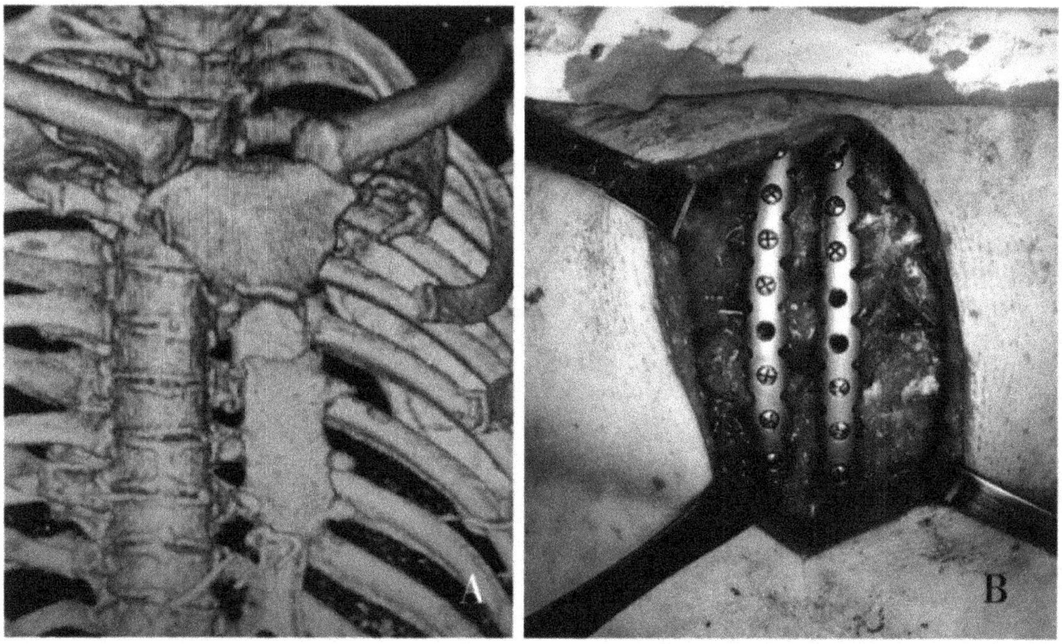

Figure 5-5-2 Using MatrixRIB to fix sternal fractures (A. 3D reconstruction of sternal fractures. The fracture is located in the sternum body, and the fracture ends are obviously dislocated. B. First, expose the fracture site, reduce the fracture, and then use MatrixRIB to fix the sternum locally)

Although sternal fracture fixation Surgery involves a midline incision, it does not include sawing open the sternum and therefore is completely different from a true median sternotomy. Through this type of incision, it is impossible to manage injuries inside the thoracic cavity. If such management is required, there are two basic methods: one is to open the sternum and expose the intrathoracic structures through the mediastinum; the other is to expose these structures through an additional lateral chest wall incision. When a sternal fracture is accompanied by injury to major mediastinal blood vessels or the heart, a vertical sternotomy is essential. The mediastinal injury must be treated first, followed by the management of the sternal fracture. Originally, the sternum would have only been transversely fractured, but in this case, it must be completely sawn open along the midline, causing even more severe damage, an outcome that is unfortunately unavoidable. Since the sternal fracture threatens the patient's life, such treatment becomes necessary to save it, and the further damage to the sternum is simply the price of survival, a helpless but

essential measure.
After the sternum is split, additional steps are required for fixation. To ensure optimal stability, the fixation technique used for a median sternotomy can be followed: first, the split portion is firmly secured with steel wires, and then the fracture ends are fixed. Although these procedures may appear very complex on the surface, they are actually not. As long as attention is paid to the Surgical details, the fixation outcome is generally quite satisfactory.
When a sternal fracture is accompanied by injury to intrathoracic organs, considering issues related to skin incisions and postoperative scarring, it is also possible to opt for a median sternal split, followed by management of the intrathoracic injuries through the mediastinum. Although this approach is feasible, it can sometimes be quite challenging. Another method is to access the thoracic cavity through the intercostal space alongside the sternum. However, this approach offers limited exposure and presents significant Surgical difficulty. To simplify the procedure, a lateral chest wall incision may be considered, with the specific method adjusted according to the severity of the injury. A decision must be made based on the severity of the injuries. Since both the sternum and intrathoracic injuries need to be addressed and the incisions may require different patient positions it is necessary to consider the order in which the injuries are treated.
Typically, the more severe injury should be managed first. Once that is completed, the incision should
be closed, the patient's position changed, and then the other injury can be addressed. Due to the need for repositioning and re-sterilization, a detailed and well-planned Surgical workflow must be designed before the operation. Only with such preparation can optimal outcomes be achieved.

8. Prognonsis

The prognosis of sternal fractures largely depends on the severity of the injury and the presence of associated damage to internal organs. Isolated, non-displaced sternal fractures generally have a good outcome with conservative treatment. However, in cases involving severe displacement, multiple fractures, or associated injuries such as to the heart, lungs, or major blood vessels, the prognosis can be more serious and requires timely and effective Surgical intervention. Proper fixation, meticulous Surgical technique, and postoperative care are essential to ensure good healing and functional recovery. With appropriate treatment, most patients can expect a favorable prognosis.

REFERENCES

[1] Klei, D. S., M. B. de Jong, F. C. Oner, et al. 2019. "Current Treatment and Outcomes of Traumatic Sternal Fractures: A Systematic Review." *International Orthopaedics* 43 (6): 1455–1464.

[2] Schulz-Drost, S., A. Mauerer, S. Grupp, et al. 2014. "Surgical Fixation of Sternal Fractures: Locked Plate Fixation by Low-Profile Titanium Plates—Surgical Safety through Depth-Limited Drilling." *International Orthopaedics* 38 (1): 133–139.
[3] Audette, J. S., M. Emond, H. Scott, et al. 2014. "Investigation of Myocardial Contusion with Sternal Fracture in the Emergency Department: Multicenter Review." *Canadian Family Physician* 60 (2): e126–e130.
[4] Schulz-Drost, S., P. Oppel, S. Grupp, et al. 2015. "Surgical Fixation of Sternal Fractures: Preoperative Planning and a Safe Surgical Technique Using Locked Titanium Plates and Depth-Limited Drilling." *Journal of Visualized Experiments* (95): 52124.
[5] Sesia, S. B., F. Prüfer, and J. Mayr. 2017. "Sternal Fracture in Children: Diagnosis by Ultrasonography." *European Journal of Pediatric Surgery Reports* 5 (1): e39–e42.
[6] Zhao, Y., Y. Yang, Z. Gao, et al. 2017. "Treatment of Traumatic Sternal Fractures with Titanium Plate Internal Fixation: A Retrospective Study." *Journal of Cardiothoracic Surgery* 12: 22.
[7] Byun, C. S., I. H. Park, W. J. Hwang, et al. 2016. "Analysis of Sternal Fixation Results According to Plate Type in Sternal Fracture." *Korean Journal of Thoracic and Cardiovascular Surgery* 49 (5): 361–365.
[8] Xu, S., J. Zhu, Q. Yu, et al. 2021. "Surgical Treatment of Sternum Comminuted Fracture with Memory Alloy Embracing Fixator." *Journal of Thoracic Disease* 13 (4): 2194–2202.
[9] Park, J. B., H. P. Lee, D. G. Yoo, et al. 2013. "Fixation of Traumatic Sternal Fractures Using Sternum Lock Plating System." *Korean Journal of Thoracic and Cardiovascular Surgery* 46 (4): 309–311.

Flail chest is the most severe type of chest wall trauma. It is termed "flail" because the fractured chest wall segment resembles a flail in appearance and behavior after injury [1]. Clinically, flail chest is often defined as a condition caused by multiple ribs fractured in multiple places, creating a free-floating segment of the chest wall. While this definition is generally accepted, it has limitations. For example, when a sternal fracture is accompanied by bilateral structural injuries, it can also result in a flail chest [2]. Therefore, a more accurate definition of flail chest should be a condition caused by extensive fractures of the chest wall, and it does not necessarily refer only to rib fractures.

1. Cause of injury

Compared to isolated rib fractures or sternal fractures, flail chest represents a more severe form of chest wall trauma. The occurrence of this type of injury is fundamentally due to two key reasons: first, the injuring force must possess specific characteristics; second, the structural bones involved must have relatively poor resistance to such force. Typically, sharp-force injuries may cause significant localized damage, but they rarely result in extensive destruction of bony structures and thus are not the main cause of flail chest. Blunt force trauma is the main injuring factor for flail chest, as it affects a large area and can cause extensive damage to bony structures, leading to the formation of a flail segment. Other complex injuries such as those caused by falls, crushing incidents, or impacts can also result in widespread bone damage and are important causes of flail chest. In addition to the external force involved, the occurrence of flail chest is also closely related to the nature of the patient's own bony structures. Elderly individuals, whose bones are more fragile and less capable of withstanding impact, are particularly susceptible to developing flail chest.

2. Pathophysiological Manifestations

The most fundamental pathological feature of flail chest is the extensive destruction of the bony structure of the chest wall [3]. This destruction directly affects the integrity and stability of the thoracic cage, impacting all functions related to the chest. The most visible effect is the appearance of the chest wall. Due to the loss of structural support, the injured area becomes sunken. However, as intrathoracic pressure changes with respiratory movement, the chest wall also moves with breathing, leading to what is known as a floating chest wall. The direction of movement of the floating chest wall is exactly opposite to that of the normal chest wall, and is therefore referred to as paradoxical breathing movement (Figure 5-6-1) [4,5].

The maintenance of normal respiratory movement requires many factors, among which an important one is the supportive function of the thoracic cage. If the thoracic cage loses its normal rigidity, it may consume the mechanical work of breathing, not only making respiration more laborious but also potentially impairing respiratory function, leading to respiratory insufficiency or even failure. Therefore, patients with flail chest experience varying degrees of respiratory function impairment.

When a flail chest occurs, the pressure within both sides of the thoracic cavity changes. If this change is asymmetrical, it can lead to mediastinal shifts. Similar to the flail chest itself, mediastinal shift consumes respiratory effort and impairs respiratory function. Additionally, because it directly affects the heart and blood vessels, it may also impair the functioning of the circulatory system

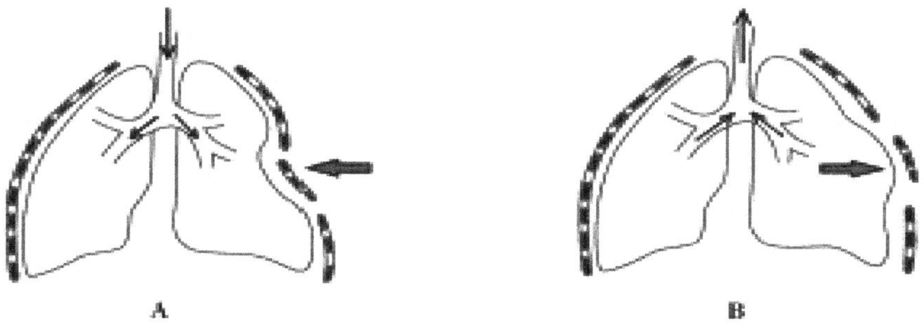

Figure 5-6-1 Mechanism of Paradoxical Respiration Formation:(A. During inhalation, the negative pressure inside the thoracic cavity increases, causing an increased pressure difference across the chest wall. When this pressure difference exceeds the chest wall's own stress resistance, a localized inward movement of the chest wall occurs, forming a local depression. (B. During exhalation, the negative pressure inside the thoracic cavity decreases, reducing the pressure difference across the chest wall, allowing the chest wall to return to its original position or even causing a localized bulge. Because the local chest wall movement during inhalation and exhalation is opposite to the normal movement direction of the thorax, this phenomenon is called paradoxical respiration)

3. Clinical Manifestations

The clinical manifestations of simple flail chest are related to chest wall trauma, mainly including the following: ① Pain [4]. This is the most common symptom. The pain comes from the fracture itself and also from the stimulation of the intercostal nerves. Since the fracture ends may rub with breathing, the pain will be aggravated by breathing movements. ② Dyspnea. This is the most common and most serious clinical manifestation. The reason for dyspnea first comes from chest wall pain. Patients often dare not breathe because of the severe pain when breathing. The second reason comes from the consumption of respiratory work by the floating chest wall. Since patients must resist the consumption of work, breathing will be very difficult. The third reason may come from damage to lung tissue. Since patients with flail chest often have lung tissue damage, it can directly increase the difficulty of breathing. The fourth reason may come from blood or air accumulation in the chest cavity. When hemothorax and pneumothorax exist, the expansion of lung tissue is restricted, which may also cause dyspnea. In general, when flail chest occurs, respiratory function can be affected through various mechanisms, leading to dyspnea. ③ Palpitation. Palpitation is directly related to increased heart rate. The increased heart rate may be caused by pain stimulation, changes in blood volume, or direct damage to the heart. When multiple factors affect the heart, the heart rate may increase, leading to panic. ④ Cough. The occurrence of cough is related to the stimulation of the lungs or pleura. When flail chest occurs, the stimulation of the pleura is difficult to avoid. If the injury is deep, it will also cause damage to the lung tissue. Therefore, coughing is a common symptom. ⑤ Hemoptysis. Hemoptysis is a manifestation of damage to the lung tissue or airway. Once hemoptysis occurs, it means that the internal organs of the chest cavity are damaged.

The clinical manifestations of simple flail chest are relatively singular, primarily presenting as symptoms localized to the chest. In reality once a flail chest occurs, the patient. The injuries are usually serious and often accompanied by damage to other organs.

The patient will show more and more complex symptoms, which are very painful for the patient and require urgent treatment. The injuries are usually serious and often accompanied by injuries to other organs. The patient will show more and more complex symptoms, which are very painful for the patient and need to be treated as soon as possible.

The signs of flail chest are first the manifestation of the local injury. In addition to the signs of the fracture itself, there may be typical signs such as a floating chest wall and abnormal breathing. From the appearance, there may be clear wounds. These signs are conducive to the diagnosis of flail chest.

4. Examination

Flail chest first requires a physical examination. Through an initial physical exam, the location, nature, and severity of the trauma can be determined, and a preliminary understanding of any associated injuries can be obtained. Further evaluation must be carried out using imaging studies. X-ray examination is the 1 simplest and also a very effective diagnostic method. It can clearly show the 2 general location and extent of fractures, and also provide a rough view of 3 injuries within the thoracic cavity. For cases of 4 isolated flail chest, X-ray is usually sufficient. However, considering the possibility of 5 associated injuries, further diagnostic evaluation is necessary. 6 CT scans can provide more detailed information, not only revealing injuries to the chest wall but also showing details of 7 intrathoracic injuries. However, for fractures of the chest wall, 8 CT scans have limitations as they cannot fully display the overall structure of the 9 thoracic cage. The most ideal examination method is 10 3D reconstruction, which can show both the complete structure of the thoracic cage and details of internal thoracic injuries [6,7]. If conditions permit, the corresponding examinations should be performed. It must be pointed out that a flail chest is often a very severe injury, and in some cases, the patient may even require mechanical ventilation. Such patients cannot be moved freely, so apart from X-ray examination, many other types of imaging are not feasible. In such situations, X-ray examination becomes the most useful and practical diagnostic method.

If conditions permit, the corresponding examinations should be performed. It must be pointed out that a flail chest is often a very severe injury, and in some cases, the patient may even require mechanical ventilation. Such patients cannot be moved freely, so apart from X-ray examination, many other types of imaging are not feasible. In such situations, X-ray examination becomes the most useful and practical diagnostic method.

The trauma of flail chest is not limited to the chest wall and chest, but may also affect other parts of the body. In order to avoid missing trauma, while completing the chest wall physical examination, a full body examination should be performed according to the situation, so that all injuries can be discovered and treated in time.

5. Diagnosis

The diagnosis of flail chest is relatively easy. It can be readily made based on the history of trauma, symptoms, physical signs, and relevant examinations. For patients with flail chest, however, the key focus of diagnosis should also include ruling out associated injuries, as this is directly related to the formulation of an appropriate treatment strategy. The first thing that needs to be clarified is whether there are any associated injuries within the thoracic cavity. The second is to determine whether there are injuries to other parts of the body. The third is to assess whether there is any impairment of vital organ function. Only after these three conditions have been ruled out can treatment focus solely on the flail Chest itself

6. Treatment

The treatment of flail chest can be divided into two types: conservative treatment and Surgical treatment [8-10]. Since the greatest hazards of flail chest are the floating chest wall and paradoxical respiration, the fundamental principle of whether using conservative or Surgical treatment should be to correct these issues. Advocate for Surgical treatment, especially in cases where conservative methods fail to effectively stabilize the chest wall. The primary goal remains to eliminate the floating chest wall as soon as possible, restore the integrity of the thoracic cage, and enable early recovery of lung function [8-11]. While early approaches favored conservative management due to the risks and complications associated with Surgery, recent advances in Surgical Techniques and material have made been operative intervention a more viable and often preferred option.

(1) Conservative Treatment

Conservative treatment is a non-Surgical treatment for flail chest. Conservative treatment is required in some special cases. These cases include: ① Poor medical conditions and lack of Surgical capability: Flail chest represents a severe injury to the bony structure of the chest wall. Surgical treatment requires appropriate medical facilities and technical support. If such conditions are unavailable, conservative treatment is the only option. ② Extremely critical condition that does not permit immediate Surgery: Surgical intervention means introducing additional trauma. If the patient is in a critically severe state especially with a poor general condition immediate Surgery is not advisable, and conservative treatment must be administered temporarily.③ Combined with other major organ injuries that preclude Surgical treatment: If flail chest is accompanied by other severe injuries such as traumatic brain injury, massive bleeding, or serious trauma in other areas, priority must be given to managing those injuries. If flail chest Surgery cannot be performed simultaneously, conservative treatment is required. ④ Severely contaminated open wounds: Since Surgical fixation involves the placement of various fixation materials, using them in contaminated wounds may lead to infection. Therefore, Surgical treatment is not appropriate in such cases.

Conservative treatment methods for flail chest include the following key points [4,5,9,10]: ① Pain relief. Pain is the main symptom, causing significant suffering and affecting breathing, so effective pain control must be given first. ② Assisted respiration to improve the patient's hypoxia. The greatest harm of flail chest is respiratory dysfunction, and patients often have severe hypoxia. Passive oxygen therapy is usually insufficient, so active assisted respiration is needed as an initial essential treatment step. The affected lung cannot fully expand; this method may limit respiratory function. The second method is mechanical ventilation with positive pressure. Positive pressure ventilation can counteract the chest wall collapse caused by flail chest, reduce paradoxical breathing, and help restore chest wall stability. ③ Management of associated injuries. Flail chest is often accompanied by other injuries such as hemothorax, pneumothorax, or lung contusions. These associated injuries should be actively treated to improve overall respiratory and circulatory function. Reduction in thoracic cavity volume may worsen respiratory distress, so the method must be applied based on the patient's condition. If respiratory difficulty intensifies, the

method should be abandoned in favor of alternative approaches. The second technique is suspension fixation. Typically, towel clamps are used to hook the ribs of the flail segment, which is then suspended from an external frame to achieve stabilization. This method eliminates the flail movement of the chest wall without reducing the thoracic cavity volume, making it a relatively better option. However, since it requires external suspension, it restricts patient mobility and causes considerable discomfort.
Conservative treatment has a certain effect on eliminating the floating chest wall of patients with flail chest, which can improve their respiratory function and buy time for the recovery of trauma. However, since it does not completely fix the fractured ribs, it will cause various problems, which will not only affect the healing effect but also bring great pain to the patient. Therefore, more and more people recommend Surgical treatment! [9,11]

(2) Surgical treatment
Flail chest is a serious injury to the bony structure of the chest wall. Generally speaking, Surgical treatment should be actively implemented as long as conditions permit. Before the operation, adequate preoperative preparation is required: the first preparation is to establish a fluid channel; the second preparation is to establish a monitoring channel; the third preparation is to improve the general condition. Preoperative preparation should be intensive and orderly, and should not be too complicated. If the condition is critical, it should be simplified as much as possible.
Chest Surgery refers to the fixation operation performed on the fracture [10-13]. These operations themselves are not complicated. However, the clinical situation is often much more complicated than the fracture. The patient may have injuries in other parts of the body or injuries in the chest cavity. Some injuries are obviously more serious than chest wall fractures. Therefore, when performing Surgery, it is necessary to have a global view, make overall arrangements, and implement treatment in an orderly manner.
Generally speaking, the basic principles of Surgery are: ① Prioritize life-threatening injuries; ② Prioritize injuries to important organs; ③ Prioritize injuries that endanger the functions of important organs. It is the most reasonable operation to consider the fixation of fractures under the premise of strictly abiding by the three priority principles.
The functions of flail chest Surgery are: ① It can help restore the shape of the thorax and restore the normal function of the thorax. The most direct effect is to eliminate floating chest wall and abnormal breathing, so that respiratory function can be restored. ② It can eliminate the friction of the fracture ends, reduce or even eliminate pain. ③ It can eliminate the dislocation of the fracture ends, avoid the fracture ends from damaging the viscera in the chest cavity, and avoid abnormal healing. ④ During the flail chest Surgery, due to the use of endotracheal intubation, sputum can be suctioned through the intubation, so that

the atelectasis part of the lung can be re-expanded, reducing the occurrence of pulmonary complications. ⑤ Through the incision of the flail chest Surgery, the damage in the thoracic cavity can be explored, providing a Surgical approach for intrathoracic Surgery.

The methods for fixing fractures are simple and can be done using various materials [2,4, 5, 13]. Fixation should be as thorough, effective, and secure as possible. Only when the bony structure of the thorax is properly stabilized can the thorax restore its normal structure and function properly

7. Prognosis

The fixation techniques for flail chest are very mature, and Surgical outcomes for isolated flail chest are generally satisfactory. However, whether these patients receive satisfactory treatment often does not depend solely on the fracture fixation itself but largely on the management of associated injuries. One of the most critical associated injuries is severe cardiac trauma. Once such trauma occurs, the situation becomes extremely urgent, requiring Surgery to be performed as quickly as possible. If the response is delayed or the approach is inappropriate, the chances of successful treatment may fail. For these patients, timely and effective management of associated injuries is crucial. There is no doubt about the necessity of fracture fixation during the emergency rescue phase. For example, in cases of brain injury or spinal cord injury, simply fixing the ribs without addressing these injuries will lead to a poor prognosis.

Overall, once flail chest occurs, it not only indicates severe chest wall trauma but also often involves multiple serious injuries throughout the body. At this time, it is essential not only to recognize the presence of flail chest but also to maintain a comprehensive, global perspective. Only by doing so can successful treatment be ensured.

REFERENCES

[1] Getz, P., P. Mommsen, J. D. Clausen, et al. 2019. "Limited Influence of Flail Chest in Patients with Blunt Thoracic Trauma: A Matched-Pair Analysis." *In Vivo* 33 (1): 133–139.

[2] Lee, S. K., and D. K. Kang. 2016. "Nuss Procedure for Surgical Stabilization of Flail Chest with Horizontal Sternal Body Fracture and Multiple Bilateral Rib Fractures." *Journal of Thoracic Disease* 8 (6): E390–E392.

[3] Naidoo, K., L. Hanbali, and P. Bates. 2017. "The Natural History of Flail Chest Injuries." *Chinese Journal of Traumatology* 20 (5): 293–296.

[4] Xia, H., D. Zhu, J. Li, et al. 2020. "Current Status and Research Progress of Minimally Invasive Surgery for Flail Chest." *Experimental and Therapeutic Medicine* 19 (1): 421–427.

[5] Lodhia, J. V., K. Konstantinidis, and K. Papagiannopoulos. 2019. "Surgical Management of Multiple Rib Fractures/Flail Chest." *Journal of Thoracic Disease* 11 (4): 1668–1675.

[6] de Jong, M. B., G. Allain, P. C. M. van Yle, et al. 2015. "Flail Chest in Polytraumatized Patients: Surgical Fixation Using Stracos Reduces Ventilator Time and Hospital Stay." *BioMed Research International* 2015: 624723.
[7] Qiu, M., Z. Shi, J. Xiao, et al. 2016. "Potential Benefits of Rib Fracture Fixation in Patients with Flail Chest and Multiple Non-Flail Rib Fractures." *Indian Journal of Surgery* 78 (6): 458–463.
[8] Beks, R. B., D. Reetz, M. B. de Jong, et al. 2019. "Rib Fixation versus Non-Operative Treatment for Flail Chest and Multiple Rib Fractures after Blunt Thoracic Trauma: A Multicenter Cohort Study." *European Journal of Trauma and Emergency Surgery* 45 (4): 655–663.
[9] Ingoe, H. M., E. Coleman, W. Eardley, et al. 2019. "Systematic Review of Systematic Reviews for Effectiveness of Internal Fixation for Flail Chest and Rib Fractures in Adults." *BMJ Open* 9 (4): e023444.
[10] Wuffels, M. M. E., T. Hagenaars, D. Latifi, et al. 2020. "Early Results after Operatively versus Non-Operatively Treated Flail Chest: A Retrospective Study Focusing on Outcomes and Complications." *European Journal of Trauma and Emergency Surgery* 46 (3): 539–547.
[11] Schuurmans, J., J. C. Goslings, and T. Schepers. 2017. "Operative Management versus Non-Operative Management of Rib Fractures in Flail Chest Injuries: A Systematic Review." *European Journal of Trauma and Emergency Surgery* 43 (2): 163–168.
[12] Guernelli, N., R. B. Bragaglia, A. Briccoli, et al. 1979. "Technique for the Management of Anterior Flail Chest." *Thorax* 34 (2): 247–248.
[13] Paris, F., V. Tarazona, E. Blasco, et al. 1975. "Surgical Stabilization of Traumatic Flail Chest." *Thorax* 30 (5): 521–527.

The chest wall is composed of three basic components: bone, soft tissue, and skin [1]. These three components are closely connected to form an integrated whole. When the chest wall is subjected to external trauma, any of these components can be damaged. While previous sections primarily focused on injuries to the bony structures, this section introduces injuries to the skin and soft tissues.

1. Structure and basic functions

The skin is located on the surface of the body, serving as both a protective barrier and a key component of physical appearance. Damage to the skin can lead to numerous issues. Beneath the skin lies the subcutaneous tissue, followed by various other soft tissues. The soft tissues of the chest wall mainly include muscles, fat, and subcutaneous tissue. In addition to their specific functions, these soft tissues also play other important roles. First, they serve a filling function while the human skeleton forms the basic framework of the body, it is not a completely seamless structure; there are considerable gaps between bones, which must be filled by tissue, a role that soft tissues effectively fulfill [1]. ①Filling function: The human skeletal structure contains numerous gaps between bones, which must be filled to maintain structural integrity. In the chest wall, the intercostal spaces (spaces between the ribs) are especially numerous and wide, requiring a large amount of soft tissue to fill them. Additionally, soft tissue is present in all other structural gaps, playing a crucial role in maintaining the overall integrity of the chest wall. ② Connecting function: The rib cage is primarily composed of bones, which are inherently separate structures. However, soft tissue surrounds and connects each bone, creating an integrated whole. These connective tissues allow the chest wall to function as a unified structure.③Aesthetic function: Beyond structural roles, soft tissues contribute significantly to the appearance of the chest wall. They cover the underlying bones and shape the external contour, playing an important role in the overall physical appearance. The bones of the chest wall have irregular shapes and cannot form a smooth surface on their own. If these bony contours were exposed on the skin's surface, they would significantly affect the aesthetic appearance. However, soft tissue covers the surface of these bones, and this covering serves several important functions:3. Aesthetic function: The soft tissues overlay the uneven surfaces of the skeletal structures, concealing the unattractive contours and giving the chest wall a full and visually pleasing appearance.④ Cushioning function: Since bones are rigid, any collision with external objects can easily cause damage. The soft tissue, located on the surface of the bones, provides excellent cushioning. This cushioning effect helps to absorb and mitigate external forces.⑤ Protective function: In addition to cushioning, soft tissues also serve to protect underlying structures. They form a barrier that reduces the risk of injury to both the bones and the internal organs housed within the chest. Soft tissues not only protect the bones of the chest wall from impact, but also safeguard important structures such as blood vessels and nerves within the chest wall, thus serving a strong protective function. ⑥ Blood supply function: The soft tissue contains a large number of blood vessels, which not only supply blood to the soft tissue itself, but also to all other structures of the chest wall, providing an excellent blood supply. ⑦ Nutritional function: The soft tissue is closely connected with all the structures of the chest wall, forming a unified whole. Because it provides an abundant blood supply, it also performs a strong nutritional function. From the above analysis, we can see that skin and soft tissue have important functions, and various problems will occur after being damaged.

Therefore, injuries to the skin and soft tissues must also be given due attention. However, in past literature on thoracic trauma, skin and soft tissue injuries have been rarely mentioned [2], and this aspect is almost entirely absent in specialized thoracic Surgery textbooks. Thoracic wall Surgery focuses on diseases affecting the entire chest wall; therefore, skin and soft tissue injuries are also a subject of study within thoracic wall Surgery.

2. Pathological changes

The skin is the body's first line of defence. When the skin is damaged, if the injury is mild, it may be limited to the skin alone, but if the injury is severe, the soft tissues may also be affected. There are many factors that can lead to skin and soft tissue injuries. Any factor that causes trauma to the chest wall can result in damage to the skin and soft tissues. Therefore, the causes of such injuries are not specific.

In terms of the nature of the injury, skin and soft tissue injuries have traditionally been classified into three types: contusions, lacerations, and contused lacerations. This classification has been widely accepted for many years and is still commonly used in most textbooks today. However, this classification is incomplete, as it lacks the most severe type of tissue loss. When the chest wall is subjected to extremely severe external force, the skin and soft tissues may be completely torn away, leaving a clear defect on the chest wall [1]. Such injuries are clearly different from other types of trauma and require greater attention from thoracic wall Surgeons.

A contusion is a specific type of injury primarily caused by lateral external force. While the skin is being compressed, there is also lateral friction, resulting in a relatively large area of damage. This type of injury can be quite deep, but there is no obvious structural tearing. The injury mainly disrupts the fine structures of the skin, while the main framework remains intact, and the basic shape of the skin can still be seen. After a contusion occurs, the wound surface may show signs such as petechiae, bruising, exudation, and swelling, but there is typically no major bleeding. The wound is often contaminated; if treated promptly, it will scab over quickly. Otherwise, it may lead to infection of the wound, with the potential to invade deeper tissues.

A laceration is a more localized type of injury, typically caused by sharp objects. The skin structure is cut open, forming a deep groove in which the full thickness of the skin is severed [3]. The damage is mainly concentrated within the wound itself. Due to the rich blood supply, there is often bleeding from the wound. Compared to contusions, lacerations are generally more severe.

A contused laceration falls between a contusion and a laceration. The injuring force is usually more intense, causing both bruising and a structural break in the skin, thereby combining features of both contusions and lacerations. As such, a contused laceration is essentially a compound type of injury. When a contused laceration occurs, the wound may show a combination of symptoms, including extensive surface bleeding and exudation, along with bleeding from the laceration itself. Although it lies between a contusion and a laceration in classification, it is not merely a transitional form from one to the other; it is the sum of both injuries. Therefore, it is considered more severe.

Soft tissue lies beneath the skin, and when it is damaged especially in cases of open trauma it is usually accompanied by severe skin injury, often with clearly visible skin loss. Therefore, contusions, lacerations, and contused lacerations of the soft tissue are generally more severe than those affecting only the skin.

In addition to open injuries, soft tissue damage can also occur in cases of closed chest wall trauma, primarily caused by the direct impact of strong external forces. Due to the skin's high elasticity, no external wound may be visible, but deeper soft tissues can still be injured. In such cases, contusions may also occur, although they are not visible on the surface. Local symptoms may include significant swelling and the presence of localized hematoma. Almost all closed chest wall injuries involve soft tissue damage, which may occur alongside damage to bony structures or independently. In addition to open injuries, soft tissue damage can also occur in cases of closed chest wall trauma, primarily caused by the direct impact of strong external forces. Due to the skin's high elasticity, no external wound may be visible, but deeper soft tissues can still be injured. In such cases, contusions may also occur, although they are not visible on the surface. Local symptoms may include significant swelling and the presence of localized hematoma [4]. Almost all closed chest wall injuries involve soft tissue damage, which may occur alongside damage to bony structures or independently.

Defect is the most severe type of skin and soft tissue injury. This type of injury can be caused by a variety of factors, but they all share one common feature: the force involved is sufficiently intense. The extent of skin and soft tissue loss can vary in both size and depth. Since blood vessels exist in all layers of the chest wall, when a local defect occurs, these vessels are torn, resulting in bleeding. At the edges of the defect, different tissue layers can be observed.

3. Clinical manifestations

The primary symptom of skin and soft tissue injury is pain [1]. Since the injury is located on the body surface, it can be accurately localized. If the injury is severe, the pain may worsen during respiratory movements. In cases of significant tissue loss, especially when the thoracic cavity is involved, symptoms such as difficulty breathing and chest tightness may occur. If there is substantial local bleeding, signs of circulatory dysfunction may also appear. The physical signs of skin and soft tissue injuries are usually quite apparent, with varying degrees of damage visible on the chest wall, making them generally easy to identify.

4. Inspection

When patients with skin and soft tissue injuries are seen in clinical settings, a diagnosis can generally be made based on symptoms and physical signs. However, such a diagnosis is clearly insufficient, as skin and soft tissue injuries are often only superficial manifestations. The patient may also have underlying injuries involving deeper layers of the chest wall or even the thoracic cavity [4], which must be diagnosed concurrently. Additionally, in cases of extremely severe trauma, the possibility of injuries to other distant parts of the body must also be considered.

5. Diagnosis

When patients with skin and soft tissue injuries are seen in clinical practice, a diagnosis can generally be made based on symptoms and physical signs. However, such a diagnosis is clearly not sufficient, as skin and soft tissue injuries are often just surface manifestations. The patient may also have injuries involving the deeper layers of the chest wall or even the thoracic cavity, which must be diagnosed simultaneously [1]. Furthermore, in cases of extremely severe trauma, it is important to consider the possibility of injuries to other, more distant parts of the body.

6. Treatment

The treatment of skin and soft tissue injuries is influenced by many factors. The therapeutic approaches vary greatly depending on the severity of the injury; therefore, in clinical practice, it is essential to assess each case carefully to determine the most appropriate treatment strategy.

In the specific treatment process, appropriate treatment must be made according to the specific situation [1].

1. Simple skin contusion: Such injuries do not require Surgical treatment,

only the wound surface needs to be cleaned and the dressings changed regularly. Since there are a lot of exudations in the early stage of the wound, it can be considered to cover it with vaseline gauze. In the treatment process, the wound surface must be thoroughly decontaminated and the principle of aseptic treatment must be paid attention to. This is the key to wound healing. When the wound surface is large, the patient may have systemic symptoms and need to be treated accordingly.

2. Simple skin laceration: Although skin laceration injures the entire skin layer, it is only a relatively shallow trauma to the chest wall. The key to treatment is to thoroughly clean the wound and then suture it directly.
3. Simple skin contusion and laceration: This type of injury covers a larger area, but only the local skin is completely torn, with an obvious crack. The first step in treatment is to thoroughly clean the wound, the second step is to suture the crack, and the third step is to cover it with vaseline gauze and change the dressing regularly.
4. Skin and soft tissue contusion: When the contusion is severe and extends into the soft tissue, there may be localized skin loss. If the defect is small, primary wound closure can be performed after debridement. If direct suturing is difficult, wound dressing changes can be used initially to allow gradual healing of the skin defect. If healing remains problematic in the later stages, flap techniques may be required for treatment.
5. Skin and soft tissue laceration: When a skin laceration extends deeply into the soft tissue, it may cause more profound damage within the wound. In such cases, the first step is still thorough debridement, during which the interior of the wound must be carefully explored. If no critical structures are damaged especially after ruling out deep bony injuries direct suturing can be performed.
6. Contusion and laceration of skin and soft tissue: This type of injury is more severe, often involving skin defects, significant soft tissue contusion, and localized lacerations. Treatment in such cases is more complex and must be tailored to the specific circumstances. The first step remains thorough debridement. After debridement, if the wounds are relatively localized, the skin can be pulled together and sutured directly. However, if the affected area is extensive, skin flap techniques will be required for proper reconstruction and healing.
7. Skin and soft tissue defect: When a true defect occurs, it indicates severe damage to the surrounding structures. The first step in management is thorough debridement, which includes four key tasks: removing contaminated foreign materials, excising necrotic tissue, eliminating fully detached tissue, and trimming the wound edges.

After debridement, if the defect is relatively small, direct suturing may be possible. However, if direct closure is too difficult or not feasible, reconstructive Surgery will be necessary. Due to the risk of contamination, reconstructive procedures are often performed at a later, planned stage.

8. Soft tissue injury in closed chest wall trauma: If the injury is accompanied by damage to bony structures, the soft tissue issues such as local hematomas can be addressed during the related Surgical procedure. If the soft tissue damage is severe, partial removal of the affected tissue may be necessary. If the damage is not serious, no additional intervention is required. In cases of isolated soft tissue injury without associated bone damage, conservative treatment is usually sufficient.
9. Skin and soft tissue injuries combined with intrathoracic organ damage: In such cases, priority must be given to treating the intrathoracic organ injuries. Once those are managed, appropriate treatment for the skin and soft tissue injuries should be carried out based on their condition.

Except for closed soft tissue injuries, all other types of skin and soft tissue injuries are open wounds, and thus require debridement. On this basis, if there are lacerations or defects in the skin or soft tissue, reconstructive procedures must be performed to manage the wound. In previous thoracic Surgeries, this aspect was rarely emphasized, leading to inconsistent treatment methods and generally unsatisfactory outcomes. However, if managed with the principles of plastic and reconstructive Surgery, the results can be significantly improved.

This is the biggest difference between chest wall Surgery and traditional thoracic Surgery.

The purpose of plastic Surgery is to achieve a more aesthetic effect. This effect is often more significant for skin and soft tissue injuries. In order to achieve this goal, it is essential to fully apply the principles of plastic and reconstructive Surgery during the actual procedures. Only by doing so can the quality of trauma care be significantly improved.

The skin and soft tissue serve as the gateway to the chest wall and thoracic cavity, and many injuries to the chest wall and thoracic organs involve damage to these tissues. Compared to other injuries, skin and soft tissue injuries are often underestimated due to their seemingly less severe nature. However, this can undoubtedly affect the overall management of related injuries. As outlined above, treating such injuries requires considerable effort. By giving adequate attention to skin and soft tissue damage alongside the treatment of other injuries the overall effectiveness of chest wall trauma care can be significantly improved.

REFERENCES

[1] Wang, W. L. 2021. "Skin and Soft Tissue Injuries in Chest Wall Trauma." *Toutiao Today*, November 4.
[2] Dogrul, B. N., I. Kiliccalan, E. S. Asci, et al. 2020. "Blunt Trauma-Related Chest Wall and Pulmonary Injuries: An Overview." *Chinese Journal of Traumatology* 23 (3): 125–138.
[3] Swann, I. J., R. Macmillan, and A. A. Watson. 1985. "A Study of Stab Wounds." *Archives of Emergency Medicine* 2 (1): 31–36.
[4] Oikonomou, A., and P. Prassopoulos. 2011. "CT Imaging of Blunt Chest Trauma." *Insights into Imaging* 2 (3): 281–295.

When traditional thoracic Surgery treats chest trauma, the main consideration is to cure the disease, that is, to save lives, and less consideration is given to aesthetic issues. There is almost no professional book that specifically focuses on aesthetic issues when discussing the treatment of chest trauma. However, the work of chest wall Surgery is completely different. Chest wall trauma Surgery belongs to chest wall Surgery, so it must follow the chest wall Surgery procedure. The general principle of Surgery is to both treat the injury and perform reconstruction [1,2]. Treating the injury primarily refers to trauma management, while reconstruction aims to achieve a cosmetically pleasing result. In the face of trauma care, aesthetic considerations may seem secondary. However, for milder injuries or those that do not pose a threat to the patient's life, the patient has the right to expect a more aesthetically satisfying outcome. Therefore, in the management of chest wall trauma. During the process, chest wall Surgeons should have a completely new concept and should not use the traditional thoracic Surgery concept to deal with chest wall trauma. This is also the biggest difference between chest wall Surgeons and thoracic Surgeons

1. The Relationship Between Treatment and reconstruction

After a chest wall injury occurs, the harm caused by the trauma itself is a matter of utmost concern. At this stage, the fundamental purpose of Surgery is to treat the injury, that is, the therapeutic aspect of chest wall Surgery. When the trauma is extremely critical, saving the patient's life becomes the overriding task, and in such cases, cost and consequences become secondary considerations. The "cost" mentioned here includes the aesthetic appearance of the chest wall. For example, in cases of chest wall trauma combined with cardiac rupture, due to the urgency of the situation, immediate thoracotomy is required to stop the bleeding. In such scenarios, the chest can be opened using the most primitive method at the fastest speed to address the cardiac rupture [3]. This is the most effective life-saving measure. At this point, it is impossible to give much consideration to cosmetic outcomes. If hesitation arises due to aesthetic concerns, it could result in a missed opportunity to rescue the patient, ultimately leading to loss of life. This clearly shows that when trauma is extremely severe, saving the patient's life takes precedence, and aesthetic considerations can be completely disregarded. However, such urgent cases are relatively rare. Especially for most chest wall injuries, there is usually enough time for the Surgeon to take postoperative aesthetics into account. Therefore, it is very necessary to consider cosmetic outcomes [4]. When weighing the relationship between treatment and aesthetics, life-saving must come first, followed by aesthetic concerns; this is the basic principle in the management of chest wall trauma.

2. Specific embodiment of plastic surgery concept

The concept of plastic Surgery is a habit. For a well-qualified chest wall Surgeon, this habit should be reflected in every operation at any time, without the need for regulations, reminders, or mandatory implementation. Every step in the trauma treatment process should be guided by the principles of reconstructive Surgery.

(1) Emphasis on Proper Incision Technique

The implementation of the incision is the most direct reflection of reconstructive principles. Since every incision results in a postoperative scar, focusing on aesthetic outcomes requires careful design and execution of the incision. In traditional thoracic Surgery trauma care, doctors often focus solely on treating the injury and rarely give much thought to the choice or technique of the Surgical incision. If aesthetic concerns are ignored and only treatment is considered, certain incisions might facilitate the Surgical procedure. However, overly careless incisions can leave very unattractive scars, which can significantly impact the postoperative appearance of the chest wall. Within reasonable limits, if Surgeons incorporate more reconstructive considerations into their incision planning and execution, the results can be drastically different. This approach undoubtedly offers many benefits to the patient.

(1) Incision considerations for open wounds [2] for open chest wall trauma, since the skin is already broken and the wound itself requires trimming, the existing wound should be used as much as possible to make the incision. Such an incision is often located near the deeper injured structures, which facilitates exposing the damaged area. If the wound is far from the site of deeper Surgical intervention, the incision can be made elsewhere; however, it is still advisable to utilize the skin wound whenever possible, as it may aid in exposure or assist with other Surgical manoeuvres.

(2) The problem of incision for closed trauma [2]. The location of closed chest wall trauma is uncertain, and the implementation of the incision should first be determined according to the operation site. If the plastic Surgery issue is not taken into consideration, the incision must be made directly on the surface of the injury, but this may cause extremely serious plastic Surgery problems. For example, for a fracture of the manubrium sternum, if the incision is made through the median sternum, the top of the incision should exceed the suprasternal fossa, which is the best incision position to expose the fracture. However, the incision here is just above the collar, and most of the clothes you wear on a daily basis cannot cover the postoperative scar. Such an incision is

obviously not an ideal incision. If you want to avoid such scars, the design can be done from two aspects. One is to move the upper end of the incision downward as much as possible, and the other is to use a transverse incision. This can ensure that the postoperative scar is as hidden as possible and does not cause a big aesthetic problem. For example, the treatment of rib fractures on the anterior chest wall of adult women. Due to the cover of the breast, it is not easy to reveal the fracture site. If the postoperative aesthetic problem is not considered, the incision can be made from any part above or around the breast. Such an incision is definitely closer to the operation site. However, such an incision is not ideal because it may not only damage the breast structure, but also cause obvious scars on the anterior chest wall. These are not aesthetically pleasing operations, so they should not be performed at will. The principle of closed chest wall trauma Surgery is to make the incision as short and hidden as possible while ensuring exposure. The most hidden part of the chest wall is the armpit, followed by the lateral chest wall. The more hidden parts of women also include the folds of the skin under the breast. These parts are the incision locations that need to be given priority. Only when there are problems with the incision at these locations are incisions at other locations considered.

(3) Wound trimming [2]. Open wounds have clear skin wounds. If the wound is caused by a sharp object, the edges of the incision are relatively neat; if the wound is caused by an irregular object, the wound may have irregular edges. Such wounds must be trimmed when they are finally sutured, otherwise a very unsightly scar will remain. When trimming the wound, the shape and position of the postoperative scar need to be considered to obtain the most aesthetically pleasing effect.

(4) Protect the incision as much as possible during the operation. When making an incision through a wound, the wound itself has already damaged the skin. If the skin is not well protected, the incision may be damaged during the pulling process, which will not only affect the healing of the incision, but also may cause larger scars after the operation.

(5) Suturing issues. Many Surgeons pay little attention to suturing the incision after treating trauma, and generally use ordinary silk thread for intermittent suturing. If there is no special need for the healing of the incision, this suturing method will undoubtedly cause more obvious scars. If the doctor has some plastic Surgery ideas, he will not be suturing so carelessly. This is actually a basic reflection of the doctor's habits or quality.

(2) Focus on preserving the organization

Chest wall trauma can affect various chest wall tissues and structures, which may not only be damaged, but also contaminated, necrotic and other changes. During Surgery, these structures and tissues need to be handled decisively. However, as part of the chest wall structure, the existence of any structure and tissue is necessary. If not handled properly, it will also affect the effect of postoperative plastic Surgery, so special attention must be paid.

1. Preserve soft tissue to the maximum extent [2]: Soft tissue plays a very important role in the chest wall. During trauma treatment, if soft tissue needs to be removed due to problems with the soft tissue itself, it is necessary to be extremely cautious and preserve as much soft tissue as possible. This is not only related to the healing of the incision, but also directly affects the appearance of the chest wall after Surgery. This is an issue that must be highly valued during plastic Surgery.
2. Do not remove bone easily [2]: In chest wall trauma, fractures sometimes committed can lead to segments of bone becoming completely detached. Some believe these segments should be removed without hesitation, but this approach is debatable. The bony structure of the thoracic cage is an organically integrated whole, and no part of it is redundant. Arbitrarily removing a section of bone can result in a localized defect, which is a major taboo in chest wall Surgery. Therefore, when conditions permit, bone should be preserved as much as possible not only to help maintain the structural integrity of the thoracic cage after Surgery but also to avoid defects that could affect the chest wall's appearance.
3. Preserve the skin as much as possible [2]: In chest wall trauma, skin damage is common. The skin may suffer from lacerations, contusions, or even large-scale tears, resulting in irregular skin flaps with narrow bases at the wound site. In cases of laceration, the wound edges are usually neat, making treatment relatively straightforward. However, in cases of severe contusion, the skin structure may be seriously damaged. Inexperienced doctors may remove the affected skin, but this is actually a major mistake in treating contusions. Even though the skin is contused even though the skin is contused, it does not mean it is completely necrotic. Its basic structure still exists, and with proper treatment, it can be fully repaired. Therefore, such skin must not be removed. Likewise, skin flaps caused by tearing should not be excised lightly. On the basis of thorough debridement, all skin should be preserved as much as possible. This not only promotes wound healing but also contributes to achieving a better cosmetic outcome

(3) Focus on the overall contour of the chest wall

The purpose of plastic Surgery is to achieve as normal or aesthetically pleasing a chest wall appearance as possible. The core structure for maintaining the appearance of the chest wall is the chest wall itself. The thoracic cage, which is the bony structure of the chest wall, is the core component in maintaining the chest wall's appearance, and must therefore be given special attention during trauma management. In addition to the thoracic cage, the soft tissue and skin of the chest wall also contribute to the overall appearance, so they must likewise be given sufficient attention during Surgery.

1. Bone fixation must not result in deformity [2]. One of the key aspects of chest wall trauma is damage to the bony structure of the chest wall, commonly referred to as fractures. Fracture fixation must follow basic orthopaedic principles. If these principles are violated, various issues may arise, one of which is malunion (deformity during healing). Such deformities inevitably affect the contour of the entire chest wall. Malunion can occur during Surgical treatment or conservative management. A typical example is the conservative treatment of flail chest. Some practitioners use localized compression to eliminate paradoxical breathing. This method essentially acts as an external fixation for the fracture, but the result of such fixation may still lead to deformity. However, it is not ideal and will inevitably cause local secondary concave deformity, which will undoubtedly seriously affect the appearance of the chest wall. It can be seen that when implementing fracture fixation, the fixed bone must be restored to its original shape. This is the most basic requirement, otherwise the fixation will not be perfect. The fixation of the flail chest is a helpless move. If you want to avoid concave deformity, you must decisively implement Surgical fixation and completely abandon conservative treatment.
2. If there is a defect, reconstruction is required [2]. Chest wall trauma may cause complete destruction of various structures and tissues. These damaged components sometimes need to be entirely removed. After removal, defects may remain in the chest wall. These defects not only affect the appearance but also impair the patient's physiological function and can significantly impact their quality of life. Therefore, if a defect exists, reconstruction should be performed whenever possible. The reconstruction may involve rebuilding the bony
3. structure alone or include reconstruction of soft tissue and skin. For soft tissue and skin reconstruction, the use of flaps must be considered. If adjacent soft tissue and skin are insufficient for Surgical needs, other flap options should be explored for reconstruction.

3.Aesthetic Considerations

Plastic Surgery is the modification of the chest wall shape in order to obtain an ideal shape. Since the clinical manifestations of various chest wall injuries are relatively complex, the effects of plastic Surgery are bound to be different. According to the different plastic Surgery effects, it can be divided into different levels [2]. Primary plastic Surgery can ensure basic physiological functions and make the chest wall shape close to normal. Intermediate plastic Surgery can make the chest wall shape basically normal on the basis of ensuring physiological functions. The highest level of plastic Surgery has additional aesthetic requirements, so that the final chest wall appearance is not only normal but also more beautiful. Such plastic Surgery is actually equivalent to beauty treatment.

In the process of trauma treatment, if the trauma is serious, primary plastic Surgery is a more reasonable plastic Surgery. If the trauma is not serious, the intermediate level of plastic Surgery should be achieved as much as possible. of course, if the highest level of plastic Surgery can be achieved, it will be the most satisfactory result, but such an effect is generally difficult to obtain.

REFERENCES

[1] Wang Wenlin. The Fundamental Nature of Chest Wall Surgery. Toutiao (Jinri Toutiao), 2021-10-31.

[2] Wang Wenlin. Issues In The Management of Chest Wall Trauma Wounds. Toutiao (Jinri Toutiao), 2021-11-04.

[3] González-Hadad A, Ordonez C A, Parra M W, Et Al. Damage Control In Penetrating Cardiac Trauma. Colomb Med (Cali), 2021, 52 (2): E4034519.

[4] Dogrul B N, Kiliccalan I, Asci E S, Et Al. Blunt Trauma Related Chest Wall and Pulmonary Injuries: An Overview. Chin J Traumatol, 2020, 23 (3): 125-138.

Section 9

APPLICATION OF THORACOSCOPIC IN CHEST WALL TRAUMA SURGERY

The development of thoracic Surgery has entered the era of minimally invasive Surgery, the main feature of which is the use of thoracoscopy. A thoracoscope is a device used to perform intrathoracic operations. The chest wall is located on the surface of the chest cavity, and almost all operations can be performed directly through the body surface. Therefore, a thoracoscope is generally not required in chest wall Surgery. However, since chest wall trauma is often accompanied by damage to the thoracic organs, this provides the possibility for the use of thoracoscopy [1,2]. Theoretically, there is only one situation in which a thoracoscopy is suitable for chest wall trauma, that is, when there is an open wound on the chest wall accompanied by damage to the thoracic organs. In this case, if thoracoscopy is not used, a long open incision would be required to perform operations inside the thoracic cavity. If such a long incision is made solely for thoracic procedures, the trauma from the incision itself may exceed the trauma from the original chest wall injury. This is highly unfavorable for the patient, thus providing sufficient justification for the use of thoracoscopy. Apart from this scenario, there seemed to be no other suitable indications for thoracoscopy. This viewpoint was once widely accepted. However, any concept can evolve with technological advancements, and the application of thoracoscopy has also changed accordingly. Once rib fracture Surgeries under thoracoscopy became feasible, thoracoscopy. The concept of mirror use has finally changed [2-6]. Today's concept believes that the following situations are suitable for thoracoscopy: ① Simple rib fractures; ② Rib fractures combined with thoracic organ injuries;③ Chest wall trauma is relatively limited, but combined with thoracic organ injuries.

Chest wall trauma is located on the body surface, so performing operations directly from the external surface is the most logical choice. However, it was discovered some time ago that rib fixation can be performed on the inner surface of the rib. This kind of procedure reconnects chest wall Surgery with thoracic cavity Surgery, giving a new justification for the use of thoracoscopy. On this basis, if thoracic organ injuries are also present, the rationale for using thoracoscopy becomes even stronger. Aside from rib fractures, other types of chest wall injuries cannot be treated from within the thoracic cavity using thoracoscopy. Therefore, in cases where these other injuries are accompanied by internal thoracic organ damage, the justification for using thoracoscopy is not as strong.

1. Thoracoscopic rib fracture Surgery

(1) Feasibility

As mentioned above, there are three situations in chest wall trauma where thoracoscopy is appropriate, but there is only one case in which thoracoscopy directly participates in the treatment of chest wall trauma, that is the fixation of rib fractures. In traditional chest wall Surgery, rib fractures are always. Direct fixation through an incision on the chest wall surface, using thoracoscopy, has overturned the traditional Surgical concept [2,3]. However, if the operational details are carefully studied, it becomes evident that this type of Surgery is highly feasible [6]: ① Convenient exposure. The inner surface of the rib has only one layer of parietal pleura, and the intercostal space contains only a thin layer of intercostal muscle. These structural characteristics make exposure through the inner surface very easy, and dissection is also very convenient. Compared to exposure through the body surface, performing rib dissection from within the thoracic cavity causes less structural damage, thus better meeting the requirements of minimally invasive Surgery.② Feasible fixation.at present, rib fracture fixation. There are three methods for fixation. If fixation is performed from within the thoracic cavity, intramedullary fixation presents certain difficulties. Fixation using a steel plate on the cortical surface mainly depends on securing the screws; this procedure can be accomplished with proper design. The encircling (embracing-type)

A fixation plate is a very simple technique if applied from the inner surface, the operation is not complex. ③ Technical support.in recent years, thoracoscopic technology has developed significantly, enabling the performance of complex intrathoracic Surgical procedures with this technique. Although fixation on the inner surface of the rib presents certain challenges, it is not significantly more difficult than other intrathoracic Surgical procedures, and therefore can be performed with ease. ④ Materials and instruments assurance fixation of rib fractures within the thoracic cavity requires specialized materials and instruments. In recent years, substantial progress has been made in related research and development, which can adequately meet the needs of the Surgery. This provides an additional guarantee for the successful completion of the procedure.

(2) Advantages

The feasibility of completing rib fracture fixation assisted by thoracoscopy objectively exists. Driven by various factors, it has quickly become a clinical reality. At present, it has been used clinically with several types of materials, and many hospitals have performed such Surgeries with gratifying results. Compared to rib fracture fixation Surgery under direct vision, thoracoscopic Surgery has obvious advantages, which include [3-6]:

1. Minimally invasive: The minimal trauma of performing rib fracture fixation under thoracoscopy is not only reflected in the reduction of the incision itself but more importantly in the reduction of trauma during the exposure of the fracture. The ribs at the fracture site exposed inside the thoracic cavity do not require a large incision over the fracture surface, nor do they require transection of the muscles over the fracture, nor extensive dissection. Therefore, the trauma is significantly reduced. Additionally, because the operation can be completed entirely through the thoracoscope's working port, strong traction on the incision is not necessary, thus avoiding traction-related injury to the incision site. Overall, the trauma is significantly less than that of fixation under direct vision.
2. Aesthetic: When performing rib fracture fixation under direct vision, an incision is generally made on the surface. To facilitate exposure, the incision often needs to extend beyond the fracture site. Such incisions are not only easily exposed but also tend to be long, resulting in unsightly postoperative scars. However, when rib fracture fixation is performed using thoracoscopy, the principle of aesthetics can be fully followed by selecting the incision in a relatively concealed area of the lateral chest wall. Since the incision itself is just a small port on the chest wall, its length can be kept sufficiently short. These factors better meet aesthetic requirements, making the postoperative results more acceptable to patients.
3. Convenient exposure: When performing rib fracture fixation under direct vision, although fractures in most areas can be exposed relatively well, fractures in certain specific locations are difficult to expose for example, fractures deep within the female breast tissue or on the deep surface of the scapula. Exposure in these areas is very challenging. To expose these fractures, incisions must be made some distance away to allow for remote exposure. Although such exposure is feasible, it requires a larger incision; otherwise, exposure is nearly impossible. However, in thoracoscopic Surgery, through the thoracic cavity. The exposure of the ribs in these areas is very convenient, making the operation simple and easy to perform. This is an advantage that open Surgery cannot match.
4. High efficiency: In addition to directly treating rib fractures, thoracoscopic Surgery also allows for the examination of injuries inside the thoracic cavity. If there is damage to internal thoracic organs, it can be addressed directly. Therefore, this type of Surgery is highly efficient, and the advantages of thoracoscopic Surgery can be maximized.

(3) Disadvantages

Using thoracoscopy to perform rib fracture fixation has many advantages. However, no procedure can be perfect, especially when it comes to a newly introduced clinical technique like this one it inevitably has many shortcomings. These shortcomings include the following aspects [6]:

1. High technical threshold, hindering widespread adoption. Thoracoscopic Surgery is a technique that requires specialized training, and using this technique for fracture management also demands corresponding training. Due to the high technical requirements, it undoubtedly increases the cost of learning. Additionally, because the Surgery requires special materials and instruments, it is difficult for general hospitals to carry out this technique. However, most of the institutions currently managing rib fractures are primary-level hospitals. For such hospitals to adopt this technique, they would face even greater challenges. This represents a contradiction between technology and demand. If doctors in primary-level hospitals are unable to master the technique within a certain period, they may be more inclined to continue using traditional open fixation Surgery.
2. High Surgical costs, difficult for patients to afford. Thoracoscopic Surgery inherently involves higher expenses. Performing fracture fixation under thoracoscopy requires specific instruments and materials, all of which are relatively expensive, significantly increasing the overall cost of the procedure. If most patients cannot afford the cost of this technique, it will hinder the widespread adoption of the technology.

3. Management of rib fractures in certain areas is relatively difficult. Although thoracoscopy provides a good view within the thoracic cavity, this is a relative concept. Once the thoracoscope is fixed in position, there are still blind spots in the field of view. To expose certain specific areas, it is sometimes necessary to make incisions in unusual locations. These incision sites may affect the aesthetic appearance of the skin after Surgery. On the other hand, if incisions are kept in more concealed areas for cosmetic reasons, exposing some regions becomes problematic, which undoubtedly affects the Surgical operation in those areas. Therefore, when performing rib fracture fixation under thoracoscopy, exposing fractures in certain locations is not easy, which directly impacts the fixation procedure. Compared to open fixation under direct vision, this is a significant disadvantage.
4. Certain types of rib fractures cannot be fixed. In most cases, the fractured ends of the ribs are long enough to provide a structural basis for fixation Surgery. However, some rib fractures are extremely severe

for example, laminated fractures making fixation very difficult. For such fractures, if one insists on completing the fixation under thoracoscopy, it is unlikely to achieve satisfactory results.

5. Fixation may not be secure. Rib fixation is generally performed using instruments, but ultimately it requires significant force. When fixation is done through thoracoscopy, the operating site is relatively far from the fracture, which limits the amount of force that can be applied. Insufficient force makes it difficult to achieve secure fixation. If we also consider certain inherent flaws in the fixation materials, achieving firm fixation can sometimes become unrealistic. Additionally, the effectiveness of fixation is closely related to the physical properties of the rib itself. If the rib is relatively thin or has a porous texture, it is equally difficult to secure the fixation. When performing thoracoscopic Surgery on such rib fractures, the expected fixation results are poor. If the Surgery cannot even achieve basic stabilization, the overall outcome is inevitably compromised.
6. The procedure is relatively difficult. No matter how skilled one is in using thoracoscopic techniques, it is undeniable that this method is significantly more difficult than open fixation under direct vision. The development of any medical technique should move in a direction that facilitates its application. However, performing rib fracture fixation using thoracoscopy seems to go against this trend, and this will be another major obstacle to its widespread adoption.
7. The procedure is more complicated. Thoracoscopic Surgery itself requires more steps and preparation of additional materials and instruments. Compared to open Surgery, thoracoscopic procedures are inherently more complex. If rib fracture fixation is performed using thoracoscopy, the complexity increases even further. The development of good techniques generally follows the path of simplification, but thoracoscopic rib fracture fixation does not align with this major trend, and thus is prone to scepticism.
8. Materials cannot be removed. Currently, most materials used for rib fracture fixation require a second Surgery for removal. If materials fixed under thoracoscopy need to be removed, the difficulty of removing them through thoracoscopy is considerable; it would be a very challenging procedure. For this reason, materials used today are generally not removed. However, not removing the materials inevitably brings related issues, and if these problems cannot be resolved, they will likewise limit the use of this Surgery.

(4) Prospects

Thoracoscopic technology has developed into a highly mature technique today, and its use in rib fracture treatment has become a clear trend nothing can stop its adoption. However, since certain shortcomings still exist in the current application of this technology, it is necessary to continuously optimize it from multiple aspects and improve various conditions for its use. Only by doing so can the technique continue to mature and gain wider acceptance.

The problems that need to be improved in this technology are mainly concentrated in the following aspects [6]: ① Improvement of instruments. There are many problems with the instruments currently used in clinical practice. They can only guarantee the most basic operations, but cannot guarantee that the operations can be completed skillfully. Therefore, the improvement of instruments will be a task that needs special attention. ② Improvement of materials. Materials are directly used for fracture fixation. Since the requirements for fixation under thoracoscopic Surgery are higher, higher requirements are placed on fixation materials. This is also a content that must be continuously improved. ③ Improvement of technology. The improvement of technology is an all-round improvement, including the improvement of thoracoscopic technology itself and the improvement of fixation technology. Only when the technology is truly mature will more people accept it.

Overall, performing rib fracture Surgery under thoracoscopy has already become a trend, with many hospitals and doctors actively adopting this approach. As a new technology with numerous advantages, it is understandable that thoracoscopic Surgery is gaining popularity [6]. However, just because something is popular does not necessarily mean it is good, so it is important to stay clear-headed amidst the hype and avoid blindly following the trend. In other words, this procedure should not be used indiscriminately for every case of rib fracture. This is essentially an issue of Surgical indications. The core of this issue lies in comparing this technique with open rib fracture Surgery under direct vision. For fractures located in relatively superficial areas, the incision can be made directly over the injured site, making the Surgery extremely simple and convenient, with minimal trauma. In such cases, open Surgery under direct vision clearly has an advantage. Considering the size of the incision required for thoracoscopic Surgery and its various shortcomings, thoracoscopy does not offer any clear advantage in treating fractures in these areas. If there is no advantage, then there is no justification for using thoracoscopy. This shows that when choosing a Surgical method, one must calmly and comprehensively evaluate the situation. A comprehensive evaluation must be made to not blindly follow trends. Only by fully understanding the advantages and disadvantages of each Surgical approach can one make a rational and scientifically sound decision to achieve the most suitable outcome and ensure greater patient satisfaction. If thoracoscopic Surgery is used recklessly just to keep up with the trend, it may not only increase the cost and complexity of the procedure but also lead to Surgical failure which would be the greatest misfortune.

2. The Use of Thoracoscopy in Chest Wall Trauma Combined with Intrathoracic Organ Injury

There are two types of chest wall trauma combined with intrathoracic organ injury: one is open chest wall trauma, and the other is closed chest wall trauma. Simple open chest wall trauma requires Surgery through the chest wall wound, and such injuries cannot be treated with thoracoscopy. However, if an open trauma is combined with intrathoracic organ injury, the use of thoracoscopy may be necessary [2,6]. When the chest wall wound is large, both chest wall and intrathoracic injuries can be treated through the wound, and in such cases, there is no need for thoracoscopy. However, if the chest wall wound is small and there is intrathoracic injury, thoracoscopy may be considered in the case of closed chest wall trauma, if there are rib fractures combined with intrathoracic organ injuries, the use of thoracoscopy can also be considered. Although thoracoscopy can be used in both types of cases, its role differs significantly. In the first scenario (open trauma), thoracoscopy is used solely for managing intrathoracic organ injuries. In the second scenario (closed trauma), thoracoscopy is used not only to address intrathoracic organ injuries but also to treat rib fractures. Using thoracoscopy to manage intrathoracic organ injuries does not present special difficulties. The first step is to explore and identify the injuries, and the second step is to treat them. From a technical standpoint, this procedure generally does not

pose significant challenges. Only in cases of unusually severe and uncontrollable bleeding is an immediate thoracotomy required. Otherwise, all operations can be completed under thoracoscopy

Essentially, the management of intrathoracic organ injuries under thoracoscopy goes beyond the scope of chest wall Surgery. However, for chest wall trauma a special category within chest wall surgery, the treatment of complications is also part of the Surgeon's responsibilities. Therefore, it requires the attention of chest wall Surgeons as well.

Overall, thoracoscopy is a tool designed for intrathoracic Surgery and plays a limited role in chest wall Surgery. However, for certain chest wall injuries, if the use of thoracoscopy can provide greater benefits to the patient, its use is justified. Chest wall Surgeons should not reject it but rather actively learn to use it.

REFERENCES

[1] Fokin, A. A., N. Hus, and J. Wycech, et al. 2020. "Surgical Stabilization of Rib Fractures: Indications, Techniques, and Pitfalls." *JBJS Essential Surgical Techniques* 10 (2): e0032.

[2] Powell, L., J. Chai, A. Shaikh, et al. 2019. "Experience with Acute Diaphragmatic

Trauma and Multiple Rib Fractures Using Routine Thoracoscopy." *Journal of Thoracic Disease* 11 (Suppl 8): S1024–S1028.
[3] Bauman, Z. M., R. Beard, and S. Cemaj. 2021. "When Less Is More: A Minimally Invasive, Intrathoracic Approach to Surgical Stabilization of Rib Fractures." *Trauma Case Reports* 32: 100452.
[4] Pieracci, F. M. 2019. "Completely Thoracoscopic Surgical Stabilization of Rib Fractures: Can It Be Done and Is It Worth It?" *Journal of Thoracic Disease* 11 (Suppl 8): S1061–S1069.
[5] Bui, J. T., S. E. Browder, H. K. Wilson, et al. 2020. "Does Routine Uniportal Thoracoscopy during Rib Fixation Identify More Injuries and Impact Outcomes?" *Journal of Thoracic Disease* 12 (10): 5281–5288.
[6] Wang, W. L. 2021. "Surgical Issues in Rib Fracture Treatment under Thoracoscopy." *Toutiao Today*, November 3.

CHAPTER 6

CHEST WALL INFECTION

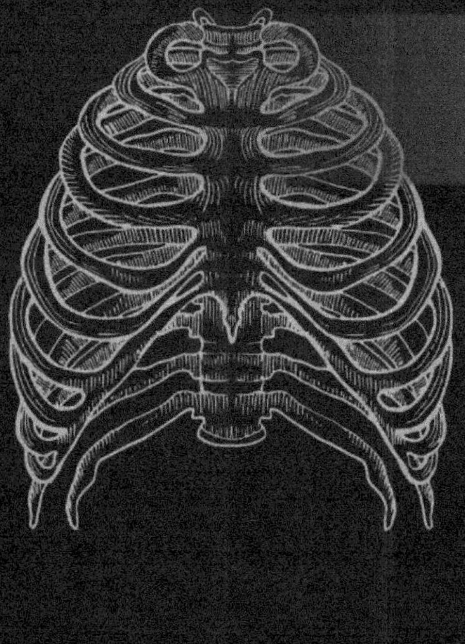

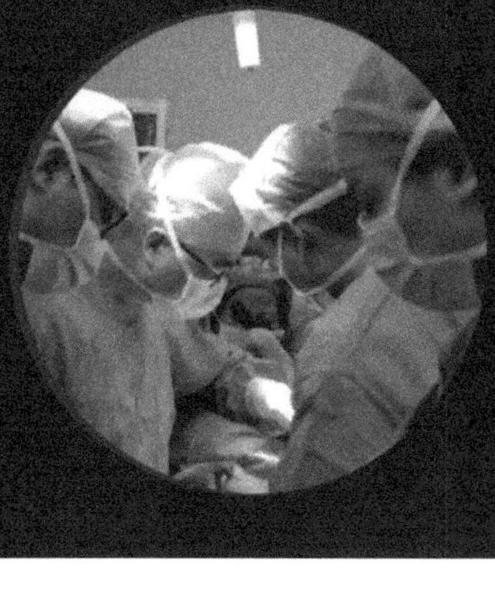

BASIC CONCEPTS OF CHEST WALL INFECTION

Chest wall infection is an important condition in chest wall Surgery, referring to infectious lesions that occur in the structures and tissues of the chest wall. The infection may be limited to the skin surface or may extend deep into the soft tissue and even the bony structures, involving the entire thickness of the chest wall [1-3]. The infection can present in various pathological forms, and in addition to local symptoms, it may also lead to severe systemic symptoms. If not treated promptly, it can result in serious consequences.

1. Classification

Chest wall infections can be classified from different perspectives. Based on the onset and course of the disease, chest wall infections can be divided into acute infections and chronic infections. Acute infections have a sudden onset with obvious local signs and systemic symptoms. Chronic infections may develop from unresolved acute infections; systemic symptoms are less pronounced, but local lesions tend to be more severe. According to the type of pathogens, chest wall infections can be classified into nonspecific infections and specific infections [2]. In most cases, the pathogens are common pyogenic bacteria, which are categorized as nonspecific infections [4,5]. In a minority of cases, the infections are caused by specific pathogens, such as tuberculosis, which is a typical example of a specific infection [3,6,7].

2. Causes

There are various causes of chest wall infection, with five being the most common: ① Trauma [2,8]. Trauma is a major cause of chest wall infection, with open chest wall injuries being the most frequent. After trauma, the wound is generally contaminated, and if debridement is inadequate, local infection may result. In some cases, infection does not appear in the early postoperative period but emerges later, which may be related to a latent lesion.② Surgery [9-12]. Surgery is another common cause of chest wall infection. An important factor is the contamination of the Surgical field by pathogens during the operation, leading to infection. If aseptic principles are not strictly followed during the procedure, or if there are issues with the sterilization of instruments, materials, or dressings, postoperative infections may occur. Postoperative infections are most commonly seen as incision infections following thoracotomy. When infection occurs, the incision typically becomes red and swollen initially. If treated promptly, the infection may be prevented from worsening. However, if the infection cannot be controlled, the incision may fail to heal and begin to produce purulent discharge.③ Occult infection [13]. Occult infections can also be considered primary infections. Their onset is insidious, with no clear cause. The most likely explanation is that an infection from another part of the body spreads through the bloodstream, although the primary source of infection is often difficult to identify. In clinical practice.

The most common is tuberculous chest wall infection, which can also be purulent. ④Direct transmission [14-16]. It is mainly caused by infection in the chest cavity. When there is an infection focus in the lungs or chest cavity, if it cannot be controlled in time, the infection may spread to the chest wall, leading to chest wall infection. This type of infection is often very serious. In addition to local symptoms, there are often obvious respiratory and even systemic symptoms. ⑤ Infection after tissue necrosis. When local chest wall tissue necrosis occurs for various reasons, it may lead to skin rupture. Once the rupture appears, the skin's protective barrier is completely lost, allowing pathogens to invade and cause infection. The most common type of tissue necrosis is the local necrosis of chest wall tumors. Tumor cells grow rapidly, and if the blood supply cannot meet the needs of cell growth, local ischemic necrosis may occur. When necrosis involves the skin, infection is likely to develop.

3. Susceptibility Factors

Under normal circumstances, the human body has strong resistance to infection. Therefore, the occurrence of chest wall infection should be considered a result of the contest between external pathogens and the body's immune defenses. Ultimately, infection arises because of a decline in immunity, accompanied by certain susceptibility factors. These factors include the following [11,17]: ① poor nutritional status nutrition directly influences the body's resistance. If a person suffers from prolonged malnutrition, their immune defenses weaken, allowing pathogens to invade. ② chronic diseases when the body suffers from chronic illnesses, resistance is reduced, increasing the likelihood of infection. For example, patients with diabetes or liver and kidney dysfunction often have significantly lower immunity, making them more prone to infection. ③ wasting diseases some cancer patients are severely debilitated, with diminished resistance, making them more susceptible to infection. ④ traumatic injury when the body undergoes trauma, resistance declines, providing an opportunity for infection. ⑤ Surgical trauma Surgery is a major stressor to the body and directly affects the patient's immune resistance, increasing the chance of infection compared to healthy individuals. ⑥ excessive fatigue when the body is overworked, immunity drops and infection risk rises significantly. In addition to the above, there are many other susceptibility factors that may reduce the body's resistance and provide an opportunity for pathogenic invasion

4. Pathology Changes

Chest wall infection lesions can start from the deep layer of the chest wall and gradually spread to the shallow layer; they can also start from the skin surface and invade the deep layer. From a pathological point of view, chest wall infection can have the following basic lesions [1,15,16]

(1) Local redness and swelling. Acute infection or early stage of infection may cause local redness and swelling, which is caused by inflammatory factors stimulating local blood vessels to increase exudation (Figure 6-1-1). If the infection is controlled in time, the redness and swelling can disappear; if the control is ineffective, other pathological changes may occur.

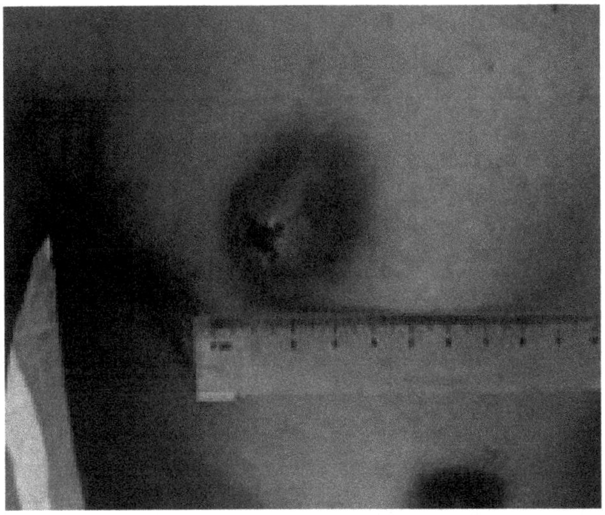

Figure 6-1-1 Localized Redness and Swelling

(2) Skin Ulceration. Infection may originate from the skin itself, either from previously healthy skin or from traumatic wounds. If superficial infections are not promptly controlled, localized skin ulceration may develop. These ulcerated areas typically exhibit purulent discharge and necrotic tissue, which are hallmark signs of skin infection. In more severe infections, the skin opening often serves as a passage between deeper infectious lesions and the external environment, with continuous purulent discharge. In serious cases, the ulceration may gradually enlarge, eventually resulting in tissue defects (Figure 6-1-2).

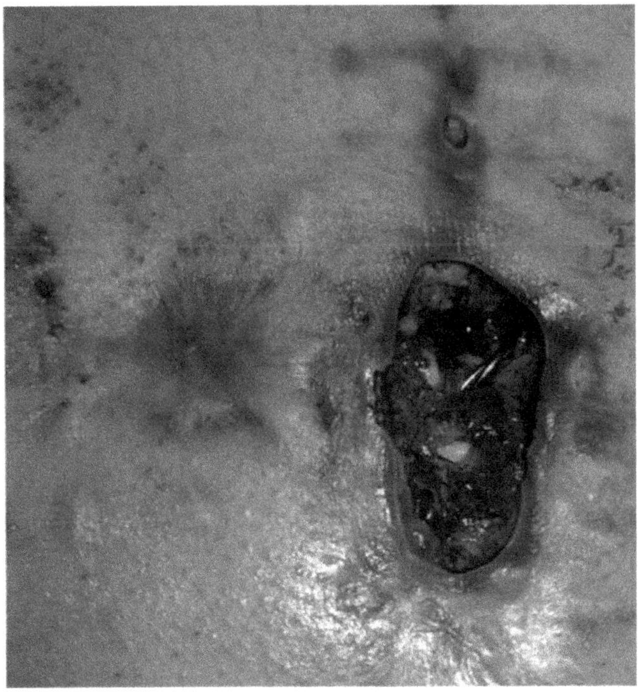

Figure 6-1-2 Skin Ulceration

(3) Fistula. A fistula is a fistula-like infection focus formed when a deep structure infection gradually breaks through the skin (Figure 6-1-3). The fistula is surrounded by necrotic tissue and infection focus, as well as fibrous tissue hyperplasia. Necrotic tissue provides

an environment for bacteria to grow, making it difficult for this lesion to heal on its own

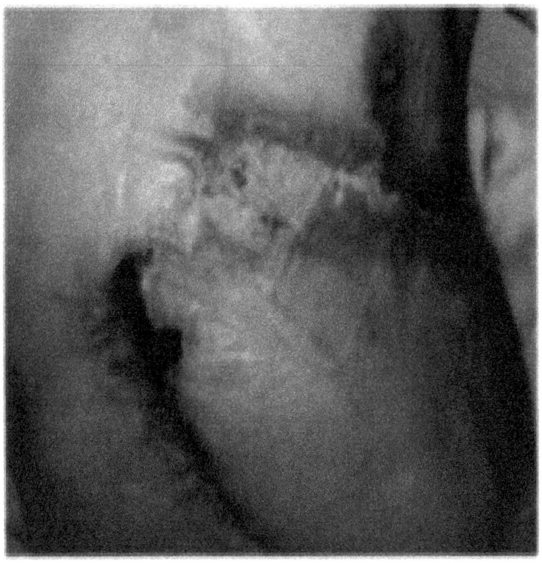

Figure 6-1-3 Fistula

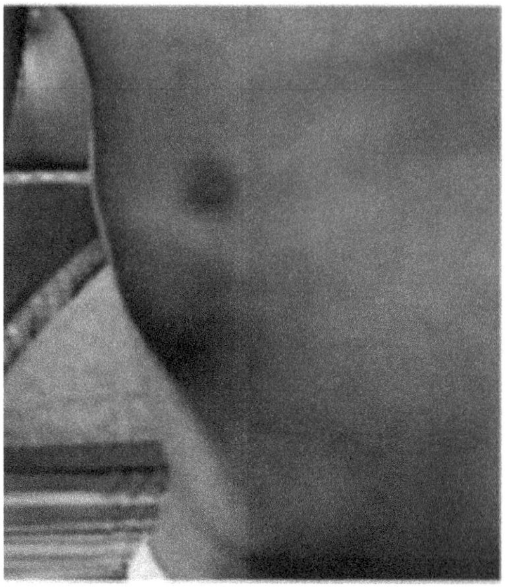

Figure 6-1-4 Abscess

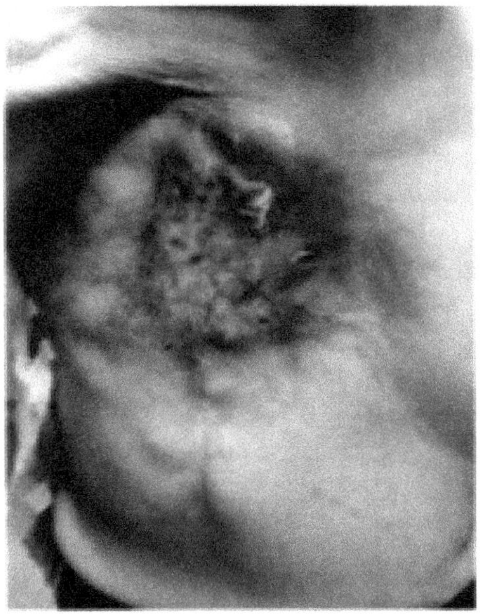

Figure 6-1-5 Local repeated infection, lesions

Invade deep structures, and form chronic osteomyelitis

(4) Abscess. An abscess is a severe, deep-seated infection in the chest wall, formed by pus and necrotic tissue encapsulated within fibrotic tissue (Figure 6-1-4). While the abscess can remain localized and persist for a long time, spontaneous absorption is nearly impossible. If the internal pus accumulates and pressure builds up excessively, the abscess may spread. The direction of spread may be inward into the chest wall, rupture into the pleural cavity, or extend outward through the skin. Once the abscess ruptures, it results in a skin breach with continuous purulent discharge, which fails to heal the cover time.
(5) Osteomyelitis. When the bony structures become infected, osteomyelitis may develop. Once osteomyelitis occurs, it often becomes a stubborn infection focus. Without thorough removal, it is very difficult for the condition to heal on its own (Figure 6-1-5).
(6) Large area defect. Chronic infection foci continue to expand and erode, causing local tissues to gradually necrotize, dissolve, and fall off, eventually forming defects at different levels of skin, soft tissue, and bone structure (Figure 6-1-6). This defect is a type of secondary chest wall defect. Since it is caused by infection, it is discussed in detail in the chest wall infection section.
(7) Neoplasm Formation. Within the infected area, some tissues continuously undergo necrosis while other tissues proliferate. If the skin cannot heal, the proliferating tissue may protrude through the opening, forming a neoplasm. The appearance of a neoplasm does not mean the infection can heal by itself. On the contrary, because the neoplasm obstructs the growth and contacts of skin cells at the center of the wound, the local opening almost cannot heal (Figure 6-1-7) To achieve healing, the neoplasm must be removed.
The pathological changes described above represent several common manifestations of chest wall infections. Each type of lesion varies in nature, severity of harm to the body, and the complexity and approach required for treatment. Therefore, when diagnosing and managing patients with chest wall infections, it is essential to have a thorough understanding of these fundamental pathological changes. Only with this knowledge can clinicians develop targeted and appropriate treatment plans, improve therapeutic outcomes, and prevent disease progression or recurrence.

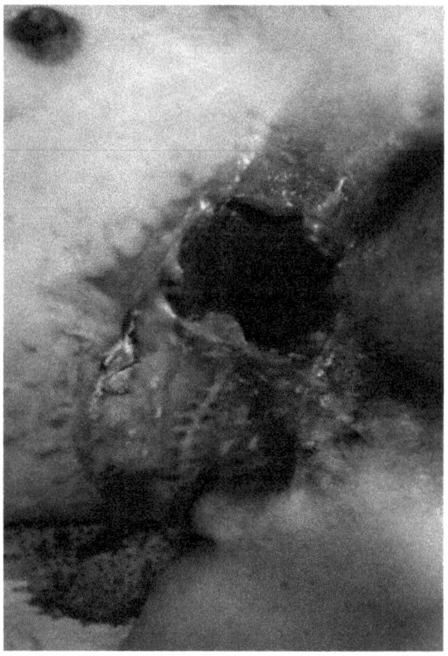

Figure 6-1-6 Large area defect

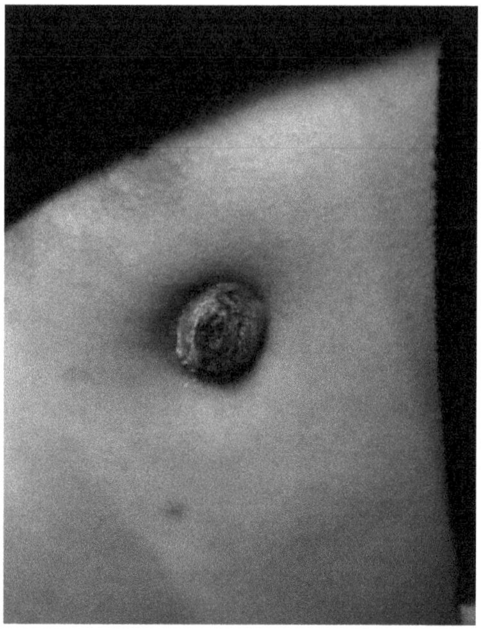

Figure 6-1-7 New growth appears in the incision and the skin cannot heal completely

5. Clinical manifestations

When chest wall infection occurs, the patient may have two clinical symptoms: local symptoms and systemic symptoms [2,13,17]. Local symptoms are mainly pain. The pain is clearly located, more severe in the acute phase, and significantly relieved or painless in the chronic phase. Systemic symptoms are mainly caused by the spread of infection or toxin secretion, and may be symptoms such as fever and general pain. The signs of chest wall infection are very clear, and there may be typical lesions. Lesions of different degrees may have different pathological changes. Lesions are the direct basis for diagnosing chest wall infection.

6. Inspection

The diagnostic approach for chest wall infections is similar to that of other chest wall Surgical diseases, beginning with a physical examination. Physical examination helps identify basic characteristics of the infection and allows for an initial assessment of the infected site. Further evaluation requires imaging studies. Both X-ray and CT scans are essential, and if conditions permit, 3D reconstruction imaging can be considered for a more detailed assessment. In certain special cases, such as infections occurring after cardiac Surgery, it is necessary to evaluate cardiac function, in which case a cardiac ultrasound should be performed. Since chest wall infection is an infectious disease, identifying the causative pathogen is crucial. Pathogen testing provides a key basis for selecting appropriate antimicrobial therapy. Before Surgery, this can be done by culturing secretions from the wound or through blood cultures.

7. Diagnosis and differential diagnosis

Diagnosing chest wall infections is relatively straightforward. Most infectious lesions exhibit typical features, making diagnosis generally uncomplicated. However, a mere qualitative diagnosis is not sufficient. It is also essential to understand detailed information about the infection site and the surrounding structures, which is crucial for effective treatment. In many cases, the surface wound on the skin is small, while the deeper infection may be more extensive. Observing surface signs alone may not reveal the full extent of the infection, so further diagnostic examinations are necessary to gather more comprehensive information. In addition to understanding the lesion itself, information about adjacent structures is equally important, especially for patients with post-Surgical incision infections, where such details can be particularly valuable. Furthermore, before confirming the final diagnosis, identifying the causative pathogen through microbiological testing is also vital. Determining the specific bacteria involved and performing antibiotic sensitivity testing can significantly aid in choosing effective antibiotic therapy.

Differential diagnosis needs to be differentiated from local ulcers caused by tumour necrosis. The latter may also have skin breaks and may be complicated by infection, but the surrounding of the breaks is tumour tissue, not normal tissue. The differentiation between the two is directly related to the scope of Surgical resection and the choice of Surgical method, so the differentiation is very necessary. There is also a very special situation that needs to be differentiated, that is, breast cancer. Local necrosis due to tumor recurrence is caused by the regrowth of malignant cells, while incision infection results from bacterial contamination. Their mechanisms are different; one is oncologic, the other infectious. Hence, treatment decisions also differ accordingly.

8. Treatment

Once a diagnosis of chest wall infection is confirmed, active treatment should be initiated. There are two main approaches to treating chest wall infection [12,13,18–20]: the first is conservative treatment, and the second is Surgical treatment. Conservative treatment mainly involves systemic and local management, while Surgical treatment requires complete excision of the infected lesion followed by further intervention as needed.

(1) Conservative treatment

Chest wall infections present with various pathological types, each differing in severity, so not all cases require Surgical treatment. For milder infections, conservative treatment can be considered. Conservative treatment mainly includes systemic antibiotic use, nutritional support, and local wound care, with local management being a key component of this approach.

For localized chest wall abscesses, conservative treatment primarily involves incision and drainage, which is the most fundamental approach [20]. Conservative management of sinus tracts includes adequate drainage and local wound care. In cases of skin ulceration, if the area is small, local dressing changes may promote gradual skin regeneration. Post-thoracotomy wound infections are the most severe type and pose a significant challenge. Conservative treatment in such cases mainly involves local wound care and adjunctive local therapies, but the results are often unsatisfactory. If conservative methods fail to completely eliminate the infection, Surgical treatment should be considered.

(2) Surgical treatment

(i) Preoperative preparation

Surgery is an important measure for treating chest wall infection. In order to ensure the success of the operation, adequate preparation is required before the operation. These preparations include [20]:① Improvement of systemic nutritional status. Some patients with chest wall infection have organic consumption, and low resistance is an important predisposing factor for infection. In order to control the infection well, the patient's systemic condition must be improved before the operation, and resistance must be enhanced to create conditions for Surgical treatment. ② Effective application of antibiotics. Antibiotics can directly kill bacteria and improve the condition of the lesion, which will be conducive to the success of the operation. Therefore, it is necessary to implement targeted treatment of pathogens before the operation. ③ Treatment of some chronic diseases. Chronic systemic diseases are seriously harmful to the human body. Due to low resistance, they are not conducive to wound healing and incision growth, so they must be effectively controlled. ④ Preparation of local lesions. The target site of chest wall infection Surgery is the lesion. In order to ensure the success of the operation, the lesion must be treated before the operation, necrotic tissue must be removed, granulation growth must be promoted, and blood circulation must be improved. Such measures play an important role in controlling infection. In recent years, some people have suggested using a negative pressure suction device to prepare the lesion before Surgery. This method can achieve satisfactory results. However, it should not be used for too long and the indications should be properly grasped, otherwise it will be counterproductive [12].

⑤Preparation of the donor flap. Many chronic infections. Some chest wall infection Surgeries require flap transplantation. Since flaps must be harvested from other parts of the body, it is essential to both design the flap properly

before Surgery and thoroughly assess the donor site conditions. This ensures comprehensive preparation for a successful Surgical outcome.
Chest wall infection is a special disease. Since the lesion itself is infected, it is easy to cause recurrence of infection after Surgery. In order to completely control the infection and obtain satisfactory results, relevant preparations must be made carefully before Surgery. Only in this way can the success rate of Surgery be improved.

(ii) Surgical principles

The clinical manifestations of chest wall infections are highly complex and can involve a variety of pathological changes. Depending on the type of lesion, the specific Surgical approach may vary. In general, Surgical treatment should follow these principles [20]:

1. Thorough removal of necrotic tissue. Necrotic tissue severely hinders wound healing. First, its presence prevents proper closure of the incision, making healing impossible. Second, necrotic tissue can harbor large amounts of pathogens; if not removed, these hidden pathogens will cause postoperative infection recurrence. Third, necrotic tissue releases various harmful factors that directly impair wound healing. Fourth, it can spread to surrounding tissues, leading to expansion of the lesion. Therefore, necrotic tissue is a major barrier to healing, and complete removal is essential for thorough recovery of the lesion.
2. Thorough elimination of the infectious focus. The infectious focus includes not only necrotic tissue but also surrounding proliferative fibrous tissue and various secretions within the lesion. These structures harbor a large number of pathogens and contain many components that hinder wound healing. Therefore, complete removal is essential.
3. Protect blood supply. For the infectious lesion to fully heal, adequate nutrition is necessary, which depends on blood supply. Therefore, sufficient blood flow is fundamental for wound healing. Without adequate blood supply, Surgery is prone to failure. Additionally, blood circulation delivers immune cells, antibodies, and intravenously administered antibiotics, all of which play a crucial role in lesion recovery.
4. Soft tissue filling. After the infectious lesion is removed, a large local defect may remain, primarily a soft tissue defect. If this defect is not effectively addressed, a large dead space may form. The presence of a dead space allows fluid accumulation, which not only directly impairs healing but also serves as an ideal environment for pathogen growth. Therefore, eliminating dead space is a critical Surgical step. There are two main ways to eliminate dead space: one is direct and

tight closure of the wound; the other is filling the defect with soft tissue. If the wound is small, direct closure is possible, but in most cases, the wound is large and requires sufficient soft tissue filling. Common soft tissues used include muscle [18-21] and omentum [22]. In practice, the choice depends on the location and characteristics of the lesion.

5. Avoid using artificial materials whenever possible [23]. Chest wall infections often involve extensive chest wall structures, and thorough removal of these infected tissues inevitably leaves large defects. If bony structures are lost, theoretically, artificial materials are needed for chest wall reconstruction. However, since all artificial materials are foreign bodies, they can easily become ideal sites for pathogen colonization and proliferation. These pathogens are difficult to eradicate and often lead to postoperative infection recurrence and Surgical failure. Therefore, the use of artificial materials is generally not recommended in most chest wall infection Surgeries. To prevent chest wall softening and paradoxical respiration caused by bony defects, alternative measures can be taken. Once the infection is controlled, if necessary, chest wall bony reconstruction can be performed as a secondary procedure, but the initial focus must be on treating the infection. It is best not to use artificial materials.

9. Prognosis

Among the five basic diseases in chest wall Surgery, chest wall infection is the most stubborn. The vast majority of thoracic Surgeons often feel helpless when facing this disease, which indicates that its prognosis has traditionally been unsatisfactory. However, since the emergence of new concepts in chest wall Surgery, the treatment of chest wall infections has greatly improved. Because the treatment concepts and methods differ from traditional thoracic Surgery approaches, the outcomes have also changed significantly. Currently, most chest wall infections can be treated satisfactorily, and even the most difficult postoperative incision infections have shown good results. It is reasonable to expect that with further advancements in various techniques, the treatment outcomes for chest wall infections will become even more favorable.

REFERENCES

[1] Brown, R. B., and J. Trenton. 1952. "Chronic Abscesses and Sinuses of the Chest Wall: The Treatment of Costal Chondritis and Sternal Osteomyelitis." *Annals of Surgery* 135 (1): 44–51.

[2] Yuan, Hongzhi, Lihong Tang, and Liang Liang Lian. 2016. "Surgical Treatment of 13 Cases of Delayed Chest Wall Abscess after Trauma." *Chinese Journal of Minimally*

Invasive Surgery 16 (2): 187–188.
[3] Anand, P., and N. Sarin. 2018. "Isolated Sternal Tuberculosis Presenting as a Chest Wall Abscess: A Case Report." *Iranian Journal of Medical Sciences* 43 (4): 440–443.
[4] Tonziello, G., R. Valentinotti, E. Arbore, et al. 2013. "Salmonella Typhimurium Abscess of the Chest Wall." *American Journal of Case Reports* 14: 502–506.
[5] Dadlani, A., S. Bandikatla, and J. A. Koch. 2021. "A Rare Case of Escherichia coli Chest Wall Abscess with Rib Osteomyelitis in a Patient with Crohn's Disease." *Cureus* 13 (3): e13860.
[6] Keum, D. Y., J. B. Kim, and C. K. Park. 2012. "Surgical Treatment of a Tuberculous Abscess of the Chest Wall." *Korean Journal of Thoracic and Cardiovascular Surgery* 45 (3): 177–182.
[7] Tanaka, S., M. Aoki, T. Nakanishi, et al. 2012. "Retrospective Case Series Analysing the Clinical Data and Treatment Options of Patients with a Tuberculous Abscess of the Chest Wall." *Interactive Cardiovascular and Thoracic Surgery* 14 (3): 249–252.
[8] Yamaoka, Y., J. Yamamura, N. Masuda, et al. 2014. "Primary Chest Wall Abscess Mimicking a Breast Tumor That Occurred after Blunt Chest Trauma: A Case Report." *Case Reports in Medicine* 2014: 620876.
[9] Dai, J., P. Greiffenstein, F. Petrella, et al. 2020. "Treatment of a Lung Lobectomy Patient with Severe Post-Surgical Infection in the Anterior Thoracic Wall by Multiple Debridement and Drainage Procedures: A Case Report." *Journal of Thoracic Disease* 12 (12): 7481–7487.
[10] Dubert, M., A. Pourbaix, S. Alkhoder, et al. 2015. "Sternal Wound Infection after Cardiac Surgery: Management and Outcome." *PLOS ONE* 10 (9): e0139122.
[11] Kubota, H., H. Miyata, N. Motomura, et al. 2013. "Deep Sternal Wound Infection after Cardiac Surgery." *Journal of Cardiothoracic Surgery* 8: 132.
[12] Fleck, T., and M. Fleck. 2014. "Negative Pressure Wound Therapy for the Treatment of Sternal Wound Infections after Cardiac Surgery." *International Wound Journal* 11 (3): 240–245.
[13] Tanaka, Y., H. Kato, K. Shirai, et al. 2016. "Sternoclavicular Joint Septic Arthritis with Chest Wall Abscess in a Healthy Adult: A Case Report." *Journal of Medical Case Reports* 10: 69.
[14] Ko, K., K. Tobino, Y. Yasuda, et al. 2017. "A Community-Acquired Lung Abscess Attributable to Streptococcus pneumoniae Which Extended Directly into the Chest Wall." *Internal Medicine* 56 (1): 109–113.
[15] Karim, S. H. A., W. Z. W. Zain, and M. N. M. Hashim, et al. 2021. "Empyema Thoracis Presented as a Giant Back Abscess." *Radiology Case Reports* 16 (5): 1061–1064.
[16] Rajput, A. K., V. Vardhan, and K. E. Rajan. 2000. "A Persistent Transpleural Fistulous Communication between Lung and Chest Wall." *Medical Journal of Armed Forces India* 56 (3): 259–261.
[17] Yang, Qinheng. 2013. "Analysis of the Causes and Prevention of Median Sternotomy Incision Infection after Cardiac Surgery." *China Health Care and Nutrition* 12 (1): 7088–7089.
[18] Borisov, V., B. Stieltjes, M. Wiese, et al. 2020. "Reconstruction of the Chest Wall with a Latissimus Dorsi Muscle Flap after an Infection of Alloplastic Material: A Case Report." *Journal of Surgical Case Reports* 2020 (8): rjaa213.
[19] Zeitani, J., M. Russo, E. Pompeo, et al. 2016. "Pectoralis Muscle Flap Repair Reduces Paradoxical Motion of the Chest Wall in Complex Sternal Wound Dehiscence."

Korean Journal of Thoracic and Cardiovascular Surgery 49 (5): 366–373.
[20] Wang, W. L. 2021a. “Treatment Principles for Chest Wall Infection.” *Toutiao*, November 1.
[21] Bakri, K., S. Mardini, K. K. Evans, et al. 2011. “Workhorse Flaps in Chest Wall Reconstruction: The Pectoralis Major, Latissimus Dorsi, and Rectus Abdominis Flaps.” *Seminars in Plastic Surgery* 25 (1): 43–54.
[22] Yasuura, K., H. Okamoto, S. Morita, et al. 1998. “Results of Omental Flap Transposition for Deep Sternal Wound Infection after Cardiovascular Surgery.” *Annals of Surgery* 227 (3): 455–459.
[23] Wang, W. L. 2021b. “Treatment Strategies for Chest Wall Abscess.” *Toutiao*, November 1.

A chest wall abscess is a form of chest wall infection or pathological change and, strictly speaking, is not an independent disease. However, due to its unique pathological characteristics and specific treatment requirements, it warrants separate discussion. A chest wall abscess refers to a purulent, encapsulated lesion that occurs between the various layers of the chest wall and is the result of an infectious process that has progressed to a certain stage. Chest wall abscesses can be caused by various factors, including trauma [1,2], Surgery [3,4], certain treatments or interventions [5,6], and metastasis from other lesions in the body [7-11]. They may present acutely or become chronic abscesses if the condition is prolonged and unresolved. Once an abscess forms, it initially causes damage to the local structures of the chest wall and may further endanger surrounding tissues and other parts of the body [12]. Therefore, an abscess represents a serious chest wall infection and must be treated with due seriousness.

1. Etiology and Pathological Characteristics

A chest wall abscess is a fundamental form of chest wall infection. Chest wall infections can be classified into specific infections and non-specific infections, and accordingly, chest wall abscesses can also be categorized as those caused by specific infections and those caused by non-specific infections. The most common type of abscess caused by specific infection is a tuberculous abscess [13], which is referred to clinically as a "cold abscess." Due to its unique pathological features, it will be discussed in a separate chapter. Non-specific abscesses are caused by non-specific pathogens, which may include pyogenic bacteria or, less commonly, other types of pathogens. Although the pathogens may vary, the pathological characteristics of these abscesses are generally similar [12,14,15].

The formation of a chest wall abscess typically originates from a specific site of infection, but it can also result from the spread of nearby lesions [8-11]. In the early stages, the lesion is localized and may present as a typical acute infectious condition, with local changes such as edema, exudation, and cellular infiltration. If promptly and effectively controlled, the lesion may gradually resolve without further progression. However, if not adequately managed, the condition can worsen, leading to increased local exudation, tissue dissolution, liquefaction, necrosis, and extensive bacterial proliferation. These bacteria are continually engulfed by white blood cells, resulting in the gradual formation of pus. Initially, the lesion may spread within a limited area. As the condition progresses, fibrous tissue proliferates around the infected site, forming an encapsulated lesion that eventually becomes a typical abscess. If treated in time, the abscess can be completely cured. If it continues to progress, it may rupture and form a sinus tract to the skin, resulting in a chronic, non-healing condition [4,11].

Chest wall abscess is a pathological change and does not necessarily exist as an independent condition. It can represent a specific stage of chest wall infection, or it may occur as a complication in other thoracic Surgical conditions, such as chest wall tumors, trauma, or defects. If these conditions become secondarily infected due to certain special factors, a chest wall abscess may develop.

2. Hazards

The hazards of a chest wall abscess come from three aspects [2,4,11], local damage at the lesion site, damage to surrounding tissues, and systemic harm. Local hazards mainly involve the destruction of tissue structures at the lesion site. Once an abscess forms in a certain area of the chest wall, soft tissues and bony structures undergo a series of characteristic changes, including dissolution, necrosis, and detachment of local structures. This leads to the gradual formation of an abscess cavity filled with pus. As the pus accumulates, the internal pressure increases and may eventually cause skin rupture. The destructive power of a localized abscess is significant, often leaving no trace of the original structures. Hazards to surrounding areas can be divided into two categories: one is mechanical damage caused by compression from the abscess, and the other is direct damage from rupture or erosion. Once formed, the abscess creates a closed space, which is highly conducive to the growth of pathogens. With increasing pus and rising pressure within the cavity, surrounding tissues may suffer from ischemia and hypoxia. This can impair their function or, in severe cases, lead to necrosis. As the abscess progresses, a fibrous capsule often forms around its periphery, which helps limit the infection. However, continued growth of the abscess may rupture the capsule, allowing the infection to invade surrounding tissues and cause further destruction and complications. Systemic hazards are generally limited since an abscess is a localized infection. However, if the abscess becomes very large or persists for a prolonged period, it may have systemic effects, leading to general symptoms of exhaustion and systemic deterioration. Some bacteria are highly invasive and may spread throughout the body via various routes, potentially triggering a strong systemic response and even posing a life-threatening risk [12].

Chest wall abscesses can occur in any part of the chest wall. Small abscesses may remain unchanged for many years, or they may gradually shrink and become organized, eventually forming a localized area of fibrosis. However, such outcomes are relatively rare. The most common scenario is progressive enlargement of the abscess followed by rupture. The rupture typically presents as a localized break in the abscess wall, through which pus leaks into surrounding areas. The direction of rupture can vary and may involve surrounding chest wall structures, the thoracic cavity, or the skin surface [10,11]. Rupture into the chest wall interior signifies further spread of the abscess. If it ruptures into the pleural cavity, it can lead to empyema and rapid dissemination of the infection, with potentially severe consequences. In comparison, rupture to the skin surface is the least harmful outcome.

3. Clinical Manifestations

The clinical manifestations of a chest wall abscess vary depending on its location and the characteristics of the lesion [2,10,15]. In the early stages, superficial lesions may present with localized redness, swelling, heat, and pain. In contrast, deeper lesions may cause no obvious discomfort (Figure 6-2-1). As the abscess enlarges and internal pressure increases, local pain intensifies and may present as severe, throbbing pain. Once the abscess ruptures, the pain typically subsides significantly, and pus begins to drain from the rupture site. Systemic symptoms of chest wall abscesses mainly include fever, which tends to occur during more severe or acute phases. Chronic abscesses may not present with any systemic symptoms. Local signs of a chest wall abscess are often distinctive and typically appear as a localized, cystic mass with well-defined borders and a fluctuant quality. Diagnostic aspiration can yield purulent material. However, if the lesion is located deep within the chest wall, local signs may be less apparent or atypical.

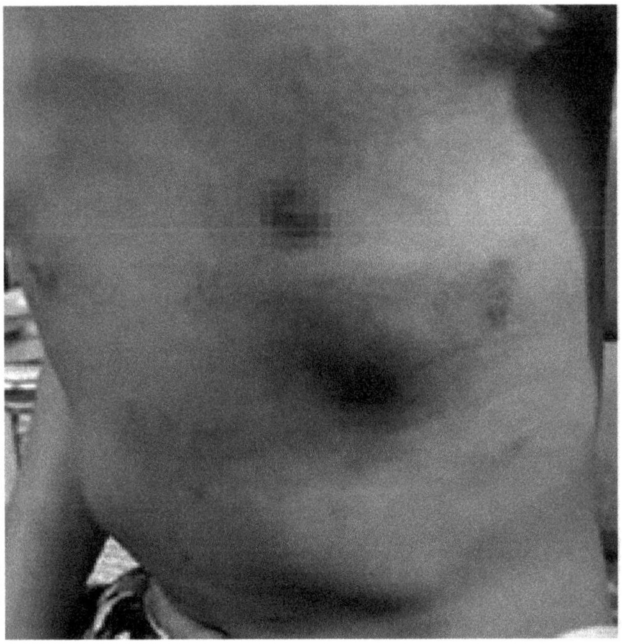

Figure 6-2-1 Left chest Wall Abscess (Local bulge,skin redness, fluctuation, tenderness. Local aspiration pus)

4. Inspection

Basic information about a chest wall abscess can be obtained through physical examination. Further evaluation should be carried out using various imaging modalities. X-ray imaging has limited sensitivity for detecting abscesses. In contrast, CT scanning not only provides detailed visualization of the abscess itself but also offers comprehensive information about adjacent structures and the thoracic cavity, making it a standard diagnostic tool in clinical practice. Ultrasound examination allows direct assessment of the lesion and is extremely helpful in determining the nature of the abscess. Three-dimensional reconstruction of chest wall structures can clearly display the abscess, bony anatomy, and surrounding tissues in a stereoscopic view, making it an advanced and informative diagnostic technique. Needle aspiration of the abscess for laboratory analysis of the pus can provide microbiological evidence, helping to identify the causative pathogen and guide targeted antimicrobial therapy.

5. Diagnosis

The diagnosis of a chest wall abscess can be established based on the patient's medical history, clinical symptoms, physical signs, and necessary diagnostic tests. In most cases, the diagnosis is not complicated. However, it is essential to differentiate it from other chest wall diseases. The first condition to differentiate from is an abscess secondary to tumor necrosis. Although an abscess may be present, the underlying pathology is actually a tumor. Therefore, a diagnosis of an abscess should not lead to missed treatment for the tumor. The second condition is a malignant tumor that mimics an abscess [16]. Some malignancies may present clinically as a chest wall abscess, but the underlying lesion is actually a cancer. The third differential is benign tumors, such as chest wall granulomas, which may present with features similar to early abscesses but lack the typical abscess structure[17]. The fourth condition to consider is parasitic infection, such as echinococcosis. This can produce imaging and clinical findings similar to an abscess in the chest wall, but can be distinguished through imaging and pathogen-specific laboratory tests [18,19].

6. Treatment

Once a chest wall abscess is diagnosed, treatment should be initiated, with the primary goal being the elimination of the abscess focus. There are two specific methods [3,4,7]: one is incision and drainage, and the other is complete excision of the lesion. Incision and drainage is a relatively conservative approach that can be considered either a standalone treatment or a preparatory step before definitive therapy. Complete excision is a more thorough approach, equivalent to a curative Surgical procedure.

(1) Incision and Drainage

Incision and drainage are the simplest and most fundamental method for treating a chest wall abscess. After the procedure, pus, necrotic tissue, and dead structures within the abscess cavity can be discharged directly, improving the local condition and laying the foundation for further healing. The procedure itself is quite straightforward; for superficial abscesses, a direct incision can be made. If the abscess is too deep, an incision can be made at an appropriate nearby location to establish a connection between the abscess cavity and the external environment.

There are three key points for performing incision and drainage [20]: ①The incision must be large enough. To ensure complete evacuation of the pus from the abscess cavity, the incision must be sufficiently wide. This is the most basic requirement for effective drainage. ②Drainage must be unobstructed. The purpose of incision and drainage is to allow the pus to flow out. Therefore, the drainage pathway must remain open and clear. If the pus cannot be fully drained, the treatment will not be effective. ③Necrotic tissue should be thoroughly removed. During the procedure, necrotic tissue inside the abscess cavity must be cleared as much as possible. Retained dead tissue can interfere with proper drainage.

After the incision and drainage procedure is completed, local treatment is generally still required. There are various methods of local treatment, with the simplest being regular wound dressing changes. During this process, it is important to keep the wound clean and promote the growth of surrounding granulation tissue to ultimately eliminate the lesion. In addition to dressing changes, topical medication can be applied; for example, the local use of antibiotics may help control infection. In recent years, some have advocated for the use of negative pressure wound therapy as a follow-up treatment for the wound, which has been shown to produce favorable outcomes [4].

For most patients with chest wall abscesses, the local lesion generally improves gradually after incision and drainage, and in some cases, it may even heal completely. However, some abscesses can be very persistent, with continuous pus discharge and a lesion that fails to resolve. In such cases, complete Surgical excision of the lesion is ultimately required.

(2) Complete Excision of the Lesion

Complete excision of the lesion refers to the thorough Surgical removal of the entire abscess focus. The procedure is relatively straightforward: an incision is made over and around the abscess, the pus is first evacuated, and then all necrotic tissue along with the surrounding fibrous capsule is completely excised until healthy tissue is exposed. If the abscess is confined to the soft tissue layer, the procedure can be performed along the surface of the bony structures. However, if the abscess involves the bone and is accompanied by osteomyelitis, the affected bone should also be removed until healthy bone is exposed.

The fibrous capsule surrounding the abscess is a dense structure that lacks blood supply. As a result, the cut surface often appears white or yellowish-white in color. A key indicator of fresh, healthy tissue is the presence of blood oozing from the cut surface. If there is no blood oozing, even if the dissection has reached the layer of healthy tissue, further excision is still necessary. Only when the cut surface shows adequate blood supply can it ensure sufficient perfusion to the wound, providing the necessary conditions for proper healing.

Complete excision of the lesion is suitable for all chest wall abscesses, but it is especially indicated for lesions with a large extent. Such lesions are difficult to heal through incision and drainage alone. Because the necrotic tissue inside the abscess cannot be completely removed by simple drainage, the abscess may instead become a chronic, open infectious lesion after incision. For these types of cases, the only effective treatment is thorough Surgical removal of the entire lesion.

Compared with incision and drainage, complete excision of the lesion is a more extensive procedure and results in significantly greater tissue damage. However, for most types of chest wall abscesses, it is almost the only effective method. If such Surgery is not performed and the infectious lesion is allowed to progress, it can cause serious harm to the patient. Therefore, despite the associated risks and costs, complete excision must be carried out.

The Surgical procedure for lesion excision includes two basic steps: the first step is to remove the lesion and convert the infected lesion into a clean one; the second step is to manage the lesion to achieve complete closure. A chest wall abscess is, by nature, an infectious lesion, and achieving a completely sterile wound through simple excision is nearly impossible. A more realistic goal is to convert it into a clean wound. Although a small number of pathogens may still be present, the replacement of necrotic tissue with healthy tissue creates a local environment that is more conducive to wound healing.

To achieve the objective of the first step, at least three aspects of work are required [20]: ①Preoperative preparation, mainly including prior incision and drainage, debridement of necrotic tissue, use of negative pressure suction devices, and local antimicrobial treatment; ②Intraoperative disinfection, including repeated and strict disinfection of the Surgical field and wound, with all procedures carried out in strict accordance with aseptic principles; ③Thorough removal of necrotic tissue during Surgery, continuing until fresh tissue is exposed.

After the above procedures, the goal of creating a clean wound can basically be achieved. The next step is to manage the wound. During the process of lesion excision, a large portion of the chest wall structure often needs to be removed, resulting in a significant defect after the operation; this is a typical case of secondary chest wall defect. To achieve proper closure of this defect, reconstruction of the involved structures is necessary. As discussed in the chapter on chest wall defects, there are three fundamental components involved: bony structures, soft tissue, and skin. If part of the bony structure is removed, in theory, reconstruction is required. However, since the wound is not sterile, the use of artificial materials for reconstruction may lead to Surgical failure. Therefore, artificial materials are generally avoided [20]. Under the condition that artificial materials cannot be used, if conservative methods can be employed to minimize the impact of bony structure loss, it will be highly beneficial for wound healing. If the defect has significant long-term consequences, reconstruction of the bony structure can be performed after the wound has fully healed.

Skin and soft tissue defects are commonly present. Soft tissue defects can be filled using other soft tissues. If there is also a skin defect, reconstruction can be considered using a musculocutaneous flap. This type of structure can simultaneously restore both the skin and soft tissue defects.

During the process of skin and soft tissue reconstruction, several technical points must be clearly understood [4,21,22]: ①Adequate blood supply must be ensured. The purpose of soft tissue filling is to allow the tissue to continue growing within the defect, thereby replacing the missing structures. For soft tissue to grow, it must have a blood supply. Therefore, when harvesting soft tissue for reconstruction, close attention must be paid to its vascular supply. This is the key to Surgical success. ② There must be no dead space. The purpose of soft tissue reconstruction is to eliminate the local defect.

A dead space means that a defect still exists, and such a space will accumulate wound exudate, providing an environment for the growth of pathogens, which is extremely unfavorable for wound healing. Therefore, when performing soft tissue reconstruction, all dead spaces must be eliminated as much as possible to create an optimal environment for healing. ③Proper drainage is essential. Any wound may produce a certain amount of exudate. If this exudate remains within the wound, it can also nourish pathogens and must therefore be removed. The way to eliminate exudate is through drainage. At the end of Surgery, an appropriate drainage tube must be placed. The more complete the drainage, the more favorable it is for postoperative healing.

(3) Postoperative Consolidation Therapy

Chest wall abscesses are infectious lesions; neither incision and drainage nor lesion excision can completely eradicate the pathogens. To increase the likelihood of Surgical success, postoperative consolidation therapy is required. This therapy includes two aspects: local consolidation treatment and systemic supportive treatment. Local treatment mainly involves wound care; in addition to routine dressing changes, methods such as infrared light irradiation can be used to promote healing. Systemic supportive treatment primarily includes overall nutritional support and the use of antibiotics. The application of these measures postoperatively can actively promote wound healing.

7. Prognosis

Chest wall abscess is a relatively common type of chest wall infection. Abscesses confined to the soft tissue involve only a limited area and are generally easier to cure as long as the treatment method is appropriate. However, if the infection involves deeper structures such as the bones, especially when osteomyelitis is present, treatment becomes very difficult, and any problem in the treatment details can affect the outcome.

REFERENCES

[1] Ichimura, H., Y. Ozawa, T. Sato, et al. 2012. "Sternal Osteomyelitis and Abscess Caused by Elbowing during a Basketball Game." *Case Reports in Medicine* 2012: 298187.

[2] Patricio, C., R. Ribeiro, R. Malheiro, et al. 2015. "A Chest Wall Pulsating Mass." *BMJ Case Reports* 2015: bcr2014207972.

[3] Ahmed, H., A. Tamburrini, M. Khan, et al. 2021. "Chest Wall Silicone Granuloma Following Ruptured Silicone Breast Implant Causing Giant Chest Wall Abscess and Osteomyelitis: The First Report." *European Journal of Breast Health* 17 (4): 383–385.

[4] Liu, Zhijun, Zhongliang He, Lifeng Shen, et al. 2019. "Analysis of the Efficacy of Free Anterolateral Thigh Musculocutaneous Flap Transplantation in the Treatment of Chronic Empyema and Chest Wall Sinus Tract." *Zhejiang Medical Journal* 41 (4): 362–364.

[5] Tang, H. L., K. K. Lau, R. Sam, et al. 2015. "Chest Wall Abscesses Due to Continuous Application of Silicone Gel Sheets for Keloid Management." *BMJ Case Reports* 2015: bcr2014206777.

[6] Gorospe, L., I. Bermudez-Coronel-Prats, C. F. Gomez-Barbosa, et al. 2014. "Parvimonas micra Chest Wall Abscess Following Transthoracic Lung Needle Biopsy." *Korean Journal of Internal Medicine* 29 (6): 834–837.

[7] Tanaka, Y., H. Kato, K. Shirai, et al. 2016. "Sternoclavicular Joint Septic Arthritis with Chest Wall Abscess in a Healthy Adult: A Case Report." *Journal of Medical Case Reports* 10: 69.

[8] Ko, K., K. Tobino, Y. Yasuda, et al. 2017. "A Community-Acquired Lung Abscess Attributable to Streptococcus pneumoniae Which Extended Directly into the Chest Wall." *Internal Medicine* 56 (1): 109–113.

[9] Rajput, A. K., V. Vardhan, and K. E. Rajan. 2000. "A Persistent Transpleural Fistulous Communication between Lung and Chest Wall." *Medical Journal of Armed Forces India* 56 (3): 259–261.

[10] Karim, S. H. A., W. Z. W. Zain, and M. N. M. Hashim, et al. 2021. "Empyema Thoracis Presented as a Giant Back Abscess." *Radiology Case Reports* 16 (5): 1061–1064.

[11] Brown, R. B., and J. Trention. 1952. "Chronic Abscesses and Sinuses of the Chest Wall: The Treatment of Costal Chondritis and Sternal Osteomyelitis." *Annals of Surgery* 135 (1): 44–51.

[12] Simmonds, N. J., and K. M. Gyi. 2008. "Cystic Fibrosis, a Burkholderia cenocepacia Chest Wall Abscess, and Rapid Clinical Deterioration." *Journal of the Royal Society of Medicine* 101 (Suppl 1): S46–S50.

[13] Tanaka, S., M. Aoki, T. Nakanishi, et al. 2012. "Retrospective Case Series Analysing the Clinical Data and Treatment Options of Patients with a Tuberculous

Abscess of the Chest Wall." *Interactive Cardiovascular and Thoracic Surgery* 14 (3): 249–252.
[14] Dadlani, A., S. Bandikatla, and J. A. Koch. 2021. "A Rare Case of Escherichia coli Chest Wall Abscess with Rib Osteomyelitis in a Patient with Crohn's Disease." *Cureus* 13 (3): e13860.
[15] Tonziello, G., R. Valentinotti, E. Arbore, et al. 2013. "Salmonella Typhimurium Abscess of the Chest Wall." *American Journal of Case Reports* 14: 502–506.
[16] Shin, Y. S., C. H. Choi, Y. J. Kim, et al. 2015. "Primary Squamous Cell Carcinoma in the Chest Wall Mimicking Abscess." *Journal of Thoracic Disease* 7 (7): E179–E181.
[17] Lee, H. S., K. J. Seo, and J. J. Kim. 2015. "Chest Wall Granuloma Associated with BCG Vaccination Presenting as Hot Abscess in an Immunocompetent Infant." *Journal of Cardiothoracic Surgery* 10: 29.
[18] Salih, A. M., D. M. Ahmed, F. H. Kakamad, et al. 2017. "Primary Chest Wall Hydatid Cyst: Review of Literature with Report of a New Case." *International Journal of Surgery Case Reports* 41: 404–406.
[19] Durhan, G., A. A. Tan, S. A. Duzgun, et al. 2020. "Radiological Manifestations of Thoracic Hydatid Cysts: Pulmonary and Extrapulmonary Findings." *Insights into Imaging* 11: 116.
[20] Wang, W. L. 2021. "Management Strategies for Chest Wall Abscess." *Toutiao*, November 1.
[21] Zheng, Shaoyi, Wen Lai, Zhifeng Huang, et al. 2015. "Clinical Efficacy of Bilateral Pectoralis Major Muscle Flaps in the Treatment of Post-Thoracotomy Sternal Osteomyelitis." *Chinese Journal of Burns* 31 (1): 61–63.
[22] Tang, Pei, Zhengyong Li, and Ying Cen. 2021. "Research Progress on Chest Wall Reconstruction for Deep Sternal Wound Infections." *Chinese Journal of Plastic Surgery* 37 (7): 810–816.

CHEST WALL TUBERCULOSIS

Chest wall tuberculosis is a localized manifestation of tuberculosis in the chest wall. It may exist solely in the chest wall or be part of systemic tuberculosis, often accompanied by tuberculosis in other areas, with pulmonary tuberculosis being the most common. Chest wall tuberculosis can result from the direct spread of pulmonary tuberculosis or be transmitted through lymphatic or hematogenous routes [1,2]. After its onset, various pathological changes may occur locally, causing varying degrees of impact on the chest wall and thus requiring treatment.

1. Pathological Changes

In the early stage, the chest wall tuberculosis lesions are small and the characteristics are not obvious. As the lesions enlarge, caseous necrosis, abscesses, fistulas, and osteomyelitis may appear. Tuberculous abscesses generally do not present with local heat; thus, they are called cold abscesses [2]. The lesions can be located in the superficial soft tissue or invade deeper structures, and may even extend beyond the bony structures to form lesions inside the thoracic cavity. When lesions span across the chest wall and exist both inside and outside the thoracic cavity, the lesion can present a dumbbell shape [3]. The fistulas in chest wall tuberculosis have no specific pattern and can develop in any direction. This characteristic causes chest wall tuberculosis to exhibit extremely diverse pathological features and is the fundamental reason why lesions in some locations are difficult to detect [4,5].

2. Harm

After the occurrence of chest wall tuberculosis, its main harm is initially confined to the local lesion, which can lead to tuberculous changes in the local tissues and, in severe cases, complete structural destruction, forming necrotic tissue. When the chest wall lesion spreads to the surrounding area, the harm may gradually increase. If the lesion spreads into the thoracic cavity, it can cause tuberculous empyema; if it spreads to the body surface, it can cause skin ulceration, severely affecting the patient's physical and mental health.

The chest wall is an organic whole composed of various structures, and it has its own special functions. When a local lesion occurs in the chest wall, if the lesion is small, it may not affect the function of the chest wall. However, if the lesion is extensive, especially when some important structures are involved, it can impact the function of the chest wall. The effect of chest wall tuberculosis on chest wall function can manifest in various ways, such as impairments in respiratory function, protective function, and motor function of the chest wall.

In addition to causing local effects on the chest wall, chest wall tuberculosis often has systemic harms associated with tuberculosis, and patients may exhibit severe discomfort. Moreover, the lesion can also spread to other parts of the body, leading to new sites of infection and causing further harm [6].

3. Clinical Manifestations

The clinical manifestations of chest wall tuberculosis can be divided into two types: local symptoms and systemic symptoms. Local symptoms may include discomfort at the lesion site and sometimes pain, though it may not always be obvious [2]. Systemic symptoms primarily reflect the general manifestations of tuberculosis, such as intermittent fever and night sweats. If the lesion is localized, systemic symptoms may be mild or absent [7]. The local signs of chest wall tuberculosis can present in various forms. In the early stages, the lesion may be very localized, appearing as a solid mass. If a tuberculous abscess forms, signs of a chest wall abscess will be evident.

4. Examination

The examination of chest wall tuberculosis begins with a physical examination. A general physical exam can help determine the basic information about the lesion, such as its location, size, boundaries, and characteristics. Further evaluation requires imaging studies. Among various imaging methods, CT scans are the most valuable [3,8], as they can provide a wealth of important information, including: ①The exact location of the lesion; ②The location of any sinus tracts; ③The condition of lesions within the thoracic cavity; ④The status of surrounding structures. Ultrasound also has some diagnostic value for chest wall tuberculosis. 3D reconstruction can offer a three-dimensional view of the lesion and surrounding structures, making it an ideal diagnostic tool if available.

Chest wall tuberculosis is a specific infection of the chest wall, called specific because it is caused by a specific pathogen. This pathogen is Mycobacterium tuberculosis. The presence of Mycobacterium tuberculosis is an important basis for diagnosing chest wall tuberculosis. Therefore, when examining patients, tuberculosis-related tests must be performed. These can include the tuberculin skin test or directly detecting Mycobacterium tuberculosis from the lesion; however, the positive rate may not be high, which could affect the diagnosis of chest wall tuberculosis [4,5,9].

5. Diagnosis and Differential Diagnosis

Key points for the diagnosis of chest wall tuberculosis are as follows: ①Local lesion of the chest wall. The local lesion is non-specific; if it presents as a "cold abscess," it may aid in diagnosis, but this sign is not specific. ②Detection of Mycobacterium tuberculosis within the lesion. This is the gold standard for diagnosing chest wall tuberculosis. However, it is often difficult to detect the bacteria in the lesion, so diagnosis needs to be combined with the tuberculin skin test and medical history. A positive tuberculin test and presence of tuberculosis lesions elsewhere in the body support the diagnosis of chest wall tuberculosis. Due to the low positivity rate of pathogen testing, diagnosis of chest wall tuberculosis is often challenging, and many patients are only confirmed by postoperative pathological examination [1].

Differential diagnosis mainly involves distinguishing chest wall tuberculosis from chest wall abscess and chest wall tumors [10]. Chest wall abscess is caused by non-specific bacterial infection and may present with obvious systemic infection symptoms, though chronic cases can be asymptomatic. Chest wall tuberculosis has distinctive systemic symptoms that differ from those of a typical chest wall abscess. Detection of Mycobacterium tuberculosis within the lesion helps differentiate between the two. Chest wall tumors may present with local necrosis.

When a chest wall tumor presents with local necrosis and forms a sinus tract, it must be differentiated from chest wall tuberculosis. Such lesions are surrounded by clearly identifiable tumor tissue, and tumor cells can be detected within the lesion. Combined with the patient's medical history, this allows for an easy distinction from chest wall tuberculosis.

6. Treatment

Chest wall tuberculosis is highly detrimental, and once diagnosed, it requires prompt treatment. There are two treatment methods: one is conservative treatment, and the other is Surgical treatment. Conservative treatment mainly involves systemic anti-tuberculosis therapy combined with local treatment [11]. Local treatment includes incision and drainage as well as local dressing changes. Conservative treatment is primarily used for superficial and localized lesions. If the lesion is deep and extensive, Surgical treatment is required.

1.Conservative Treatment

For patients with mild lesions, conservative treatment can be considered. Conservative treatment first requires standardized anti-tuberculosis therapy, based on which local management is performed. Local treatment mainly targets tuberculous abscesses, with the specific method being incision and drainage. An incision can be made directly on the surface of the lesion to thoroughly remove pus and necrotic tissue within the lesion, followed by dressing changes and other subsequent treatments. The specific methods are the same as those used in the management of chest wall abscesses.

2. Surgical Treatment

Severe chest wall tuberculosis responds poorly to conservative treatment and requires Surgical intervention. Considering the particularity of chest wall tuberculosis, thorough preoperative preparation must be completed before

Surgery can be performed.

(i) Preoperative Preparation

Preoperative preparation for chest wall tuberculosis can include many aspects of local management of the lesion, systemic preparation, preparation of materials, and planning of the Surgical approach but the most important aspect is preoperative anti-tuberculosis therapy. To effectively suppress the growth of Mycobacterium tuberculosis and prevent its spread after Surgery, strong anti-tuberculosis treatment is generally recommended for 2 weeks prior to Surgery. If the chest wall infection is extremely severe or shows signs of spreading to surrounding areas, treatment should be extended to over 3 months. This approach is believed to help reduce the size of the chest wall lesion and stabilize other tuberculosis foci in the body, thereby improving the success rate of Surgery. Although this method has scientific merit, it must be emphasized that once chest wall tuberculosis has progressed to the stage requiring Surgical intervention, anti-tuberculosis therapy often has limited effect and rarely achieves significant results. Overemphasis on preoperative anti-tuberculosis treatment may bring additional problems for the patient and even delay the condition. Therefore, such treatment should be applied appropriately and tailored to the specific characteristics of the disease.

(ii) Surgical Procedure

The most notable feature of chest wall tuberculosis is the unpredictability of the lesion, which means there is no fixed Surgical procedure; decisions must be made based on intraoperative findings. To ensure the smooth completion of the Surgery, certain issues require special attention: ①Incision Considerations [12]. The incision for chest wall tuberculosis Surgery differs from that of general chest wall infections, primarily due to the unique pattern of lesion spread in tuberculosis. In most cases, the lesion tends to spread downward more easily. To better expose the primary lesion, the incision is generally placed in a higher position. This helps to avoid missing any part of the lesion. On the anterior chest wall, the incision typically needs to be parallel to the direction of the ribs.
This is conducive to exposure; incisions in other areas can be selected based on the specific situation. If the local skin is invaded or has a fistula, a fusiform skin incision should be made to avoid the lesion. ②The issue of lesion tracking [13]. The path of a tuberculous sinus tract is not fixed and is often concealed, making it difficult to detect. During the process of lesion removal, a thorough examination is necessary, and every suspicious sinus tract must be traced to avoid missing any lesions. ③The issue of handling bony structures [10]. Severe tuberculosis lesions often invade bony structures, leading to varying degrees of bone destruction. Such lesions must be thoroughly removed; otherwise, recurrence may occur. ④The issue of handling intrathoracic lesions. Many chest wall tuberculosis lesions are accompanied by intrathoracic lesions, and

the internal and external lesions are connected through intercostal invasion. If a thorough examination is not conducted preoperatively or careful exploration is not performed intraoperatively, intrathoracic lesions may be missed. While removing intrathoracic lesions, the structure of the chest wall must also be carefully examined, and if the ribs or intercostal structures are affected, they must also be completely removed. ⑤Chest wall reconstruction issue. Excessive resection of the chest wall's bony structure can lead to local defects, which theoretically require chest wall reconstruction. However, since the lesion is infectious, placing artificial materials for reconstruction may cause infection recurrence, so reconstruction must be approached with caution (Figure 6-3-1). To minimize damage, tissue flaps can be considered for filling [14]. This not only partially eliminates the defect but also helps incision healing. ⑥Skin defect management issue. During lesion removal, if part of the skin is excised, a local skin defect will form. Small skin defects can be directly sutured; larger defects require reconstruction with skin flaps.

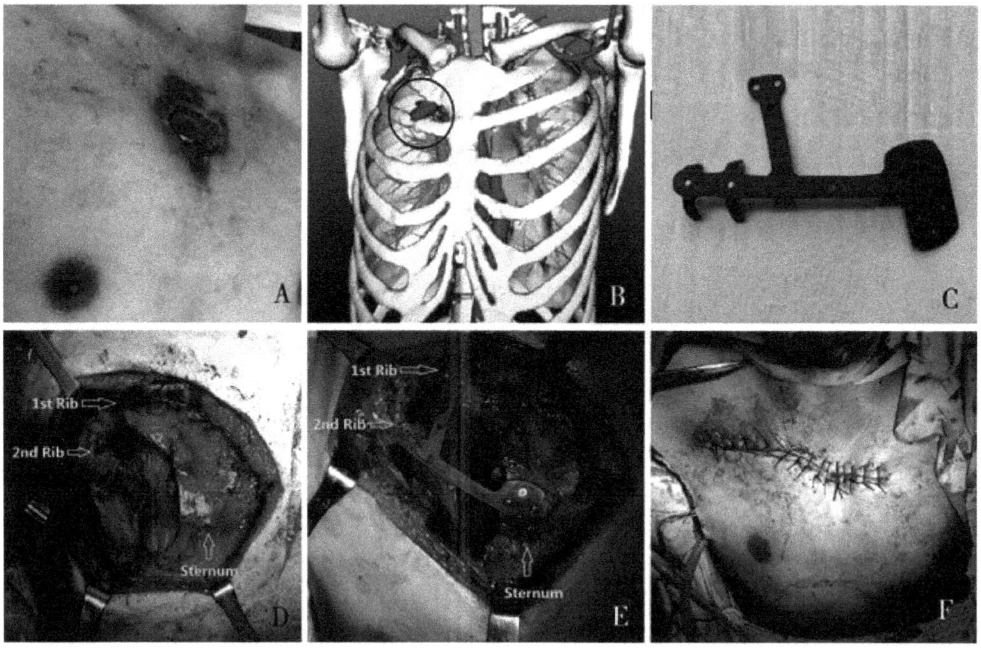

Figure 6-3-1 Chest wall tuberculosis lesion removal + chest wall reconstruction with digital material (A. Local chest wall ulceration with skin defect; B. 3D reconstruction of the thorax showing the lesion location; C. Customized digital material designed based on lesion information; D. Complete removal of the lesion; E. Implantation and proper fixation of the digital material; F. Direct suturing of the incision)

(iii) Postoperative management

After the main Surgical procedures are completed, postoperative local management is required to consolidate the Surgical results. Local management includes three aspects: Adequate drainage. Due to the large Surgical field and multiple areas of tissue involvement, there is usually considerable exudate. If the exudate is not drained, it can accumulate locally. The presence of fluid can affect incision healing and lead to Surgical failure. Therefore, fluid must be drained appropriately. Local irrigation, generally using streptomycin. Chest wall tuberculosis lesions contain a large number of tubercle bacilli. Although lesion removal eliminates the main lesion, it does not guarantee complete eradication of the bacilli. The presence of these bacteria poses a potential risk and may lead to recurrence. To eliminate the bacteria as much as possible, the wound surface can be repeatedly irrigated with streptomycin, which effectively removes residual bacilli and prevents recurrence. Local compression. After wound closure, good healing requires the elimination of dead space. One method to eliminate dead space is local compression, which is generally applied for about 3 weeks postoperatively. However, the pressure should not be too strong, as it may affect local blood circulation.

(iv) Consolidation treatment

Chest wall tuberculosis is a localized lesion of the chest wall. Although some lesions may be extensive and even invade intrathoracic structures, the lesions can generally be removed through Surgical treatment. Therefore, the success rate of Surgery is relatively high. However, Surgical success does not guarantee absolute prevention of lesion recurrence. Considering the strong infectivity of Mycobacterium tuberculosis, postoperative consolidation treatment is still necessary to achieve a complete cure. This is an important measure to prevent recurrence of the lesion.

Consolidation treatment mainly includes four basic aspects [11,13,14]: ①Anti-tuberculosis therapy. Since it is impossible to completely eliminate Mycobacterium tuberculosis during Surgery, and Surgery may also lead to the spread of tuberculosis lesions to other areas, postoperative anti-tuberculosis treatment is necessary. This treatment should last for about six months and must be carried out in a standardized manner. Standardized treatment helps completely eliminate the tuberculosis lesions. ②Systemic supportive treatment. Tuberculosis is a consumptive disease, and patients generally have poor overall health. Surgery represents an additional stress for the patient. To ensure early postoperative recovery, systemic supportive treatment must be emphasized. ③Prevention of common infections. Although chest wall tuberculosis Surgery targets tuberculous lesions, there is also the possibility of infection by non-specific pyogenic bacteria. Therefore, infection prevention measures must be taken to avoid such infections. ④Local incision care. One of the signs of Surgical success is proper incision healing. For lesions caused by specific infections, incision healing is especially important. If the incision does not heal, deeper infections may occur, leading to Surgical failure. Such recurrence due to poor incision healing is undoubtedly the greatest regret. To avoid this, various effective measures must be taken to ensure proper healing of the incision.

7. Recurrence issues

Chest wall tuberculosis is a relatively stubborn disease, but stubborn does not mean incurable. As long as effort is made in every detail, this disease is not difficult to cure. However, like many chronic infectious lesions, no matter how carefully treatment is carried out, failed Surgeries cannot be completely avoided. Some patients may have prolonged illness and develop refractory lesions. The reasons for Surgical failure or recurrence may be related to the following factors [7,10,11]:

1. Improper anti-tuberculosis treatment. Although chronic tuberculosis lesions are not necessarily sensitive to anti-tuberculosis treatment, reasonable preoperative medication can prevent the spread of bacteria, and postoperative medication can effectively prevent recurrence. If the medication is not standardized, it may lead to recurrence.
2. Incomplete Removal of Lesions. Thorough removal of lesions is key to preventing recurrence. If lesions are left behind for any reason, recurrence becomes difficult to avoid. Common causes of residual lesions include: ①Inadequate Preoperative Diagnosis or Misunderstanding of the Lesion: If the lesion is misdiagnosed as a general infection due to insufficient diagnosis or poor understanding, parts of the lesion may remain. ② Inadequate Treatment of Dumbbell-Shaped Abscesses: If only the chest wall component of a dumbbell-shaped abscess is removed while the thoracic cavity portion is neglected, residual lesions will remain in the chest cavity. ③Involvement of Bony Structures: If the lesion affects bony structures and this is not promptly identified or sufficiently resected, residual disease may occur. ④Involvement of Supraclavicular Lymph Nodes by Upper Anterior Chest Wall Lesions: These lymph nodes are prone to being invaded. If not removed, residual disease may persist. ⑤Involvement of Parasternal Lymph Nodes by Parasternal Lesions: These lymph nodes must also be removed thoroughly; incomplete removal can leave behind disease. ⑥Tuberculosis of the Chest Wall and Sinus Tract Spread: Chest wall tuberculosis can spread through sinus tracts, which may be very fine, while a sizable lesion could be hidden at the other end of the tract. If not detected, such lesions can also be left behind.
3. Pathogens not eliminated. The occurrence of chest wall tuberculosis may originate from lesions in surrounding organs or structures, such as tuberculous empyema or spinal tuberculous abscesses. These lesions can directly spread to the chest wall and form chest wall tuberculosis. When performing Surgery on chest wall tuberculosis, if the primary lesion is not identified or not completely removed, it may

lead to recurrence of the disease.

4. Improper timing of Surgery. After systemic anti-tuberculosis treatment, significant improvement in toxic symptoms can be considered a basic condition for Surgical treatment. If the patient's general condition is poor and tuberculosis in other parts of the body is not well controlled, postoperative recurrence is more likely to occur.
5. Excessive dead space in the Surgical field. After lesion removal, if excessive dead space remains in the Surgical field, fluid or blood accumulation within the cavity can easily lead to reinfection and recurrence of the lesion.
6. Improper use of drainage tubes. When using drainage tubes postoperatively, it is essential to ensure that the tubes remain completely unobstructed. Poor drainage can lead to fluid retention and cause lesion recurrence.
7. Poor general condition after Surgery. Tuberculosis is a consumptive disease. If the patient's nutritional status is poor and general condition is weak after Surgery, with low immunity, recurrence of the lesion is more likely.
8. Emergence of drug-resistant tuberculosis. When drug-resistant tuberculosis bacteria appear, various anti- tuberculosis drugs become ineffective, which may lead to recurrence.
9. Distant tuberculosis lesions spread again to the chest wall, causing recurrence. Lesions around the chest wall are relatively easy to detect, but if the primary lesion is located in a distant part of the body and is not identified in time, it may spread to the chest wall again after Surgery, resulting in recurrence.
10. Tuberculous lesion within the incision. If there is a tuberculous lesion within the incision, it may lead to poor wound healing after Surgery, and the lesion may recur as a result.

When recurrence occurs after chest wall tuberculosis Surgery, the condition may worsen or be milder than before. Regardless of whether it worsens or improves, it still requires further treatment. The treatment method can be determined based on the specific characteristics of the lesion; it can be conservative treatment or another Surgery. The basic Surgical approach is similar to the first operation, but special attention must be paid to Surgical details; otherwise, failure may occur again, leading to another recurrence of tuberculosis.

8. Prognosis

Chest wall tuberculosis is a rare and specific type of thoracic Surgical disease. In earlier times, when public health conditions were poor and tuberculosis was widespread, chest wall tuberculosis occurred relatively frequently. In recent years, however, this condition has become very rare, especially in urban areas, with most current cases concentrated in remote regions. During earlier treatment efforts, a few institutions developed relatively mature treatment methods and achieved some success. However, due to the highly variable nature of the disease, its stubborn pathology, and high recurrence rate, treating chest wall tuberculosis remains a significant challenge [12,13]. To effectively treat this condition, it is essential to strictly follow fundamental treatment principles and carefully manage every detail of the therapeutic process. Only by doing so can Surgical success be ensured; otherwise, recurrence of the lesion may occur, leading to treatment failure.

REFERENCES

[1] Keum, D. Y., J. B. Kim, and C. K. Park. 2012. "Surgical Treatment of a Tuberculous Abscess of the Chest Wall." *Korean Journal of Thoracic and Cardiovascular Surgery* 45 (3): 177–182.

[2] Kabiri, E. H., E. A. Alassane, M. K. Kamdem, et al. 2020. "Tuberculous Cold Abscess of the Chest Wall: A Clinical and Surgical Experience. Report of 16 Cases (Case Series)." *Annals of Medicine and Surgery* 51: 54–58.

[3] Quan, Changbin, Guokun Ao, Hong Li, et al. 2011. "CT Diagnosis of Chest Wall Tuberculosis." *Chinese Journal of Clinical Physicians (Electronic)* 5 (20): 5925–5929.

[4] Tanaka, S., M. Aoki, T. Nakanishi, et al. 2012. "Retrospective Case Series Analysing the Clinical Data and Treatment Options of Patients with a Tuberculous Abscess of the Chest Wall." *Interactive Cardiovascular and Thoracic Surgery* 14 (3): 249–252.

[5] Zhang, W., J. Chen, X. Wu, et al. 2020. "Preoperative Ultra-Short-Course Chemotherapy Combined with Surgery for the Treatment of Chest Wall Tuberculosis." *Infection and Drug Resistance* 13: 2277–2284.

[6] Hsu, H. E., and C. Y. Chen. 2019. "Tuberculous Retropharyngeal Abscess with Pott Disease and Tuberculous Abscess of the Chest Wall: A Case Report." *Medicine (Baltimore)* 98 (27): e16280.

[7] Jin, Feng, Cheng Wang, and Baoling Yang. 2005. "Reoperation Treatment for Postoperative Recurrence of Chest Wall Tuberculosis." *Shandong Medical Journal* 45 (30): 40–41.

[8] Grover, S. B., M. Jain, S. Dumeer, et al. 2011. "Chest Wall Tuberculosis: A Clinical and Imaging Experience." *Indian Journal of Radiology and Imaging* 21 (1): 28–33.

[9] Papavramidis, T. S., V. N. Papadopoulos, A. Michalopoulos, et al. 2007. "Anterior Chest Wall Tuberculous Abscess: A Case Report." *Journal of Medical Case Reports* 1: 152.

[10] Jiang, Youding, Sui Chen, and Tao Jiang. 2014. "Summary of Treatment of 346 Cases of Chest Wall Tuberculous Abscess and Literature Review." *Chinese Journal of Thoracic and Cardiovascular Surgery* 30 (7): 417–418.

[11] Lü, Xiaowu, Chiyu Jia, Shengjuan Feng, et al. 2014. "Advances in Surgical Treatment of Chest Wall Tuberculous Wounds." *Infection and Inflammation* 15 (2): 122–124.

[12] Xie, Jichen, Liu'an Sun, Yajie Ma, et al. 2009. "Clinical Study on Radical Surgery for Chest Wall Tuberculosis." *Chinese Journal of Tuberculosis and Respiratory Diseases* 31 (10): 605–607.

[13] Wang, Haihong, Zhaohua Xia, and Hongchun Li. 2010. "Discussion on Surgical Treatment of Chest Wall Tuberculosis." *Chinese Modern Doctor* 48 (18): 127–130.
[14] Xu, Chengcheng, and Xiangning Fu. 2011. "Application of Pedicled Greater Omentum Transplantation in Surgical Treatment of Refractory Chest Wall Tuberculosis." *Journal of Clinical Surgery* 19 (6): 411–413.

Section 4

POST-THORACOTOMY INCISIONAL INFECTION

Thoracotomy is generally a major Surgical procedure, and traditional operations in the past involved relatively long incisions. In recent years, with the advancement of minimally invasive Surgery, traditional thoracotomies have become less common. However, for certain specific intrathoracic diseases, long incisions are still necessary to complete the treatment. Longer incisions mean greater trauma and an increased risk of infection. Incisional infection is a specific and serious complication after thoracotomy. Once an infection occurs, it not only affects wound healing but may also lead to involvement of the deep Surgical field, with very serious consequences. Therefore, incisional infection is an important issue that must be taken seriously after thoracotomy [1,2]. However, due to the complexity of managing such infections, many thoracic Surgeons have a strong fear of them. This mindset can actually hinder effective treatment. In recent years, some experts have devoted themselves to the study of incisional infections and have accumulated a wealth of experience, significantly improving the treatment outcomes for this complication.

1. Causes of Onset

Incisional infection can occur after any type of thoracic Surgery, including lung Surgery, esophageal Surgery, mediastinal Surgery, and Surgeries involving the chest wall itself. It can also occur after cardiac Surgery; however, due to its unique characteristics, which will be discussed separately in the next section.

The occurrence of incisional infection is related to various factors, including both objective and subjective causes [3]. Objective factors mainly include the following: ① Poor local blood supply. Wound healing requires adequate nutrients, sufficient anti-inflammatory factors, and an optimal healing environment all of which depend on good blood circulation. If the blood supply is poor, wound healing may be compromised. ② Foreign bodies within the incision. Foreign materials such as implants, Surgical materials, and sutures, even if properly sterilized, can still irritate local tissues. This irritation can provoke adverse tissue reactions, and if pathogens are present, infection can easily develop. ③Condition of local soft tissue. Proper wound healing depends on good soft tissue coverage. If the deeper layers beneath the skin lack sufficient soft tissue, healing may be delayed, potentially leading to infection. ④Patient's general condition. When a patient has low systemic immunity, it negatively impacts wound healing and increases the risk of incisional infection.

Subjective factors are mainly related to the behavior of the patient and the Surgeon. For patients, this includes actions that damage the wound such as bathing too early, engaging in physical activity prematurely, or accidentally

injuring the incision which can all lead to wound damage and subsequent infection.
Physician-related factors are mainly technical [3], including the degree of adherence to aseptic principles, suturing techniques, drainage management, and postoperative wound care. All of these may affect incision healing. Aseptic principles are fundamental rules that must be observed at all times. If contamination occurs during the procedure, postoperative incisional infection can easily develop. Suturing technique also has a significant impact on incision healing.
It has a significant impact. During suturing, it is essential to ensure proper alignment of the incision with appropriate tension. Poor alignment can directly expose the skin edges and affect healing. Sutures that are too tight may compromise blood supply, while sutures that are too loose may lead to excessive exudate, both of which can impair incision healing. The healing of the incision is also related to the condition of drainage. If drainage is not smooth, exudate may accumulate within the incision, potentially forcing it open or serving as a culture medium for bacteria, thereby increasing the risk of infection. After the incision is sutured, regular dressing changes are required. If dressing changes are not performed according to basic principles, infection may also occur. Among the many factors that contribute to incisional infection, the Surgeon's technical skills are often the decisive factor. Only when the Surgeon continuously improves their technical level can the likelihood of infection be reduced.

2. Pathological Changes
In the early stages, incisional infection may present with signs of acute inflammation, including redness, swelling, warmth, and pain at the incision site. If the infection is not promptly controlled, it can lead to exudation, tissue necrosis, liquefaction, and suppuration within the incision. When the pressure from the pus becomes too high, it may result in pus leakage or directly force the incision open, forming an open lesion (Figure 6-4-1).

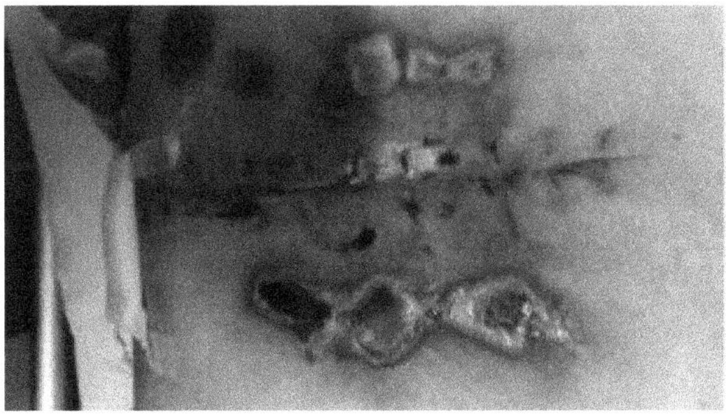

Figure 6-4-1 Incisional Infection After Thoracic Surgery

The specific pathological changes associated with incisional infection include the following [4]: ①Local Mass. In the early stages of infection, swelling occurs at the incision site, presenting as a firm mass with a texture different from the surrounding tissue. This is often accompanied by localized redness, increased skin temperature, and marked tenderness. ② Abscess Formation. As the infection progresses, pus begins to accumulate internally. If it is not discharged in time, an abscess may form. The abscess can protrude toward the body surface as a palpable mass, typically tender with a noticeable fluctuation. ③Incision Dehiscence [5]. As pressure builds inside the abscess, it may rupture through the skin incision, causing pus to leak out and potentially leading to complete separation of the wound edges. ④Sinus Tract Formation [6]. Deep-seated abscesses beneath the incision may drain through the incision itself or rupture through nearby normal tissue. The resulting drainage pathway becomes a sinus tract. Sinus tracts can discharge pus repeatedly and are difficult to heal if not properly managed. ⑤Full-Thickness Incisional Infection. If the infection is not contained, it may spread through all layers of the incision, ultimately causing complete wound dehiscence with continuous purulent discharge. ⑥Osteomyelitis [7]. The chest wall bones lie in the deepest layer. In severe soft tissue infections, the infection can spread to the bone, leading to suppurative osteomyelitis. ⑦Infection Spread: If the incisional infection is not effectively controlled, it may spread beyond the incision site. The infection can extend to surrounding chest wall structures and even deeper tissues, potentially involving the thoracic cavity and resulting in a more extensive and severe infection.

3. Hazards

Any disease requiring thoracotomy is not an ordinary condition and often carries significant risks. For such patients, the sole purpose of Surgery is to treat the disease. The incision is made solely to allow Surgical access. If the incision heals smoothly after Surgery, it has fulfilled its purpose. However, if an incisional infection occurs, it is equivalent to developing a new chest wall disease after treating the intrathoracic condition. This not only increases the cost of Surgery but also introduces additional harm. If the infection becomes chronic or spreads to surrounding areas or even into the thoracic cavity, the patient may face greater complications, and in severe cases, it can be life-threatening. Therefore, once an incisional infection occurs, every possible measure must be taken to control it; this is the only way to minimize the cost and consequences of Surgery.

4.Clinical Manifestations

The clinical manifestations of incisional infection are mainly localized but can also include systemic symptoms [3]. In the early or acute stages, infection typically presents as redness, swelling, warmth, and pain around the incision site. If not effectively controlled, the pain may worsen and evolve into throbbing pain, accompanied by progressive swelling at the incision. As the swelling advances, the incision may split open, allowing pus to drain, which may lead to temporary relief of pain. Systemic symptoms reflect generalized infection and may include fever, chills, fatigue, and general malaise. If the infection spreads into the thoracic cavity, respiratory symptoms may occur, such as cough, chest pain, and shortness of breath. When the infection involves the intrathoracic Surgical site, additional symptoms may appear depending on the affected structure.

5.Examinations

When incisional infection is suspected, the first step is a physical examination to directly assess the incision and surrounding tissue. This provides preliminary information about the wound and the underlying lesion. If the incision has already dehisced, it should be fully opened to allow further inspection of deeper tissue involvement. For localized incisional infections, imaging is of limited value. However, if there is a need to evaluate the surrounding area or check for intrathoracic involvement, imaging becomes essential (Figure 6-4-2).X-ray: Simple and quick, but not highly accurate. CT scan: More valuable; it helps visualize the lesion, surrounding structures, and the thoracic cavity.3D reconstruction: Can be performed if conditions permit, providing a clearer spatial understanding of the lesion.

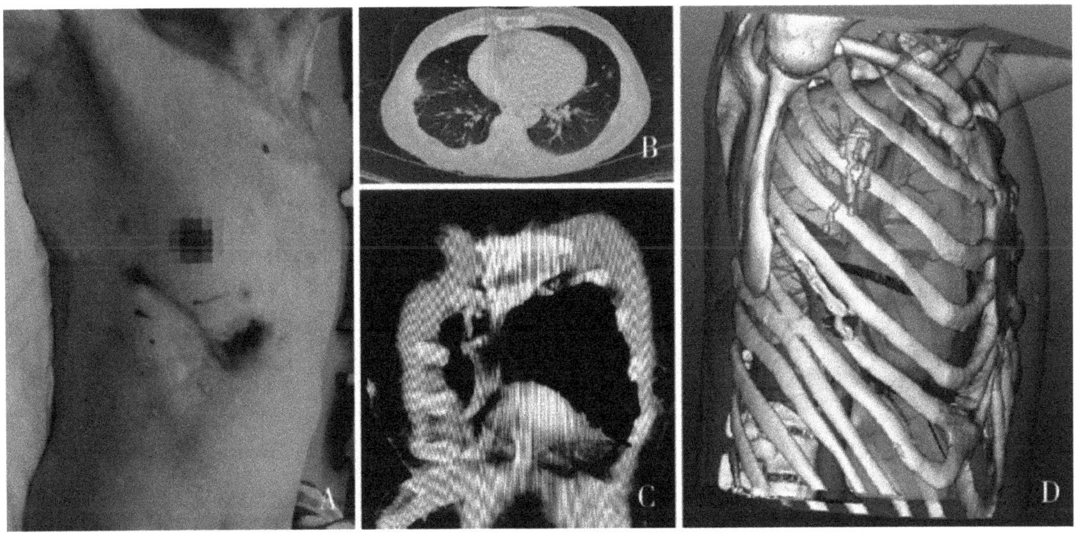

Figure 6-4-2 Imaging examinations of incision infection (A. Persistent incision infection after chest Surgery with repeated pus discharge; B. CT cross-section showing a chest wall lesion; C. CT image displaying lesions in the right chest wall and thoracic cavity; D. 3D reconstruction image indicating abnormal bony structures in the right chest wall, with obvious lesions in the middle and anterior parts of the 6th rib)

6. Diagnosis

The diagnosis of incision infection is relatively straightforward, but two key points must be emphasized: ①A recent thoracotomy (open chest Surgery) has been performed; ②Infection occurs before the incision has healed. Emphasizing the recent Surgery highlights the causal relationship between the incision and the infection.

Emphasizing the timing of the infection also underscores this causal link. If the infection appears after the incision has healed, it is not considered an incision infection but rather a general chest wall infection. Since the principles and methods of treatment for these two conditions are completely different, it is essential to differentiate between them.

7. Treatment

Wound infections can present in various forms, but the treatment principle is singular: first, convert the infected wound into a clean wound, then perform secondary suturing.

The basic method to convert an infected wound into a clean wound is dressing changes. The purpose of dressing changes is to remove pus, foreign bodies, and necrotic tissue from the wound, turning the purulent wound into a clean wound that gradually heals. If the infection is not severe, after dressing changes, granulation tissue around the wound will gradually proliferate and continuously fill the wound. Skin tissue can also grow steadily toward the center of the wound, eventually possibly achieving complete healing.

If the wound is too large and cannot be cleared by dressing changes alone, Surgical excision of the lesion is required (Figure 6-4-3). The specific procedure is [4]: ①Thorough disinfection. Before formal disinfection, perform initial debridement; after debridement is complete, carry out thorough disinfection.

Disinfect and drape, then remove the lesions inside the incision and in the deep layers. After completing the removal, disinfect and drape again, and then proceed with further operations. ②Thoroughly remove necrotic tissue. Necrotic tissue includes both soft tissue and bony structures, and all diseased tissues must be completely removed. ③Thoroughly eliminate the infection foci. Both superficial and deeply hidden infection sites must be cleared. ④Completely remove all foreign bodies. All foreign materials within the incision must be fully removed, including various shaping plates, fillers, wires, sutures, and so on.

After the above treatments, the lesion is essentially completely removed. During the process of lesion removal, a large amount of necrotic tissue may be excised, potentially resulting in local tissue defects. If the wound is closed directly, it may be difficult to achieve proper closure due to the presence of these defects. At this point, the use of autologous tissue for filling can be considered. The most commonly used autologous tissues are the greater omentum[8]and surrounding tissue flaps [9]. If there is a skin defect, skin flaps are needed for reconstruction.

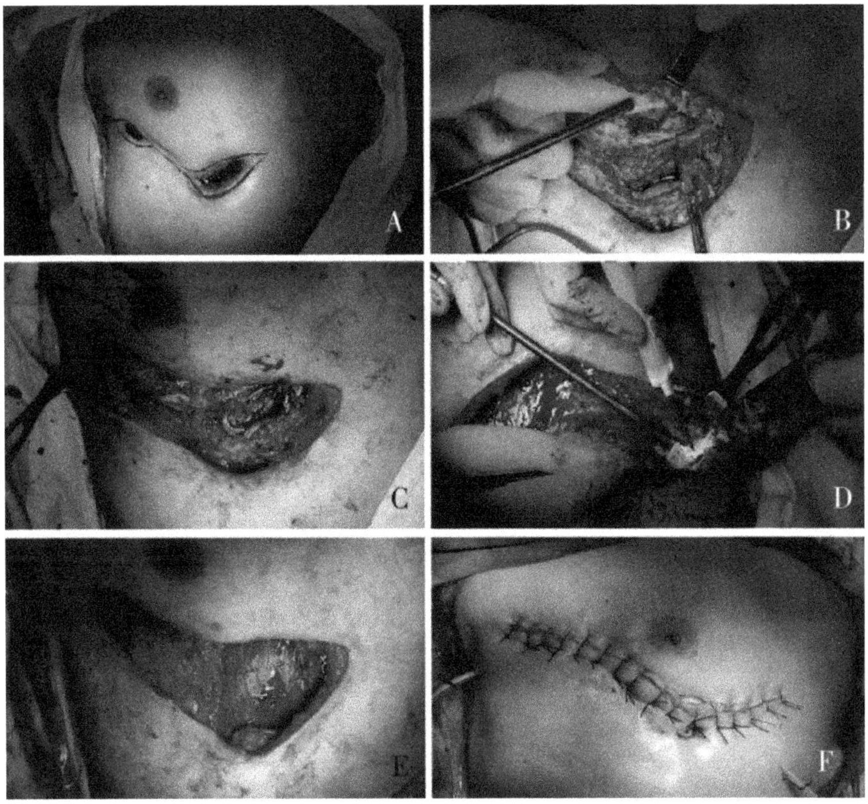

Figure 6-4-2 Imaging examinations of incision infection (A. Persistent incision infection after chest Surgery
with repeated pus discharge; B. CT cross-section showing a chest wall lesion; C. CT image displaying lesions in
the right chest wall and thoracic cavity; D. 3D reconstruction image indicating abnormal bony structures in
the right chest wall, with obvious lesions in the middle and anterior parts of the 6th rib)

During the above procedure, several issues need to be noted [4]: ①When reconstructing defects, it is not recommended to use artificial materials for reconstruction. After thorough removal of necrotic tissue and infectious foci, many normal tissues are also removed, often resulting in relatively large local defects.

These defects. According to the principles of defect reconstruction, these structures need to be rebuilt to restore the integrity of the chest wall. However, reconstruction means that new materials must be used, and most of these materials are foreign bodies. The use of foreign bodies provides a carrier for the persistence of pathogens and is therefore not recommended. ②Thoroughly eliminate dead space. Dead space will lead to the retention of exudate, which not only serves as a culture medium for bacteria but also prevents wound edges from closing, which is extremely detrimental to healing. Therefore, it must be completely eliminated. ③Ensure adequate drainage. The presence of fluid accumulation inside the incision is unfavorable for wound healing and must be smoothly drained. To achieve this, drainage tubes should be placed not only inside the incision but also in the deep spaces to ensure all possible fluid is drained outside the body. ④Full-thickness interrupted skin sutures. This method effectively stops bleeding, prevents exudation, and reduces the use of sutures. It is the most reasonable suturing technique, and during this stage, impractical cosmetic intradermal suturing should not be used for aesthetic reasons. ⑤Tension-reducing sutures. Because skin defects may exist, tension during suturing can be high. Excessive tension affects blood supply and compresses the local skin, which easily leads to skin necrosis. Once necrosis occurs, the incision faces risk again, so tension-reducing sutures must be applied to minimize local tension on the incision as much as possible. ⑥Enhance nutrition. The overall nutritional status directly relates to infection control, especially for patients with incision infections who have undergone previous Surgeries and reoperations for infectious foci. The patient's general condition may be affected and thus relevant measures must be taken to improve it. ⑦ Anti-infective treatment. Incision infections are generally local infections, but the Surgery itself may cause infection spread. Therefore, it is necessary to use powerful antibiotics postoperatively to effectively cooperate with local incision treatment.

During the treatment of incision infection, it is often necessary to compromise the integrity of the thoracic cage. This can not only lead to secondary chest wall deformities but may also affect chest wall function, even causing complications such as flail chest and paradoxical breathing. Such conditions are very unfavorable for the patient's postoperative recovery. However, controlling the infection is the primary mission at this time, and changes to the thoracic structure must be accepted as a necessary sacrifice to achieve infection control. To mitigate these adverse effects, external compression can be applied postoperatively to eliminate paradoxical breathing, helping the patient smoothly get through the perioperative period. If the deformity is significant, or if local depressions compress important deep structures, corrective or reconstructive Surgery of the thoracic cage may be considered after the infection has been completely eradicated. This essentially divides the Surgery for incision infection into two separate procedures.

8. Prognosis

Surgical site infection is a highly challenging condition that requires great effort to manage successfully. Mild infections can achieve satisfactory results with appropriate treatment. However, some infections are extremely stubborn, and despite tremendous efforts, the outcomes are unsatisfactory, with the incision becoming infected again. In such cases, it is necessary to carefully summarize experiences, deeply reflect on the procedural details, and after thorough preparation, perform Surgical treatment again until success is achieved [4].

REFERENCES

[1] Schiraldi, L., G. Jabbour, P. Centofanti, et al. 2019. "Deep Sternal Wound Infections: Evidence for Prevention, Treatment, and Reconstructive Surgery." *Archives of Plastic Surgery* 46 (4): 291–302.

[2] Reiss, N., U. Schuett, M. Kemper, et al. 2007. "New Method for Sternal Closure after Vacuum-Assisted Therapy in Deep Sternal Infections after Cardiac Surgery." *Annals of Thoracic Surgery* 83 (6): 2246–2247.

[3] Wang, W. L. 2021a. "The Harm and Clinical Manifestations of Median Sternotomy Incision Infection." *Today's Headlines*, November 1.

[4] Wang, W. L. 2021b. "Issues in Debridement of Chest Wall Surgical Wound Infection." *Today's Headlines*, November 1.

[5] Nadir, A., M. Kaptanoglu, E. Sahin, et al. 2013. "Post-Thoracotomy Wound Separation (Dehiscence): A Disturbing Complication." *Clinics (São Paulo)* 68 (1): 1–4.

[6] Yuan, Tianzhu, Qi Wang, Yuhong Jia, et al. 2011. "Surgical Repair of Refractory Chest Wall Incision Sinus Tract." *Chongqing Medical Journal* 40 (2): 207.

[7] Wyckman, A., I. Abdelrahman, I. Steinvall, et al. 2020. "Reconstruction of Sternal Defects after Sternotomy with Postoperative Osteomyelitis Using a Unilateral Pectoralis Major Advancement Muscle Flap." *Scientific Reports* 10: 8380.

[8] Yasuura, K., H. Okamoto, S. Morita, et al. 1998. "Results of Omental Flap Transposition for Deep Sternal Wound Infection after Cardiovascular Surgery." *Annals of Surgery* 227 (3): 455–459.

[9] Spindler, N., S. Kade, U. Spiegl, et al. 2019. "Deep Sternal Wound Infection: Latissimus Dorsi Flap Is a Reliable Option for Reconstruction of the Thoracic Wall." *BMC Surgery* 19: 173.

Cardiac Surgery can be performed through a variety of incisions, including median sternotomy, lateral thoracic wall incisions, and some minimally invasive incisions in special locations. Among these, the median sternotomy is the most commonly used. Due to its special anatomical location, infection of this incision can be particularly severe once it occurs. The incidence rate of median sternotomy infection is relatively high. Different studies report varying rates depending on the observed population, with figures in the literature ranging from 0.1% - 10% [1-7]. Surgical site infection is influenced by many factors, including the Surgical method, the Surgeon's operating habits, and the patient's physical condition. Median sternotomy infection is a very dangerous complication. Once it occurs, it often leads to serious consequences, and many patients die due to a lack of effective treatment. Literature statistics show a mortality rate of 30% -50% [8-10]. Due to the complexity and highly specialized nature of its treatment, many cardiac Surgeons are not proficient in managing this condition and ultimately have to refer patients to thoracic Surgeons. However, this condition also presents a major challenge for thoracic Surgeons. In recent years, with the collaborative efforts of multidisciplinary teams, treatment of this infection has gradually improved, and some effective methods have been developed and achieved promising outcomes.

1. Conceptual Issues

Postoperative cardiac incision infection is a general concept. Due to the many types of incisions, infections of all incisions should belong to this category. However, because management of the median sternotomy incision is more challenging, when referring to incision infection, it mostly means infection of the median sternotomy incision. This infection is also called (sternal wound infection, SWI) [1], (postoperative osteomyelitis) [2], (post- sternotomy mediastinitis) [3,11], (post-sternotomy dehiscence) [12], (sterno-mediastinitis) [13], and (deep sternal wound infection, DSWI)[4,5], etc. Although the names are different, the connotations are basically the same, all referring to infectious complications occurring at the incision site after cardiac Surgery. Therefore, the term postoperative sternal incision infection after cardiac Surgery is more representative. For convenience, it will be abbreviated as postoperative cardiac incision infection.

2. Classification

Due to different research perspectives, postoperative sternal wound infections can be classified in various ways. One classification is based on the depth of infection: superficial and deep incisional infections, the latter referring to the deep sternal wound infections mentioned above [10]. The infectious focus is located in the subcutaneous or soft tissue layer and does not involve the sternal wound. This type of infection is easier to control. Deep incision infections have lesions that extend deeply, involving the sternal wound and even reaching the mediastinum, which is the most severe type. This is the main focus of this section. Some authors divide postoperative cardiac incision infections into three types [12]: Type A is skin and soft tissue infection; Type B is skin and soft tissue infection reaching the sternum but not involving the sternum; Type C is infection of the sternum and mediastinum. Other authors classify them into three different types [14]: Non-infectious sternal instability, deep incision infection without sternal instability, and deep incision infection with sternal instability. This classification emphasizes internal stability. Additionally, some authors classify based on the time of infection onset [12]: Type I occurs within the first postoperative week; Type II occurs 2-6 weeks postoperatively; Type III occurs from 6 weeks to several years postoperatively. The different classification methods emphasize different aspects and have distinct clinical significance.

3. Causes of Onset

The occurrence of postoperative cardiac incision infection is related to many factors, but can be summarized into two: one is the decline of the body's resistance, and the other is pathogen infection. These two factors interact and complement each other, ultimately leading to infection.

The decline in the body's resistance is the result of multiple factors [2,7,11]. The first factor is the damaging effect of cardiopulmonary bypass on blood cells. Cardiac Surgery is generally performed under cardiopulmonary bypass. During this process, the body’s blood is circulated through various tubes for a long time; these tubes are not part of the human vascular system, and circulating blood through such tubes causes damage to its components. The destruction of blood cells reduces the body’s resistance through related mechanisms. The second factor is the trauma caused by the cardiac Surgery itself. Cardiac Surgery is generally major Surgery; although the concept of minimally invasive Surgery has become quite popular, absolute avoidance of trauma is impossible. These injuries also reduce the body's resistance. The third factor is the trauma from the Surgery itself. The Surgical field of median sternotomy is large, and the scope of invasion is wide, causing especially severe damage to the body, which also significantly lowers the body's resistance.

The decline in the body's resistance provides the possibility for incision infection to occur. If pathogens are present at this time, the probability of infection will greatly increase. The sources of pathogens for median sternotomy incision infection come from multiple channels: on one hand, they may originate from the environment; on the other hand, they may come from various instruments and materials, as well as from cardiopulmonary bypass. During Surgery through a median sternotomy incision, the entire mediastinum needs to be fully opened. The wide exposure to the air inevitably increases the chance of infection. Cardiac Surgery is a very special type of Surgery that requires a large number of instruments and materials, such as valves, patches, artificial blood vessels, sutures, etc. These materials are all artificial and foreign bodies. Although these materials undergo strict sterilization before Surgery, excessive use undoubtedly increases the risk of infection. Additionally, because cardiopulmonary bypass is used and the priming fluid for the bypass comes from outside the body, this becomes another possible source of pathogens.

After the decline of the body's resistance, infection can easily occur under the attack of various pathogens. The occurrence of infection also requires certain susceptibility factors, such as diabetes, liver and kidney dysfunction, and general malnutrition, all of which increase the chance of infection [7,11]. In addition, another important factor is the healing of the postoperative sternal wound itself. If the sternal incision can heal quickly, the incidence of incision infection will be greatly reduced. If the sternal wound fails to heal, it may lead to poor wound healing or even infection.

The healing of the sternal incision is affected by multiple factors [15]: ① Blood supply issues: The main blood supply to the sternum comes from the internal thoracic artery. The integrity of this artery is critical for satisfactory healing of the sternal incision. However, in some cardiac Surgeries, the internal thoracic artery needs to be harvested, and during almost all Surgeries, steel wires are used to fix the sternum. The placement and tightening of the fixation wires may also damage the internal thoracic artery. Once this artery is cut or damaged, the blood supply to the sternum is affected, and the sternum must rely on some small surrounding nourishing vessels, which may sometimes be insufficient for healing. ②Fixation condition: Good sternal healing depends on satisfactory fixation. In some cases, achieving satisfactory fixation is difficult. If the sternotomy cut deviates from the midline, fixation is hard to guarantee. Additionally, unsatisfactory placement of the steel wires may also affect fixation. In cases of osteoporosis, the sternum is difficult to fix firmly. Unsatisfactory fixation inevitably affects healing. ③Use of bone wax: Bone wax is used to stop bleeding at the sternal edges. A small amount of bone wax does not significantly affect healing. However, excessive use may cause liquefaction of the bone wax, which also impairs healing. ④Effect of subcutaneous tissue: Sternal healing requires sufficient soft tissue coverage. If there is too little soft tissue, the sternum and fixation wires lie directly beneath the skin, which is unfavorable for healing.

The healing of the sternal wound itself is the fundamental guarantee for the healing of the entire incision. If the sternum cannot heal, local looseness and friction occur at the incision, causing fluid leakage, which ultimately becomes a susceptibility factors for incision infection.

4. Pathological Changes

Postoperative cardiac incision infection is similar to incision infection after ordinary thoracotomy. In the early stage, acute inflammation may appear, characterized by redness, swelling, heat, and pain. As the infection worsens, a local abscess may form at the incision. The abscess contains increasing pus, and the pressure can cause the incision to rupture, allowing pus to overflow. Sinus tracts may form locally at the incision, or the incision may be forcibly opened. There can be extensive tissue necrosis inside the incision, and the sternum may show signs of osteomyelitis. Severe infection can spread to the surrounding chest wall or extend into the mediastinum, eventually resulting in mediastinitis [13].

5. Harm

Postoperative cardiac incision infection is a very difficult complication to treat. Many cases cannot be cured despite multiple treatments or Surgeries. This infection not only causes a great psychological impact on patients but also affects their physiological functions. In summary, these impacts mainly include three aspects[15]: ①Impact on thoracic function: The sternum is an important component of the thorax and a key structure for maintaining thoracic stability. A median sternotomy requires splitting the sternum down the middle. If the incision cannot heal properly, the sternum cannot close normally, which severely affects the stability and integrity of the thorax. Abnormal thoracic structure further leads to functional abnormalities, causing various functional problems for the patient. ②Impact on cardiac function: Infection of the cardiac Surgical incision can gradually develop into mediastinal infection. Various infectious factors will directly affect the heart. Cardiac Surgery itself already impacts heart function, and postoperative infection inevitably further impairs cardiac function. Further effects. ③Impact on respiratory function. After the occurrence of incision infection, because the incision must be opened, abnormal breathing may occur locally at the incision site. This is the most direct effect on respiration. In addition, the integrity of the thorax is damaged, which also affects breathing.

6. Clinical Manifestations

The clinical manifestations of postoperative cardiac incision infection are divided into two types: local symptoms and systemic symptoms [15]. Local symptoms mainly refer to characteristic signs at the incision site. Early on, there may be redness, swelling, heat, and pain. If the infection is uncontrolled, symptoms may gradually worsen, mainly with increased pain. If the incision dehisces or pus spontaneously drains, the pain may lessen, and systemic symptoms may not necessarily appear. If the infection spreads or toxins are released, fever, fatigue, chills, and other symptoms may occur. Since the infection may affect cardiopulmonary function, respiratory and circulatory symptoms can also be present.

The signs of postoperative cardiac incision infection are mainly localized to the incision area. Early signs include redness and swelling. As the infection worsens, a local abscess may form. Continued development of the abscess can cause incision dehiscence with large amounts of pus drainage. Severe infection can cause complete opening of the incision, tissue liquefaction, and necrosis within the wound, with continuous discharge from the incision (Figure 6-5-1).

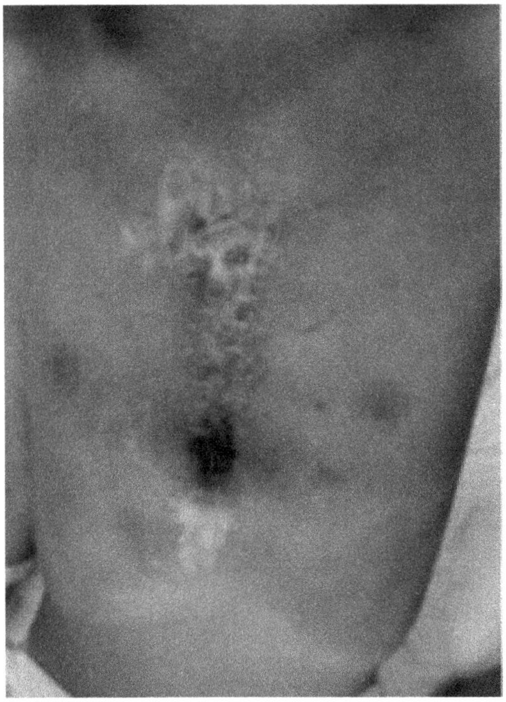

Figure 6-5-1 Postoperative Cardiac Incision Infection.

7. Examinations

The focus of postoperative cardiac incision infection examination is on the lesion itself and the surrounding structures. The most effective method is direct exploration of the incision site to understand the extent of the lesion, involved structures, and mediastinal infection. Imaging examinations provide limited information about the local incision area but play an important role in showing the surrounding structures, especially within the mediastinum. The most useful imaging method is CT scanning, which can be combined with 3D reconstruction of relevant structures for clearer visualization. Ultrasound can show local incision information and can also be used to examine the heart, clarifying the infection's impact on cardiac structures and function.

8. Diagnosis

In most cases, the diagnosis of postoperative incision infection after cardiac Surgery is relatively straightforward. Any infectious lesion occurring within the

Surgical incision after cardiac Surgery falls into this category. However, some infections are more insidious and may present no symptoms in the early stages. If the infection begins in the mediastinum or within the sternum, imaging examinations are required for a definitive diagnosis.

9. Treatment

Once a postoperative incision infection after cardiac Surgery is diagnosed, prompt treatment is necessary. There are two treatment approaches: conservative treatment and Surgical treatment. Infections confined to the superficial layer of the incision without sternal involvement can be effectively managed with conservative treatment. The main components of conservative treatment include local wound care and topical therapy. In recent years, some authors have applied negative pressure wound therapy in the treatment of postoperative incision infections after cardiac Surgery[11,16,17]. This technique can serve as a transitional treatment before Surgery or be used independently, though its effectiveness remains uncertain.

When large-area or deep infections cannot be effectively treated with conservative methods, Surgical treatment becomes necessary. The fundamental principles of Surgical treatment are generally the same as those for managing incision infections after standard thoracic Surgery: first, convert the infected wound into a clean wound, and then proceed with wound closure.

(1) Preoperative Preparation

Surgical treatment for postoperative incision infections after cardiac Surgery is a complex and extensive process. To ensure the success of the Surgery, thorough preoperative preparation is essential. The preparation includes:① Systemic preparation: After cardiac Surgery, patients are often in a weakened state. Recurrent incision infections can lead to significant physical depletion, resulting in poor overall condition. Performing Surgery under such circumstances is far from ideal. Therefore, various measures must be taken preoperatively to improve the patient's general condition. ②Pathogen identification: It is important to identify the type of pathogen and its antibiotic sensitivity before Surgery, to guide subsequent treatment. ③ Anti-infection treatment: Targeted anti- infective therapy should be administered preoperatively. This helps eliminate pathogens from other parts of the body and partially controls the local infection at the incision site, which is crucial for the success of Surgery. ④ Local incision preparation: Since the Surgical focus is the infected area around the incision, thorough local preparation is vital. This typically includes wound dressing changes, removal of necrotic tissue, and adequate drainage. These measures aim to clean the wound as much as possible and promote the growth of granulation tissue, laying a solid foundation for successful Surgery.

(2) Surgical Treatment

Surgical treatment of postoperative incision infections after cardiac Surgery primarily focuses on managing the local lesion, consisting of two main aspects: first, thoroughly removing the infectious focus; second, treating the wound. The specific procedures are as follows:

(i) Removal of the Infectious Focus

The purpose of removing the infectious focus is to convert the infected wound into a clean incision. The following steps are required [17,18]: ①Repeated disinfection. Strictly adhere to aseptic principles to disinfect the area around and inside the Surgical field repeatedly. Every detail, step, and local area of the operation must be disinfected multiple times to eliminate pathogens to the greatest extent possible. ②Thoroughly remove foreign bodies. All steel plates, wires, patches, and sutures in the Surgical field may harbor pathogens and must be completely removed. ③Completely excise necrotic tissue. All necrotic tissue, including suspicious areas, must be fully removed, especially any suspicious necrotic parts of the sternum. If the sternal lesion extends to involve the costal cartilage or ribs on either side, these structures must also be removed. Additionally, necrotic tissue within the mediastinum must be completely cleared. ④ Thoroughly remove infected tissue. All pus, purulent debris, and infection-related tissues and structures within the Surgical field must be fully removed, leaving no dead space or residual infection. ⑤Treat materials on the surface of the heart. Artificial vessels, patches, pledgets, and exposed sutures on the heart and major blood vessels are common hiding places for pathogens. Since these materials cannot be removed, special sterilization and disinfection measures must be taken to minimize the risk of reinfection.

(ii) Closed wound

After the infection focus is eliminated, the wound basically reaches a clean or even sterile state. Next, the wound needs to be closed. At this time, the wound is a defect of varying degrees, essentially falling within the category of secondary chest wall defects, and the treatment principles are basically the same as those for general secondary chest wall defects. However, due to the special context involving cardiac Surgery, higher Surgical technical requirements are needed and must be specifically addressed.

(iii) The issue of handling bony structures.

The most critical step in wound closure is the handling of the bony structures within the lesion. This involves two main aspects: first, the treatment of the sternal wound, and second, the management of bony structure defects. The sternum and surrounding bony structures are essential components of the thoracic cage, playing a crucial role in its stability. Therefore, in theory, the sternal wound should not only be closed and fixed, but all defects involving bony structures should also be reconstructed. However, since infections at the Surgical site often involve the sternal wound, direct closure and fixation may lead to recurrence of the infection. If the wound is extensive and requires resection of the sternum and the adjacent costal cartilage or ribs, residual infection may still be present around the defect. Given that reconstruction of the defect would necessitate the use of artificial materials, which significantly increases the risk of infection recurrence, the use of such materials must be abandoned to completely eliminate that possibility. Reconstructing chest wall bony defects is almost entirely dependent on artificial materials. Forgoing them means such reconstruction cannot be carried out, which negatively affects the stability of the thoracic cage. However, since the primary goal of the Surgery is to eliminate the Surgical site infection, stability of the thoracic cage must not be overemphasized at this stage. That said, not overemphasizing does not mean ignoring it completely. If the defect significantly impairs respiratory function, it becomes a more serious issue, and efforts should be made to address it whenever conditions allow. The proper approach is to use autologous soft tissue for filling. While this method is not as effective as using artificial materials, it can minimize the defect as much as possible and help avoid adverse outcomes.

(iv) The issue of autologous tissue filling.

As mentioned above, since the sternum cannot be directly closed and there may be defects in the bony structures, soft tissue is required to fill the defect. Clinically, two main types of soft tissue are used: one is the greater omentum[19], and the other is muscle flap [20-22]. The greater omentum is effective for lesions in the lower part of the sternal incision. However, due to the limited amount of tissue it provides, it cannot meet the needs of larger defects and is therefore not an ideal filling material. Muscle flaps are the most commonly used and most effective filling tissue. There are three types of muscle flaps available for use [4,20-22]: first, the rectus abdominis flap; second, the latissimus dorsi flap; and third, the pectoralis major flap. The rectus abdominis flap can be used for filling operations in the lower part of the incision, but this flap also has certain drawbacks [4,23]. First, a relatively long incision must be made in the abdomen, which adds additional trauma; second, the amount of tissue in this flap is sometimes limited and insufficient to fill larger defects. The latissimus dorsi flap is located relatively far from the incision and requires extensive mobilization to be effective, so it is rarely used in clinical practice [20]. The pectoralis major flap is the most commonly used filling tissue in clinical practice [17,21,22]. It can be harvested directly through the median incision itself, which reduces additional trauma. The flap provides a large amount of tissue and can be harvested bilaterally, thus meeting the requirements of almost all filling procedures.

In clinical practice, there are three methods for using the pectoralis major muscle flap for filling. The first method is the anterograde muscle flap.

Specifically, this involves severing the pectoralis major from its attachments to the sternum and costal cartilages to mobilize the muscle as much as possible, then placing the free end of the muscle into the sternal gap for filling (Fig. 6-5-2). The pectoralis major receives its blood supply primarily from the pectoral branch of the thoracoacromial artery, with additional contributions from branches of the lateral thoracic artery, thoracodorsal artery, and subscapular artery. Its medial blood supply comes from branches of the internal thoracic artery. Once the medial attachment is severed, the internal thoracic artery no longer supplies the muscle, but the lateral vessels are able to provide sufficient blood flow, which justifies the use of this muscle flap. This flap technique is relatively simple to perform and can meet the needs for filling the middle and upper parts of the incision. If combined with a greater omentum flap in a joint procedure, defects in all regions can be effectively filled. The main limitation of this muscle flap is its length of extension. Because its lateral base is fixed, it cannot be pulled significantly toward the midline for central filling, which clearly limits its applicability. If a large amount of tissue is required for the filling, this muscle flap may not be sufficient.

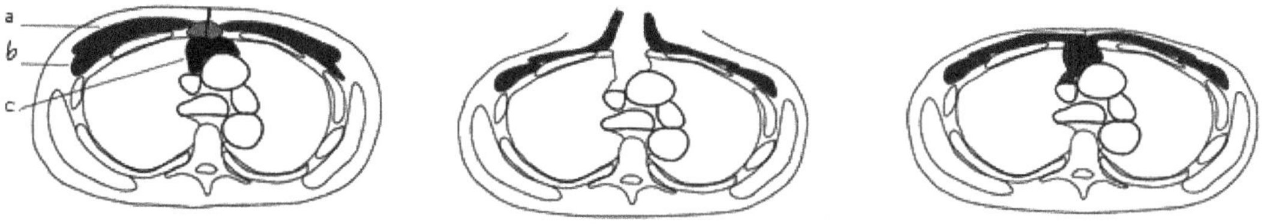

A B C

Figure 6-5-2 Pectoralis Major Muscle Flap Filling the Lesion (A. Lesion location. a. Pectoralis major; b. Pectoralis minor; c. Lesion site.B. Begin mobilizing the pectoralis major from the midline and pull it toward the lesion to ensure sufficient flap length.C. Fill the muscle flap into the lesion and secure it properly.)

The second method is the retrograde pectoralis major muscle flap. Specifically, this involves severing the muscle at an appropriate point on its lateral side, then rotating the muscle to fill the incision site (Figure 6-5-3). At this point, all of the lateral blood vessels are cut off, and the only remaining blood supply comes from the internal thoracic artery. Because the resected tissue volume is sufficiently large and the remaining tissue lies close to the incision, it can meet the filling needs of all areas of the incision, making it an ideal filling material. However, this muscle flap also has its drawbacks. Since the blood supply relies solely on the internal thoracic artery, in Surgeries where this artery is damaged, the viability of this muscle flap is compromised. Fundamental guarantee.

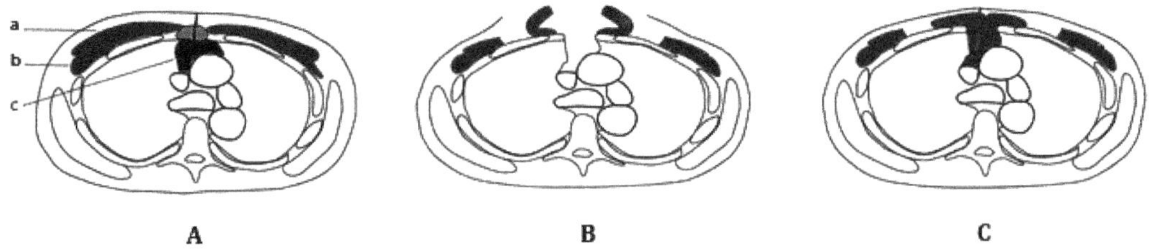

Figure 6-5-3: Retrograde Pectoralis Major Muscle Flap Filling the Lesion (A. Lesion location. a. Pectoralis major; b. Pectoralis minor; c. Lesion. B. The pectoralis major is transected from the lateral side of the midline, and the medial half is rotated toward the midline. C. The muscle flap is used to fill the lesion and is securely fixed.)

The third method is the separation of the muscle flap [24]. Specifically, the pectoralis major muscle flap is divided into two parts: the upper portion is used as an anterograde muscle flap, and the lower portion as a retrograde muscle flap. This design allows for meeting different filling requirements.

When using the pectoralis major muscle flap, the range and method of flap resection should be designed based on the location to be filled and the amount of tissue required. If the filling requirement is relatively small, a unilateral pectoralis major flap can be used [2,7]. If a larger volume of muscle is needed for filling, bilateral muscle flaps may be considered [7,19]. Some advocate for using a unilateral pectoralis major flap, with the main reasons being [2]: ①It avoids affecting the function of both upper limbs due to the use of bilateral pectoralis major flaps. ②It preserves the contralateral pectoralis major as a backup flap in case the initial Surgery fails, allowing for a secondary operation using the opposite side. Regardless of which method is used for filling, several general principles must be observed: Every gap must be filled as completely as possible to avoid leaving dead space. The flap must be securely fixed to prevent loosening.

Adequate drainage must be placed in the mediastinum and thoracic cavity to prevent fluid accumulation. Hemostasis must be thorough and appropriate to prevent hematoma formation. To minimize irritation from sutures, coarse Prolene sutures may be considered for closure. These principles are fundamental to ensuring the success of the filling procedure and must be strictly followed during Surgery, as they are the essential safeguards for a successful outcome.

(v) Closure of the skin incision.

Under the guidance of the above principles, the space and defects between both sides of the sternum can generally be eliminated. The next step is the closure of the skin incision. In cases of postoperative sternal wound infection after cardiac Surgery, there is usually no significant skin defect, so direct suturing is often possible. To minimize suture-related reactions, interrupted full-thickness sutures may be considered. If the tension is too high, tension-reducing sutures should be used.

(3) Postoperative Management

Cardiac Surgery itself imposes significant trauma on the patient, and a Surgical site infection further increases the physical burden. When Surgical intervention is used to treat the infection, the body endures yet another major insult. As a result, patients are often extremely weakened postoperatively and require robust supportive measures to improve their overall condition. This comprehensive support is fundamental to the success of the Surgery.In addition to supportive measures, necessary anti-infection treatment must be performed; this is an essential measure to consolidate the therapeutic effect. If there is no clear pathogenic target, broad- spectrum antibiotics can be used. Additionally, proper local treatment of the incision is required. Local treatment includes regular dressing changes and appropriate physiotherapy, which greatly helps incision healing.

(4) The Issue of reoperation

Postoperative incision infection after cardiac Surgery is a highly challenging complication. Although good results can be achieved through the above-mentioned treatments, such as surgeries inherently carry many uncertainties, and thus, reoperation failure may occur. Generally speaking, as long as the procedures are strictly followed as described above, even if failure occurs again, the patient's condition will significantly improve, manifesting as a marked reduction in the extent and severity of the infection. Such cases can often achieve satisfactory outcomes through local treatment. Even if reoperation is necessary, the difficulty will be greatly reduced.

The principles of reoperation are roughly the same as those of the first Surgery. However, an important requirement is not to easily completely remove parts that were satisfactorily repaired during the first Surgery. Doing so would not only cause excessive damage but also result in a passive situation with no available tissue for filling. of course, if the first Surgery not only failed to improve the incision condition but also worsened the infection, the extent of removal cannot be too conservative.

10. Prognosis

Although postoperative incision infection after cardiac Surgery is not a common complication, it is an extremely challenging one. Once it occurs, it becomes very difficult to manage [7,19]. To this day, major cardiac Surgery centers regard this complication as one of the most troublesome, and overall treatment outcomes have remained unsatisfactory. With the emergence of thoracic wall Surgery concepts, understanding of this complication has gradually deepened, providing theoretical support for improvements in treatment methods. After continuous exploration, the treatment of this complication has seen significant improvement. However, due to the remaining uncertainties, related techniques still require further refinement.

REFERENCES

[1] Dubert, M., A. Pourbaix, S. Alkhoder, et al. 2015. "Sternal Wound Infection after Cardiac Surgery: Management and Outcome." *PLOS ONE* 10 (9): e0139122.

[2] Wyckman, A., I. Abdelrahman, I. Steinvall, et al. 2020. "Reconstruction of Sternal Defects after Sternotomy with Postoperative Osteomyelitis Using a Unilateral Pectoralis Major Advancement Muscle Flap." *Scientific Reports* 10: 8380.

[3] van Wingerden, J. J., D. T. Ubbink, C. M. van der Horst, et al. 2014. "Poststernotomy Mediastinitis: A Classification to Initiate and Evaluate Reconstructive Management Based on Evidence from a Structured Review." *Journal of Cardiothoracic Surgery* 9: 179.

[4] Li, Y. H., Z. Zheng, J. Yang, et al. 2017. "Management of Extensive Thoracic Defects after Deep Sternal Wound Infection with the Rectus Abdominis Myocutaneous Flap: A Retrospective Case Series." *Medicine (Baltimore)* 96 (16): e6391.

[5] Schiraldi, L., G. Jabbour, P. Centofanti, et al. 2019. "Deep Sternal Wound Infections: Evidence for Prevention, Treatment, and Reconstructive Surgery." *Archives of Plastic Surgery* 46 (4): 291–302.

[6] Morgante, A., and F. Romeo. 2017. "Deep Sternal Wound Infections: A Severe Complication after Cardiac Surgery." *Giornale di Chirurgia* 38 (1): 33–36.

[7] Torto, F. L., G. Turriziani, C. Donato, et al. 2020. "Deep Sternal Wound Infection Following Cardiac Surgery: A Comparison of Monolateral and Bilateral Pectoralis Major Flaps." *International Wound Journal* 17 (3): 683–691.

[8] Kobayashi, T., A. Mikamo, H. Kurazumi, et al. 2011. "Secondary Omental and Pectoralis Major Double-Flap Reconstruction Following Aggressive Sternectomy for Deep Sternal Wound Infection after Cardiac Surgery." *Journal of Cardiothoracic Surgery* 6: 56.

[9] Deschka, H., S. Erler, L. El-Ayoubi, et al. 2013. "Suction-Irrigation Drainage: An Underestimated Therapeutic Option for Surgical Treatment of Deep Sternal Wound Infections." *Interactive Cardiovascular and Thoracic Surgery* 17 (1): 85–89.

[10] Jones, G., M. J. Jurkiewicz, J. Bostwick, et al. 1997. "Management of the Infected Median Sternotomy Wound with Muscle Flaps: The Emory 20-Year Experience." *Annals of Surgery* 225 (6): 766–778.

[11] Kaul, P. 2017. "Sternal Reconstruction after Poststernotomy Mediastinitis." *Journal of Cardiothoracic Surgery* 12 (1): 94.

[12] Anger, J., D. C. Dantas, R. T. Arnoni, et al. 2015. "A New Classification of Post-Sternotomy Dehiscence." *Revista Brasileira de Cirurgia Cardiovascular* 30 (1): 114–

118.
[13] Ennker, I. C., and J. C. Ennker. 2012. "Management of Sternomediastinitis." *HSR Proceedings in Intensive Care & Cardiovascular Anesthesia* 4 (4): 233–241.
[14] Rupprecht, L., and C. Schmid. 2013. "Deep Sternal Wound Complications: An Overview of Old and New Therapeutic Options." *Open Journal of Cardiovascular Surgery* 6: 9–19.
[15] Wang, W. L. 2021. "The Hazards and Clinical Manifestations of Median Sternotomy Infection." *Jinri Toutiao (Today's Headlines)*, November 1.
[16] Dohmen, P. M., T. Markou, R. Ingemansson, et al. 2014. "Use of Incisional Negative Pressure Wound Therapy on Closed Median Sternal Incisions after Cardiothoracic Surgery: Clinical Evidence and Consensus Recommendations." *Medical Science Monitor* 20: 1814–1825.
[17] Song, F., and Z. Liu. 2020. "Bilateral Pectoralis Major Muscle Advancement Flap Combined with Vacuum-Assisted Closure Therapy for the Treatment of Deep Sternal Wound Infections after Cardiac Surgery." *Journal of Cardiothoracic Surgery* 15: 227.
[18] Zhang, H., J. Lin, H. Yang, et al. 2020. "Bilateral Partial Pectoralis Major Muscle Turnover Flaps for the Management of Deep Sternal Wound Infection Following Cardiac Surgery." *Journal of Thoracic Disease* 12 (10): 6010–6015.
[19] Yasuura, K., H. Okamoto, S. Morita, et al. 1998. "Results of Omental Flap Transposition for Deep Sternal Wound Infection after Cardiovascular Surgery." *Annals of Surgery* 227 (3): 455–459.
[20] Spindler, N., S. Kade, U. Spiegl, et al. 2019. "Deep Sternal Wound Infection: Latissimus Dorsi Flap Is a Reliable Option for Reconstruction of the Thoracic Wall." *BMC Surgery* 19: 173.
[21] Pairolero, P. C., P. G. Arnold, and J. B. Harris. 1991. "Long-Term Results of Pectoralis Major Muscle Transposition for Infected Sternotomy Wounds." *Annals of Surgery* 213 (6): 583–590.
[22] Bakri, K., S. Mardini, K. K. Evans, et al. 2011. "Workhorse Flaps in Chest Wall Reconstruction: The Pectoralis Major, Latissimus Dorsi, and Rectus Abdominis Flaps." *Seminars in Plastic Surgery* 25 (1): 43–54.
[23] Hever, P., P. Singh, I. Eiben, et al. 2021. "The Management of Deep Sternal Wound Infection: Literature Review and Reconstructive Algorithm." *JPRAS Open* 28: 77–89.
[24] Parisi, P., F. Lo Torto, B. Carlesimo, et al. 2018. "The Split Pectoralis Flap: Combining the Benefits of Pectoralis Major Advancement and Turnover Techniques in One Flap." *Plastic and Reconstructive Surgery* 141 (1): 191e–192e.

Negative pressure wound therapy (NPWT) [1-3] is known by various names, such as vacuum-assisted closure (VAC) [4-6] or vacuum sealing drainage (VSD) [7,8]. In foreign literature, the first two terms are more commonly used, while most Chinese authors prefer to use VSD [7,8]. Although the names differ, they refer to exactly the same technique. NPWT was first proposed by Morykwas et al. [2] in 1997. Due to its significantly better outcomes compared to conventional infection management methods, it was quickly adopted. Over many years of clinical practice, this technique has been used in various medical specialties, including for acute and chronic wounds, infectious lesions, etc., all with relatively satisfactory results [1,4-6]. In recent years, this technique has started to be applied in thoracic Surgery, especially in cases of Surgical incision infections [9,10], and clinical experience has shown that its efficacy is also superior to conventional treatment methods.

As previously mentioned, the basic principle in managing infectious lesions is to first convert them into clean or even sterile wounds before proceeding with suturing. In this entire process, the initial treatment step is the most critical. Traditional methods have been relatively singular, primarily relying on simple dressing changes[11,12]. Dressing changes require the incision to be completely opened, all steel plates, wires, sutures, or other foreign bodies to be removed, necrotic tissue to be cleared, and the wound to be repeatedly flushed with disinfectant and antibacterial solutions, followed by placement of drainage. Although dressing changes are the simplest and most commonly used method, they come with many problems[12]: ①Infectious lesions often produce large amounts of exudate and necrotic tissue, necessitating frequent dressing changes and constant replacement of wound materials, which significantly increases the workload. ②The procedure requires debridement of necrotic and infected tissue, often involving direct cutting and trimming of tissue within the incision, which causes considerable pain to the patient. ③Drainage is typically achieved through tubing, but due to the limited drainage area, it often fails to achieve satisfactory results. ④The need to keep the incision fully open creates a large wound surface, which can have a negative psychological impact on the patient. ⑤It often takes a very long time to achieve any meaningful effect, and even then, the outcomes are frequently uncertain. These issues make it clear that although dressing changes are a simple procedure, they come with many drawbacks. If other, more reasonable methods could replace traditional dressing changes, it would lead to significant improvements in wound management.

1. Basic Components of the NPWT Device

NPWT (Negative Pressure Wound Therapy) is a technique that treats infectious lesions using a specialized mechanism. The essence of this technique is to transform an open, infected wound into a closed, relatively clean one, thereby creating a local environment that promotes tissue regeneration and is conducive to antibacterial activity ultimately allowing the infection to be controlled in the shortest possible time[11,12]. To achieve this, NPWT requires specific materials and devices. Its basic components consist of three main parts [13-15]: ①Special sponge-like material with multi-sided hole drainage tubes: This material is made from a high-polymer synthetic substance, featuring numerous tiny pores. It offers excellent biocompatibility, water permeability, and malleability. It is non-toxic and causes no irritation to human tissue; a rigid drainage tube is embedded within the sponge material, and the tube contains numerous side holes, allowing for convenient drainage. ②Bio- permeable adhesive film: This structure is a semi-permeable membrane with good oxygen permeability and water resistance, capable of preventing bacterial invasion. ③Negative pressure suction device: This device can continuously apply negative pressure suction through a drainage tube (Figure 6-6-1).

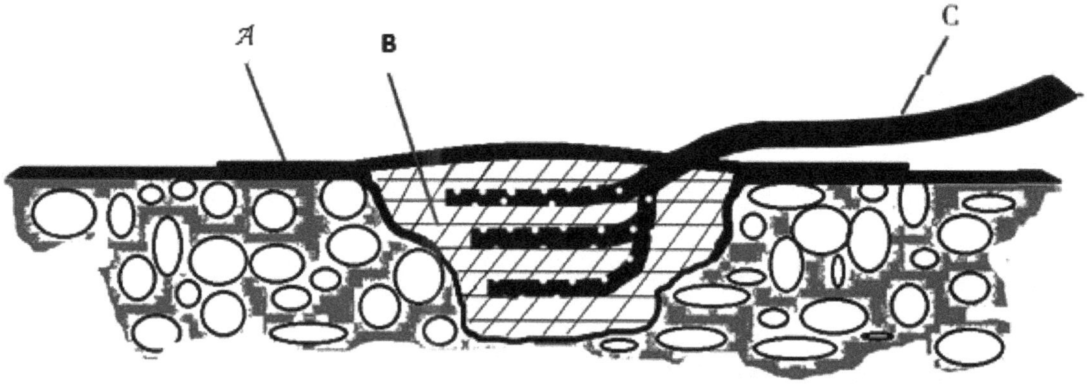

Figure 6-6-1 Basic Components of NPWT (A. Bio-permeable adhesive film; B. Sponge material; C. Suction tube one end is placed in the sponge material and has side holes, while the other end is connected to the negative pressure suction device)

2. Specific Operation of NPWT Technology

NPWT (Negative Pressure Wound Therapy) is a specialized drainage technique with strict operational requirements (Figure 6-6-2). The specific steps are as follows [5,7,13,15,16]: ①Debridement: This procedure can be performed under local anesthesia in a general dressing room. If the lesion is too large, deep, or severely damaged, it must be performed under general anesthesia in an operating room. The infected area must be fully exposed, and all necrotic tissue, purulent secretions, wires, sutures, drainage materials, and other foreign bodies must be thoroughly removed to eliminate any dead space. The wound should then be repeatedly irrigated with povidone-iodine, hydrogen peroxide, and normal saline to ensure the wound surface is as clean as possible. ② Placement of NPWT filler material:

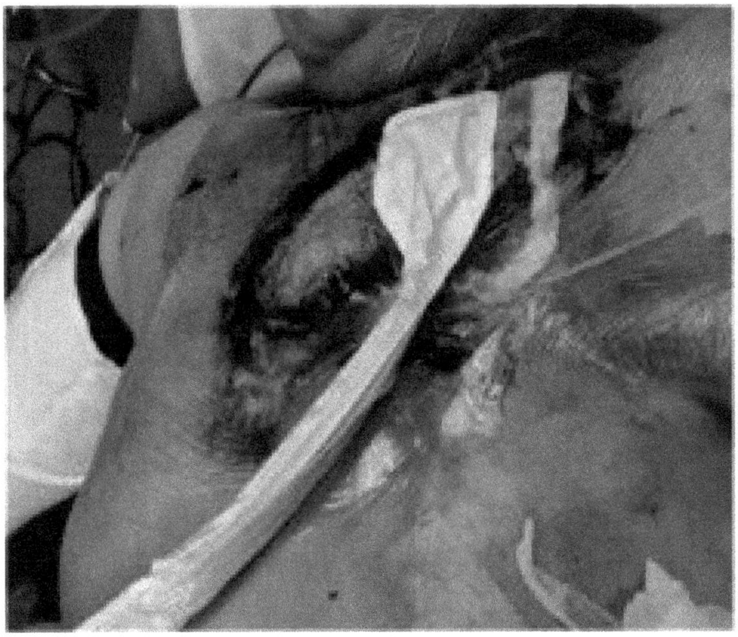

Figure 6-6-2: Patient undergoing wound suction using technology

The NPWT filler is made of specially designed material, which is commercially available for clinical use. The material should be trimmed according to the size, extent, and depth of the wound so that it slightly exceeds the area of the lesion and completely fills it. ③ Connection of the negative pressure drainage tube: Placement of the drainage tube is one of the critical steps in the procedure. The NPWT materials used in clinical practice generally come with pre-made drainage tubes. During the procedure, the components must be connected according to the design requirements, brought out through the incision, and connected to the negative pressure suction device connection. ④ Membrane covering: Seal the entire wound area with a bio-permeable adhesive film, ensuring the area around the drainage tube is properly sealed to prevent air leakage, thus creating a completely enclosed space around the wound. ⑤ Connection of the drainage tube to the negative pressure suction device: Currently available commercial negative pressure suction devices are intelligent systems that operate in an intermittent suction mode. The negative pressure is adjustable, typically set at -125 mmHg, operating for 5 minutes followed by a 2-minute pause.

3. Key Points in the Operation of NPWT Technology

1. Debridement

Debridement is the first crucial step in NPWT technology. To achieve optimal results, the procedure must follow the principles below [12,16]. ①Thoroughness: For the soft tissues of the chest wall, thorough debridement is not very difficult, but it is more challenging for bony structures, especially cartilage. The main difficulty lies in distinguishing necrotic tissue. Incomplete debridement due to unclear identification may affect treatment outcomes. Additionally, debridement of deeper or more hidden areas is also difficult and requires careful exploration to find and completely remove necrotic tissue. ②Appropriateness: This principle may seem contradictory to the first but actually represents a balance between the two. Appropriateness limits the extent of debridement based on thoroughness. This is very important. The chest wall is a vital structure with limited thickness; excessive or too deep debridement may lead to significant loss of chest wall integrity, causing two adverse outcomes: first, it may cause paradoxical respiration. If NPWT cannot effectively eliminate this, respiratory function may be compromised, possibly causing more harm than the infection itself; second, overly extensive debridement may allow the infection to spread into the thoracic cavity, which goes against the original intent of using NPWT to treat or control infection. Therefore, debridement must be carefully balanced to thoroughly remove the infected area while preserving healthy tissue to achieve the best results. ③Safety: Although the chest wall may not seem to contain critical structures, some infections may involve important anatomy, such as the internal thoracic artery used in coronary artery bypass grafting, which is extremely important. If incision infection occurs after such Surgery and NPWT is necessary, debridement must be done with extra caution to avoid damaging these structures. Besides such critical structures, inherent elements within the incision such as the heart and major vessels in post-cardiac Surgery infections must also be carefully protected, as injury could lead to serious consequences. In summary, safety during debridement is essential; without it, the procedure loses its meaning.

2. Filling

When placing the filler material into the infected area, certain technical aspects must also be carefully considered [16]: ① The filler must be appropriately sized, neither too small nor too large. If too small, it cannot fill the infected area, and the filler will not be in close contact with the surrounding structures, potentially leaving residual cavities, which significantly hinders the effectiveness of NPWT. If too large, it may cause compression, which is also detrimental to the proper functioning of NPWT. ②The shape of the filler is very important, and it must basically match the shape of the lesion, so that the filler can be filled. Properly filled. ③Complete filling must be ensured, with no potential dead space left. Due to tissue compression or deep location, some dead spaces may be hidden and difficult to detect and fill. Careful exploration during Surgery is necessary to fully identify the location of dead spaces and ensure their complete elimination.

3. Drainage

The core function of NPWT is drainage; therefore, the placement and connection of the drainage tube are especially important throughout the entire procedure [16]. Commercially available materials generally include specially designed drainage tubes. During the procedure, the tubing must be connected strictly according to the product instructions; incorrect connections will prevent effective drainage. The placement of the drainage tube involves two parts: one is the connection between the drainage tube and the filler material, which must be completed according to the product design requirements; the other is securing the drainage tube on the body surface, which usually requires routing it out through a skin incision and firmly fixing it in place.

4. Covering

When covering with a membrane structure, sterile technique must be strictly observed. Generally, the surrounding skin should first be thoroughly disinfected, and then the membrane is applied. The basic

The requirement for covering is that it must be airtight no air leaks or gaps are allowed, as this is the foundation for the proper functioning of the entire device [16].

5. Negative Pressure Suction

The parameters of the negative pressure suction device can generally be set manually. Intermittent suction is an important method; continuous, uninterrupted suction should be avoided, as it can not only fail to produce good results but also cause problems. During use, attention must be paid to the negative pressure settings, and excessive pressure should not be applied in pursuit of better suction effects. Another issue to note is the temporary disconnection of the negative pressure device. After a period of suction, the device can be temporarily detached, the tubing sealed, allowing the patient to leave the ward for appropriate activity, which is beneficial for recovery [16].

6. Duration of Use

The typical duration for NPWT treatment is generally 7 - 10 days, during which it can be combined with anti- infection and other supportive therapies. After one cycle, the wound should be reassessed, and if necessary, the treatment can be repeated [16].

4. Advantages of NPWT Technology

NPWT technology has many advantages [1,3,5,13,15]: ①It completely changes the nature of drainage. NPWT converts passive drainage into active drainage, point drainage into surface drainage, and regional drainage into comprehensive drainage, greatly improving the quality of drainage. ②It thoroughly eliminates dead space. NPWT can completely remove spaces that retain secretions and necrotic tissue, significantly improving the local environment of the wound and further promoting healing. ③ It removes inflammatory exudate and bacterial toxins. The secretions from infected lesions contain large amounts of inflammatory exudate and bacterial toxins, which are key factors causing local damage and impeding healing. NPWT technology can effectively remove these substances.

These substances are thoroughly drained from the wound, playing an important role in healing. ④ Eliminates local edema. Infected lesions often have tissue edema, which is unfavorable for healing. NPWT effectively improves capillary circulation and blood flow velocity, increases local blood volume and tissue oxygen content, and effectively reduces tissue edema. The reduction of edema promotes wound healing. ⑤Improves microcirculation. NPWT effectively enhances microcirculation, not only increasing local oxygen levels and nutrient supply but also raising local antibiotic concentrations, thereby improving anti-infection effects. ⑥Stimulates cell and tissue growth. The negative pressure of NPWT generates mechanical stress on cell membranes, converting physical traction into biochemical changes that promote cell proliferation, angiogenesis, and tissue repair, ultimately accelerating wound healing. ⑦Effectively controls infection. NPWT effectively controls local infection, preventing its spread and transmission, laying a foundation for complete wound healing. ⑧ Reduces workload. NPWT can replace daily dressing changes, significantly reducing workload. ⑨Increases patient confidence. After NPWT use, the wound is sealed, with no large amounts of exudate or necrotic material discharged, which quickly calms the patient's emotions and benefits recovery. ⑩ Shortens treatment duration. NPWT use significantly shortens treatment cycles, improves infection control efficiency, and reduces costs.

5. Contraindications of NPWT Technology

Although NPWT technology has many advantages, it is not suitable for every wound. The main contraindications include [2,5,7,15]: ①Wounds with cancerous lesions. Using NPWT on such wounds may stimulate tumor cell growth. ②Wounds with obvious wet gangrene. NPWT can promote the progression of wet gangrene, worsening the condition. ③Wounds with dry eschar. Dry eschar provides good protection for the wound, and NPWT may damage the eschar, removing its protective effect. ④Untreated chronic osteomyelitis. If chronic Osteomyelitis is not properly treated, the lesion is difficult to eliminate; using NPWT in this case may not help and could accelerate infection spread.

⑤Wounds with active bleeding. These wounds require thorough hemostasis first. If bleeding persists, NPWT negative pressure suction may worsen it. ⑥Wounds with directly exposed blood vessels and nerves. Continuous negative pressure suction may cause damage to these exposed structures. ⑦Wounds with excessive drainage beyond NPWT's capacity. Some wounds have persistent large amounts of drainage, such as infected incisions with empyema or esophageal fistula; the drainage volume exceeds NPWT's ability, potentially causing fluid accumulation. ⑧Patients allergic to NPWT materials. Such patients cannot use this technology.

6. Simple NPWT Devices

NPWT technology has been used clinically for many years, and there are currently various products available. However, these products are often expensive and sometimes difficult to use. To achieve effects similar to these products, simple negative pressure suction devices can be made. This type of device has also been shown to produce satisfactory results when used in certain types of wounds [17]. The specific approach involves replacing specialized NPWT components with more readily available materials: physiological saline-soaked gauze is used instead of professional filling materials; standard medical transparent adhesive film replaces the specialized membrane covering; a regular sterile gastric tube is used in place of a vacuum suction tube; and an ordinary negative pressure suction device is used instead of a dedicated NPWT machine. Although this approach is relatively simple, it essentially meets the general requirements of NPWT technology and can therefore achieve good therapeutic outcomes. In clinical practice, we have independently designed similar devices and obtained relatively satisfactory results (Figures 6-6-3 to 6-6-5) [12].

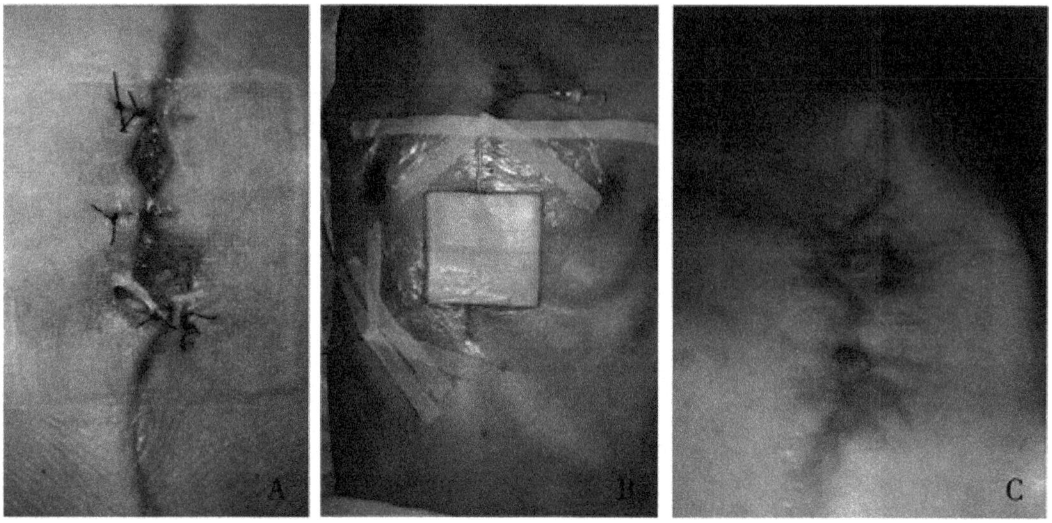

Figure 6-6-3 Case treated with a simple NPWT device: The patient had a midline sternotomy incision with poor local healing post-Surgery and repeated dressing changes were ineffective. The wound was treated with a self-made simple NPWT device, resulting in healing after 2 months. (A. Original wound, ineffective with repeated dressing changes; B. Wound treated with the simple NPWT device; C. Essentially healed after 2 months.)

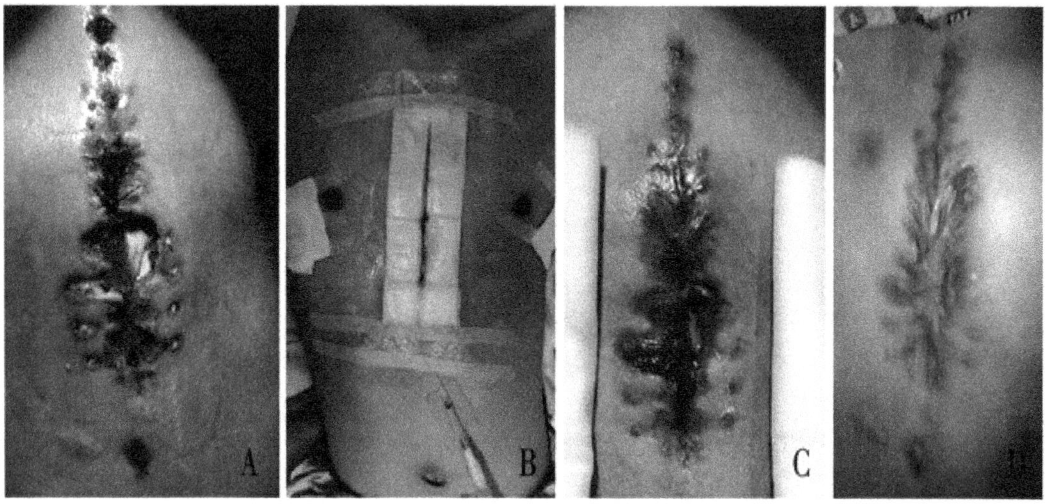

Figure 6-6-4 Case of incision infection treated with a simple NPWT device: A patient with a midline sternotomy incision infection had a non-healing postoperative wound. After multiple repeated sutures, the wound gradually enlarged. The wound was treated using a self-made simple NPWT device, achieving complete healing after 4 months. (A. Original wound; B. Wound treated with the simple NPWT device; C. Wound at 3 months; D. Wound at 4 months)

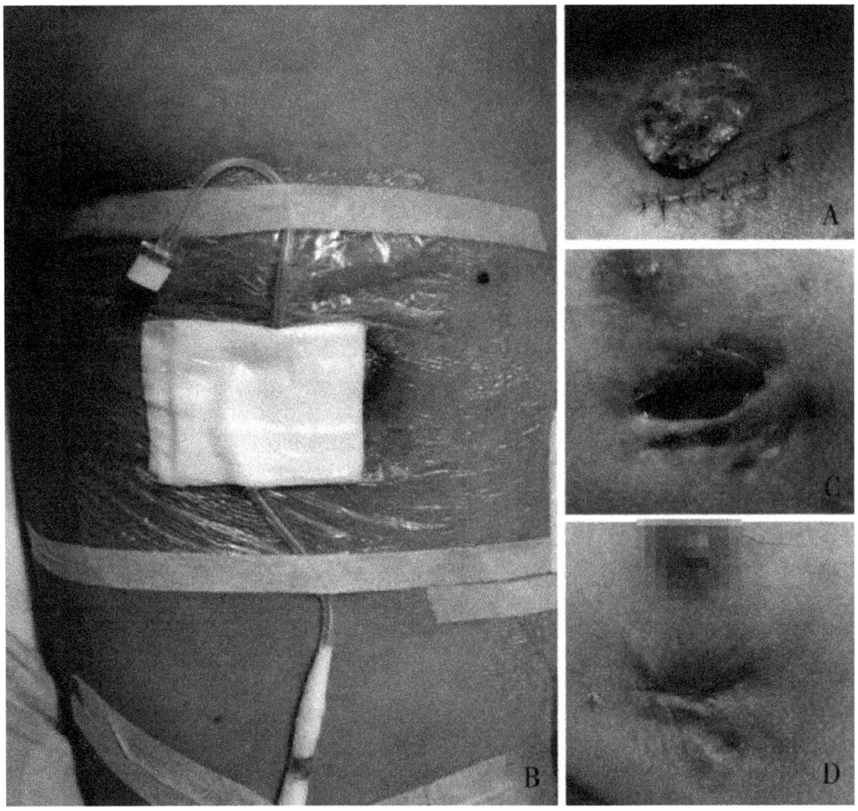

Figure 6-6-5 Case of incision infection treated with a simple NPWT device. The patient had a recurrent infection on the anterior chest wall wound that was slow to heal. The wound was treated using a simple NPWT device, and it healed after 4 months. (A. Anterior chest wound located below the right nipple; B. Wound treated with the simple NPWT device; C. Wound at 3 months; D. Healed wound at 4 months)

7 .Applications of NPWT Technology

In clinical practice, NPWT can be used as the sole treatment for infection sites or as a transitional method [12]. For smaller lesions, NPWT can be applied for the entire course of treatment. If the wound is too large and cannot heal in the short term, NPWT can serve as a transitional method; once granulation tissue has grown satisfactorily, the wound can be sutured, and NPWT then acts as an effective adjunctive therapy [1,4,5].

Controlling chest wall infections is a highly challenging task that requires a multifaceted approach to achieve good results. The application of NPWT offers a good option for infection control. However, it must be clearly understood that the effectiveness of any single technique is limited. If the infection is extremely severe or there are unfavorable objective factors, NPWT alone may not yield good outcomes. Therefore, it is essential to remember that while NPWT is valuable, it does not constitute the entirety of treatment[12]. Only by diligently addressing every aspect of treatment can stubborn chest wall infections be thoroughly overcome.

REFERENCES

[1] Lalezari, S., C. J. Lee, A. A. Borovikova, et al. 2017. "Deconstructing Negative Pressure Wound Therapy." *International Wound Journal* 14 (4): 649–657.
[2] Shine, J., J. I. Efanov, L. Paek, et al. 2019. "Negative Pressure Wound Therapy as a Definitive Treatment for Upper Extremity Wound Defects: A Systematic Review." *International Wound Journal* 16 (4): 960–967.
[3] Torbrand, C., E. Anesäter, O. Borgquist, et al. 2018. "Mechanical Effects of Negative Pressure Wound Therapy on Abdominal Wounds: Effects of Different Pressures and Wound Fillers." *International Wound Journal* 15 (1): 24–28.
[4] Banasiewicz, T., M. Borejsza-Wysocki, W. Meissner, et al. 2011. "Vacuum-Assisted Closure Therapy in Patients with Large Postoperative Wounds Complicated by Multiple Fistulas." *Videosurgery and Other Miniinvasive Techniques* 6 (3): 155–163.
[5] Agarwal, P., R. Kukrele, and D. Sharma. 2019. "Vacuum-Assisted Closure (VAC)/Negative Pressure Wound Therapy (NPWT) for Difficult Wounds: A Review." *Journal of Clinical Orthopaedics and Trauma* 10 (5): 845–848.
[6] Gabriel, A., J. Shores, B. Bernstein, et al. 2009. "A Clinical Review of Infected Wound Treatment with Vacuum-Assisted Closure (V.A.C.) Therapy: Experience and Case Series." *International Wound Journal* 6 (Suppl 2): 1–25.
[7] Dai, Qingchun, Min Zhang, and Yuanzhang Yao. 2007. "Current Status and Prospects of Vacuum Sealing Drainage in Trauma Repair." *Trauma Surgeon* 9 (4): 371–373.
[8] Huang, Q., J. T. Wang, H. C. Cu, et al. 2019. "Comparison of Vacuum Sealing Drainage and Traditional Therapy for Treatment of Diabetic Foot Ulcers: A Meta-Analysis." *Journal of Foot and Ankle Surgery* 58 (5): 954–958.
[9] Reiss, N., U. Schuett, M. Kemper, et al. 2007. "New Method for Sternal Closure after Vacuum-Assisted Therapy in Deep Sternal Infections after Cardiac Surgery." *Annals of Thoracic Surgery* 83 (6): 2246–2247.
[10] Jiang, X., F. Bu, Y. Xu, et al. 2021. "Antibiotic-Loaded Bone Cement Combined with Vacuum Sealing Drainage to Treat Deep Sternal Wound Infection Following Cardiac Surgery: The First Case Report." *Journal of Cardiothoracic Surgery* 16 (1): 292.
[11] Feng, Xiaodong, and Yuanying Xu. 2013. "Clinical Observation of 40 Cases of Continuous Negative Pressure Drainage in the Treatment of Open Pneumothorax and Chest Wall Infectious Wounds." *Zhongwai Yixue Yanjiu* 11 (29): 14–15.
[12] Wang, W. L. 2021a. "Application of Continuous Negative Pressure Drainage Technology in the Treatment of Chronic Chest Wall Infection." *Medical Technology Channel*, October 28.
[13] Gabriel, A., J. Shores, C. Heinrich, et al. 2008. "Negative Pressure Wound Therapy with Instillation: A Pilot Study Describing a New Method for Treating Infected Wounds." *International Wound Journal* 5 (3): 399–413.

[14] Campbell, P. E., G. S. Smith, and J. M. Smith. 2008. "Retrospective Clinical Evaluation of Gauze-Based Negative Pressure Wound Therapy." *International Wound Journal* 5 (2): 280–286.
[15] Scalise, A., R. Calamita, C. Tartaglione, et al. 2016. "Improving Wound Healing and Preventing Surgical Site Complications of Closed Surgical Incisions: A Possible Role of Incisional Negative Pressure Wound Therapy: A Systematic Review of the Literature." *International Wound Journal* 13 (6): 1260–1281.
[16] Wang, W. L. 2021b. "Key Technical Points of Negative Pressure Wound Therapy in Chest Wall Surgery." *Toutiao (Jinri Toutiao)*, November 1.
[17] Zuo, Jingfang, Aifeng Meng, Xiaoxu Zhi, et al. 2018. "Study on the Application of a Modified Simple Negative Pressure Suction Device in Refractory Incisions after Esophageal Cancer Surgery." *Chinese Journal of Oncologic Surgery* 10 (6): 413–416.

Verses Kindler Publication

www.ingramcontent.com/pod-product-compliance
Lightning Source LLC
LaVergne TN
LVHW070524061126
851857LV00024B/2138